Population-Based Nursing

Ann L. Cupp Curley, PhD, RN, is the Nurse Research Specialist at Capital Health in Trenton, New Jersey. In this capacity, she promotes and guides the development of clinical research and facilitates evidence-based practice. Her clinical background includes several years working in community and public health nursing. She has extensive experience teaching undergraduate, MSN, and DNP courses, including the DNP course, Principles of Epidemiology. Dr. Curley has delivered many papers and presentations on Evidence-Based Practice, Evaluation and Motivation for Nurse Educators, Teaching Effectively, Ergonomics, and the Aging Nursing Workforce. Her publications include *Urban Health Informatics, An Evidence-Based Approach to Scheduling*, and *A Nurse's Perspective on Cuba*. She authored a chapter in Fulton et al.'s textbook *Foundations of Clinical Nurse Specialist Practice on Population-Based Data Analysis*. A specialist for the Institute for Nursing, Foundation of the New Jersey State Nurses Association from 1997 to 2009, she received her BS in nursing at Boston College, an MSN in Community Health/CNS track from the University of Pennsylvania, and a PhD in Urban Planning and Policy Development at Rutgers, The State University of New Jersey.

Patty A. Vitale, MD, MPH, FAAP, holds multiple appointments, including Assistant Professor of Pediatrics and Emergency Medicine at Cooper Medical School of Rowan University and Robert Wood Johnson Medical School, New Jersey; Adjunct Assistant Professor at University of Medicine and Dentistry of New Jersey's School of Public Health, Department of Epidemiology; and Visiting Clinical Associate in the College of Nursing, Rutgers University. Dr. Vitale is an attending Pediatric Emergency Medicine physician at Cooper University Hospital in Camden, New Jersey. For over 6 years she has taught, Principles of Epidemiology to graduate and doctoral students in public health, nursing, and biomedical sciences at UMDNJ. Dr. Vitale did her residency and post doctoral training in Pediatrics and Community Pediatrics at the University of California, San Diego. During fellowship, she obtained her master's in Public Health from San Diego State University. She is certified by the American Board of Pediatrics and has served on National and Statewide Committees for the American Academy of Pediatrics in the areas of epidemiology, government affairs, and young physicians. She also sits on the editorial board for *AAP-Grand Rounds* a publication of the American Academy of Pediatrics. She volunteered as Team Physician for the U.S. National Gymnastics Team (2003–2008). She is a Junior Olympic National Elite and NCAA Women's Gymnastics Judge and former gymnastics coach and was inducted into the California Interscholastic Hall of Fame for Sports Officials in San Diego, CA (2009). Her national and local lectures (43) and publications have focused on family violence, pediatric and adolescent health, simulation as an educational tool, and homelessness. She has received many honors including the 2004 AMA Foundation Leadership Award, 2002 Fellows Award for Excellence in Promoting Children's Health (Academic Pediatric Association), 2002 Pediatric Leaders of the 21st Century (American Academy of Pediatrics), among others.

Population-Based Nursing

Concepts and Competencies for Advanced Practice

Ann L. Cupp Curley, PhD, RN

and

Patty A. Vitale, MD, MPH, FAAP

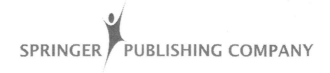

SPRINGER PUBLISHING COMPANY

Springer Publishing Company, LLC
11 West 42nd Street
New York, NY 10036
www.springerpub.com

Acquisitions Editor: Margaret Zuccarini
Composition: diacriTech

ISBN: 978-0-8261-0671-1
E-book ISBN: 978-0-8261-0672-8

15 / 8

The author and the publisher of this work have made every effort to use sources believed to be reliable to provide information that is accurate and compatible with the standards generally accepted at the time of publication. Because medical science is continually advancing, our knowledge base continues to expand. Therefore, as new information becomes available, changes in procedures become necessary. We recommend that the reader always consult current research and specific institutional policies before performing any clinical procedure. The author and publisher shall not be liable for any special, consequential, or exemplary damages resulting, in whole or in part, from the readers' use of, or reliance on, the information contained in this book. The publisher has no responsibility for the persistence or accuracy of URLs for external or third-party Internet Web sites referred to in this publication and does not guarantee that any content on such Web sites is, or will remain, accurate or appropriate.

Library of Congress Cataloging-in-Publication Data

Curley, Ann L. Cupp.
  Population-based nursing : concepts and competencies for advanced practice / Ann L. Cupp Curley, Patty A. Vitale.
       p. cm.
  Includes index.
  ISBN 978-0-8261-0671-1
  1. Public health nursing. 2. Evidence-based nursing. I. Vitale, Patty A. II. Title.
  RT97.C87 2012
  610.734--dc23
                          2011037152

Special discounts on bulk quantities of our books are available to corporations, professional associations, pharmaceutical companies, health care organizations, and other qualifying groups. If you are interested in a custom book, including chapters from more than one of our titles, we can provide that service as well.

For details, please contact:
Special Sales Department, Springer Publishing Company, LLC
11 West 42nd Street, 15th Floor, New York, NY 10036-8002
Phone: 877-687-7476 or 212-431-4370; Fax: 212-941-7842
Email: sales@springerpub.com

Printed in the United States of America by Gasch Printing.

Contents

Contributors

Barbara A. Benjamin, EdD, RN   Assistant Clinical Professor, University of North Carolina at Chapel Hill, School of Nursing, Chapel Hill, North Carolina

Ann L Cupp Curley, PhD, RN   Nurse Research Specialist, Capital Health, Trenton, New Jersey

Janna L. Dieckmann, PhD, RN   Clinical Associate Professor, University of North Carolina at Chapel Hill, School of Nursing, Chapel Hill, North Carolina

Susan B. Fowler, RN, CNRN   Nursing Leadership Consultant

Barbara A. Niedz, PhD, RN, CPHQ   Corporate Vice President for Quality Improvement, APS Healthcare, White Plains, New York; Contributing Faculty, Walden University, School of Nursing, Leadership and Management Track RN-MSN Program, Minneapolis, Minnesota

Sonda M. Oppewal, PhD, RN   Clinical Associate Professor and Associate Dean for Clinical Partnerships and Practice, University of North Carolina at Chapel Hill, School of Nursing, Chapel Hill, North Carolina

Patty A. Vitale, MD, MPH, FAAP   Assistant Professor of Pediatrics and Emergency Medicine at Cooper Medical School of Rowan University and Robert Wood Johnson Medical School, New Jersey

Foreword

Gillian Gill claims that *Notes Affecting the Health, Efficiency, and Hospital Administration of the British Army* (2004) was "probably the best thing that Florence Nightingale ever wrote" (p. 417). Nightingale's *Notes*, written in 1857, detailed morbidity and mortality findings related to the Crimean War; her findings were subsequently used by a Royal Commission that advocated reforms in the British Army Medical Department. Using statistical methods to illuminate disease atrocities experienced by her population of interest—soldiers in the British Army—Nightingale provided evidence-based research that basic sanitary measures, fresh food, good latrines, and appropriate clothing decreased the mortality rate of soldiers, a population whose mortality rate, even in peacetime, exceeded the mortality rate noted in the 1665 Great Plague. An early proponent of evidence-based practice embedded in the burgeoning science of statistics, a tool intrinsic to the scientific method; Nightingale's findings on her population resulted in implementation of dramatic changes in the British Army.

Almost 150 years later, the American Association of Colleges of Nursing (AACN) published its *Essentials of Doctoral Education for Advanced Nursing Practice* (2006). Crafted in the context of multiple Institute of Medicine reports documenting deficiencies in the U.S. healthcare delivery and health educational systems, and a severely recurrent national shortage of primary care providers, the *Essentials* offer eight fundamental outcome competencies deemed intrinsic to all advanced practice nurses prepared at the clinical doctoral degree level—that is, the Doctor of Nursing Practice (DNP) program, which is considered nursing's terminal practice entity. Of paramount importance is Essential Number Eight: *Clinical Prevention and Population Health for Improving the Nation's Health* (p. 15). The AACN defines population health to include aggregate, community, environmental/occupational, and cultural/ socioeconomic dimensions of health, with aggregates noted as a group of individuals with a shared characteristic (e.g., gender, diagnosis, age, and so forth). In the basic baccalaureate, nursing education broadly addresses health promotion and disease prevention interventions, and clinical DNP programs challenge registered nurses to employ evidence-based clinical prevention and population health services that improve health indices for individuals through direct care provision and for populations through policies and programs grounded in evidence.

Advanced practice nurses in primary care have tools at their readiness to guide individual care management decisions: recommendations of the U.S. Preventive Health Services Task Force (2009), implementation guidelines from *Healthy People 2020* (2011), statements and guidelines from a variety of organizations (e.g., American Heart Association, American Academy of Nurse Practitioners,

American Cancer Society, and others), and publications of the World Health Organization regarding social determinants of diseases. As a provider matures in practice, the information gleaned from these available resources can be reviewed intelligently, with implications for care management culled efficiently. For the DNP student or novice practitioner, these resources require context, an expansive and detailed overview within which the essential language embedded in the AACN's emphasis on clinical prevention and population health services *makes sense.* The establishment of a professional practice that integrates current evidence into daily clinical prevention and population health practice mandates a solid, thorough clinical doctoral education, one both practical and theoretical.

Ann L. Cupp Curley, PhD, RN, and Patty A. Vitale, MD, MPH, FAAP, have provided such a foundation in this book, *Population-Based Nursing: Concepts and Competencies for Advanced Practice,* a textbook written for registered nurses in DNP programs and master's programs in community health nursing. Written in the Nightingale tradition of *Notes* (1857), Curley, Vitale, and their coauthors ground graduate nursing students in the empirical tradition of the health sciences— biostatistics and epidemiology—and relate these sciences to evidence-based advanced nursing practice provided to individuals and populations. Basic constructs are explored in detail, with reference to applicability in practice. Written with a collegial tone, as if in conversation with the authors, the book engages readers to continue on, to turn pages, to learn more. Fast-paced and succinctly thorough, this book will surely find its way as a *must-read* reference on shelves of graduate nursing students. With an emphasis on healthcare disparities, Curley and Vitale provide a practical approach to managing patients suffering from specific diseases viewed as populations. A two-way lens is employed. First, there is focus on populations of individuals with poor health indices; second, there is attendant focus on diseases as populations of interest to be managed through clinical primary and secondary prevention strategies. This pan-dimensional view enables graduate nursing students to integrate individual care within both the broad context of the human population of interest and the index disease of concern. This approach anchors novice practitioners who, up to this point in their careers, have managed the individual only, with somewhat tangential references to management of the broader environments within which the individual resides.

In Chapter 5, Curley leads with a compelling statement: "Nurses in advanced practice have an obligation to improve the health of the population they serve by providing evidence-based care." Curley's mandate that advanced practice nurses are *obligated* in their role to use evidence-based care is refreshing. Inherent in this obligation is the centrality of research acumen, a full working knowledge of research tools and methodologies as critical to care delivery as clinical reasoning and physical diagnosis. The authors explicate this centrality in Chapters 3, 4, and 5. Using clinical examples, they address the full integration of research tools in determining if select findings are appropriate for use in providing individual care or in designing a primary or secondary prevention program targeting a disease as a specific population of interest. The various management perspectives obtained through qualitative and quantitative designs are explored. Beginning with a full explication of a PICO question (population, intervention, comparison, and outcomes), students are guided through the basics of question statement, literature review, and assessment of evidence. Once in practice, DNP graduates will gratefully employ published algorithms giving structure to their management regimens. The pragmatic directions provided by the Adult Treatment Panel III (2004), or those of the Joint National Committee on Prevention, Detection, Evaluation, and Treatment of High Blood Pressure (2003), guide management decisions on the basis of evidence. The authors expand on the word *evidence* as it is used in care delivery and provide readers with steps in how to assess evidence and address questions such as: *What are the grading systems used to evaluate evidence? How are levels of evidence ranked? What is best practice evidence?* Such questions, although seemingly apparent, are well nuanced from the vantage point of the novice, who is moved along in understanding from the simpler to the more complex constructs. The theme of accountability as related to research skills and to choice of appropriate evidence for guiding specific practice regimens is intermeshed throughout the text.

In Chapter 8, devoted to evaluation of practice at the population level, author Barbara A. Niedz addresses the responsibility of advanced practice nurses to achieve improved clinical outcomes at the population level. The focus on responsibility for *quality* outcomes, not just the delivery of care appropriate to the disease or community, is fully explicated in Niedz's discussion of the Centers for Medicare and Medicaid Services' (CMS) oversight of reimbursement for care delivered, as well as refusal to reimburse for occurrence of *"never events"*—preventable poor outcomes that contribute significantly to the cost of care delivered. Drilling down on the advanced practice nurse's accountability for quality individual patient or population outcomes, as well as responsibility for cost-effective care, easily recognized clinical situations is explored as examples. Discussing, for example, congestive heart failure patient discharge instructions, Niedz reviews key quality questions to be asked of such patients; emanating from these questions, quality measurement metrics can be outlined that evaluate effectiveness of care provided to the individual as well as to the population of patients with this disease. As with research tools, quality measurement tools are interwoven as skills as essential as the appropriate use of the stethoscope.

Perhaps one of the most charming and robust discussions is provided by Barbara A. Benjamin in Chapter 9: Community Assessment and Collaboration: The Foundation of a Lasting Relationship. Benjamin speaks of *bidirectional communication*, a practical tool to be used in improving population health indices. As her predecessors Nightingale, Jane Addams, and Lillian Wald had advocated, Benjamin details the *how-to's* of engaging as a partner with communities in efforts to improve that population's health indices. With meticulous attention to detail, she outlines, step-by-step, how to conduct a community assessment in partnership with community leaders and other key players of systems that interact to affect a community's health. Transportation, social and welfare systems, religious entities, schools, housing authorities, and public health departments represent complex systems implicated in communities' health indices and in care delivery patterns. Benjamin reviews how community evidence is obtained by a variety of methods, such as focus groups, windshield surveys, census and disease reports, and more. As with motivational interviewing, the techniques available to advanced practice nurses for community assessment involve listening carefully to residents and using their perspective as the orientation for further data collection, analysis, and interpretation.

An added bonus with this text is the inclusion of exercises and discussion questions providing students with opportunities for interaction on the constructs essential to the topics presented in each chapter. The exercises are complex, presenting scenarios representative of each chapter's primary focus. Very importantly, this book is written by seasoned clinicians who have spent significant portions of their careers in the academy. This text also serves as a model of a successful collaboration. Ann L. Cupp Curley, with her rich educational background in urban planning and policy development as well as community health, served in faculty roles in universities in New Jersey. As a core faculty in a newly established DNP program at the University of Medicine and Dentistry of New Jersey, Curley evolved great interest in translating the mandates for accountable, responsible advanced practice nursing in primary care into educational products—courses, books, assignments—easily consumed by the targeted student. Patty A. Vitale brings to the text her extensive experience as a faculty member with a strong clinical practice and public health background. Vitale has mentored many students over the years in their community-based fieldwork projects. She has a long history of working with communities throughout her career including outreach in the areas of domestic violence, child abuse, and violence prevention. Both fine academicians, Ann Curley and Patty Vitale have achieved what Nightingale advocated: educating nurses in the community who would transform the provision of health care and save an untold number of lives. Curley and Vitale's history of working and teaching together in a DNP program has clearly contributed to the depth and breadth of the material in the book. Accountable, evidence-based practice as detailed in this text affords DNP students the context, skills, and lexicon for novice practice contributing to the improved welfare of individuals and populations. It was a joy to read this book, and I am confident that readers will have the same reaction.

Frances Ward, PhD, RN, CRNP
David R. Devereaux Chair of Nursing
Temple University, Philadelphia, PA

Preface

The inspiration for this book grew out of our experience while co-teaching an epidemiology course for students enrolled in a doctorate in nursing practice (DNP) program. We found it difficult to find a textbook that addressed the course objectives and was relevant to nursing practice. We decided a population-based nursing textbook targeted for use as a primary course textbook in a DNP program or as a supplement to other course materials in a graduate community health nursing program would be of great benefit and value to students enrolled in these programs. This book is the result of that vision.

The chapters address the essential areas of content for a DNP program as recommended by the American Association of Colleges of Nursing (AACN), with a focus on the AACN core competencies for population-based nursing. The primary audience for this text is nursing students enrolled in either a DNP program or a graduate community health nursing program. Each chapter includes discussion questions to help nursing students use and apply their newly acquired skills from each chapter.

This textbook introduces successful strategies that nurses have used to improve population outcomes and reinforces high-level application of activities that require the synthesis and integration of information learned. The goal is to provide readers with information that will help them to identify healthcare needs at the population level and to improve population outcomes. In particular, *Chapter 1* introduces the concept of population-based nursing and discusses examples of successful approaches and interventions to improve population health.

In order to design, implement, and evaluate interventions which improve the health of populations and aggregates, APNs need to be able to identify and target outcome measures. *Chapter 2* explains how to define, categorize, and identify population outcomes using specific examples from practice settings. The identification of outcomes or key health indicators is an essential first step in planning effective interventions and a requirement for evaluation. The chapter includes a discussion of nursing-sensitive indicators, *Healthy People 2020*, national health objectives, and health disparities. Emphasis is on the identification of healthcare disparities and approaches that can be used to eliminate or mitigate them. APNs can advocate for needed change at local, regional, state, or national levels by identifying areas for improvement in practice, by comparing evidence needed for effective practice, and by better understanding health disparities. APNs have an important collaborative role with professionals from other disciplines and community members to work toward eliminating health disparities.

Epidemiology is the "basic science" of prevention (Gordis, 2008). Evidence-based practice as it relates to population-based nursing combines clinical practice and public health together through the use of population health sciences in clinical practice (Heller & Page, 2002). Programs or interventions that are designed by APNs should be evaluated and assessed for their effectiveness and ability to change or improve outcomes. This is true at an individual or population level. Data from these programs should be collected systematically and in such a manner that can be replicated in future programs. Data collection must be organized, clearly defined, and analyzed with clearly defined outcomes developed early in the planning process. Best practice requires that data are not just collected; data must also be analyzed, interpreted correctly, and if significant, put into practice. Understanding how to interpret and report data accurately is critical as it sets up the foundation for evidence-based practice. With that said, it is important to understand the basics of how to measure disease or outcomes, how to present these measures, and know what type of measures are needed to analyze a project or intervention. *Chapter 3* describes the natural history of disease and concepts that are integral for the prevention and recognition (e.g., screening) of disease. It also introduces the basic concepts that are necessary to understand how to measure disease and design studies that are used in population-based research. Disease measures such as incidence, prevalence, and mortality rates are covered, and their relevance to practice is discussed. The basics of data analysis including the calculation of relative risk, attributable risk, and odds ratio are presented with examples of how to use these measures. Study design selection is an important part of the planning process for implementing a program. A portion of *Chapter 3* is dedicated to introducing the most common study designs, as correct design selection is an essential part of sound methodology, successful program implementation, and overall success.

In order for APNs to lead the field in evidence-based practice, it is critical that they possess skills in analytic methods to identify population trends and evaluate outcomes and systems of care (AACN, 2006). They need to carry out studies with strong methodology and be cognizant of factors that can affect study results. Identification and early recognition of factors that can affect the results or outcomes of a study such as systematic errors (e.g., bias) should be acknowledged as they cannot always be prevented. In *Chapter 4*, the APN is introduced to the elements of bias with a comprehensive discussion of the complexities of data collection and the fundamentals of developing a database. Critical components of data analysis are discussed including causality, confounding, and interaction.

In order to provide care at an advanced level, nurses must incorporate the concepts and competencies of advanced practice into their daily practice. This requires that APNs acquire the knowledge, tools, and resources to know when and how to integrate them into practice. In *Chapter 5*, the APN will learn how to integrate and synthesize information in order to design interventions that are based on evidence to improve population outcomes. Nurses require several skills to become practitioners of evidence-based care. In this chapter, they will learn how to identify clinical problems, recognize patient safety issues, compose clinical questions that provide a clear direction for study, conduct a search of the literature, appraise and synthesize the available evidence, and successfully integrate new knowledge into practice.

Information technologies are transforming the way that information is learned and shared. Online communities provide a place for people to support each other and share information. Online databases contain knowledge that can be assessed for information on populations and aggregates and internet sites provide up to date information on health and health care. *Chapter 6* describes how technology can be used to enhance population-based nursing. It identifies Web sites that are available on the World Wide Web and how to evaluate them for quality. It also describes potential ways that technology can be used to improve population outcomes and how to incorporate technology into the development of new and creative interventions. APNs use data to make decisions that lead to program development, implementation, and evaluation. In *Chapter 7*, the APN will learn how to design new programs using organizational theory. Nursing care delivery models that address organizational structure, process, and outcomes are described.

Oversight responsibilities for clinical outcomes at the population level are a critical part of advanced practice nursing. The purpose of *Chapter 8* is to identify ways and means to evaluate population outcomes, evaluate systems' changes as well as effectiveness, efficiency, and trends in care delivery across the continuum. Strategies to monitor healthcare quality are addressed as well as factors that lead to success. These concepts are explored within the role and competencies of the APN.

In order for APNs to make decisions at the community level, APNs who work in the community need to be part of the higher level of care management and policy decision making in partnership with the community-based consortium of health care policy makers. *Chapter 9* describes the tools for successful community collaboration and project development. Emphasis is placed on identifying community needs and assessment of their resources. Specific examples are given in order to guide APNs in developing their own community projects.

Chapter 10 identifies barriers to change within communities and the importance of developing and sustaining community partnerships. Specific strategies for program implementation are discussed, as well as the methods to empower the community to advocate for themselves. Specific examples are given in order to guide APNs in executing a project that has community acceptance and has sustainability.

REFERENCES

American Association of Colleges of Nursing (AACN). (2006). *The Essentials of Doctoral Education for Advanced Practice Nursing*. Retrieved from http://www.aacn.nche.edu/DNP/pdf/Essentials.pdf

Gordis, L. (2008). *Epidemiology* (4th ed.). Philadelphia: Elsevier Saunders.

Heller, R., & Page J. (2002). A population perspective to evidence based medicine: "Evidence for Population Health." *Journal of Epidemiol Community Health, 56,* 45–47.

Acknowledgments

We would like to express our grateful acknowledgment to those professional colleagues who provided direction, guidance, and assistance in writing this book. We would also like to thank our family and friends for their support throughout this process. Thank you to our publisher, Margaret Zuccarini for her invaluable advice, assistance, and infinite patience. We would also like to acknowledge the following graduates of the DNP program at the University of Medicine and Dentistry of New Jersey: Debbie F. Buck, MSN, APN, BC, Noel Rosner DNP, RN, APN-C, Amy J. Sirkin, DNP, APN-C, Amy R. Weinberg, DNP, MSN, FNP-BC, and especially Margaret Conrad, DNP, MPA, RN, BC, CTN-A. We could not have completed the text without the help of the library staff of the Health Services Library of Capital Health, especially Erica Moncrief, MS, Director of Library Services, and Jennifer Kral, MLS, Capital Health Librarian.

ONE

Introduction to Population-Based Nursing

Ann L. Cupp Curley

For decades, nursing practice focused on caring for individual patients and on providing care based on a mixture of tradition and clinical experience. Nursing remains, and should remain, a practice-based and caring profession, but nursing practice is changing. There is a growing awareness of the need to provide evidence-based care and to design interventions that have a broad impact on the populations that nursing serves. Population health obligates healthcare professionals to implement standard interventions, based on the best research evidence, to improve the health of targeted groups of people. It also obligates nurses to discover new and effective strategies for providing care and promoting health. While clinical decision making related to individual patients is important, it has little impact on overall health outcomes for populations. Interventions at the population level have the potential to improve overall health across communities.

This book addresses the essential areas of content for a doctorate in nursing practice (DNP) as recommended by the American Association of Colleges of Nursing (AACN), with a focus on the AACN core competencies for population-based nursing. The goal is to provide readers with information that will help them to identify healthcare needs at the population level and to improve population outcomes. Although the focus is on the essential components of a DNP program, the intent is to broadly address practice issues that should be the concern of any nurse in an advanced practice role.

This chapter will introduce the reader to the concept of population-based nursing. The reader will learn how to identify population parameters, the potential impact of a population-based approach to care, and the importance of designing nursing interventions at the population level in advanced nursing practice.

BACKGROUND

For all the scare tactics out there, what's truly scary—truly risky—is the prospect of doing nothing.
    —President Barack Obama (2009), *The New York Times*, August 16

The first decade of the 21st century has been witness to a growing and contentious debate on healthcare reform. President Barack Obama's stated goals have been to extend healthcare coverage to the millions who lack health insurance, stop the insurance industry's practice of denying coverage on the basis of pre-existing conditions, and cut overall healthcare costs.

There is ample evidence that there is a need for healthcare reform in the United States. The gross domestic product (GDP) is the total market value of the output of labor and property located in the United States. It reflects the contribution of the healthcare sector relative to all other production in the United States. In 1960, the health sector's proportion of the GDP was 5% (i.e., $5.00 of every $100.00 spent in the United States went to pay for healthcare services). By 1990, this figure had grown to 12% and by 1996, 14%. According to a report issued by the Committee on the Budget of the United States Senate, unless changes are made in how the United States provides care to its citizens, the GDP for the healthcare sector is projected to grow to 25% by 2025 and 49% by 2089 (Orszag, 2008).

The cost of healthcare is reflected in the insurance industry. Health insurance premiums have increased 131% for employers since 1999, and employee spending for health insurance coverage (employee's share of family coverage) has increased 128% between 1999 and 2008. Studies estimate that the number of excess deaths among uninsured adults aged 25 to 64 is approximately 22,000 per year. This mortality figure is more than the number of deaths from diabetes mellitus (17,500) within the same age group (National Coalition on Health Care, 2010). The Commonwealth Fund, a private foundation which stated mission is to promote a high performing healthcare system, commissioned a survey of U.S. adults that was conducted by Princeton Survey Research Associates (Collins, Doty, Robertson, & Garber, 2010). The survey looked at the effect of health insurance coverage on health care-seeking behaviors. They found that among uninsured women aged 50 to 64, 48% say they did not see a doctor when they were sick, did not fill a prescription, or skipped a test, treatment, or follow-up visit because they could not afford it. The survey results also showed that only 67% of uninsured adult respondents had their blood pressure checked within the past year compared to 91% of insured adults. Additionally, only 31% of uninsured women aged 50 to 64 reported having a mammogram in the past two years, compared to 79% of women with health insurance.

In a report published by the Urban Institute, the authors estimate that in a worst case scenario, there could be 59.7 million people in the United States who are uninsured by 2015 if healthcare reform is not enacted. The authors estimate that this number could increase to 67.6 million by 2020. Nearly 90 million people—about one third of the population below the age of 65—spent a portion of either 2007 or 2008 without health coverage (Garrett, Buettgens, Doan, Headen, & Holahan, 2010).

Although the United States spends more money on healthcare than any other country in the world, life expectancy in the United States ranks 49th and infant mortality ranks 46th among all nations (CIA, 2011). A report issued by the Institute of Medicine (IOM) argues that the system used in the United States for gathering and analyzing health measures is part of the problem. A second problem is the inadequate system in the United States for gathering, analyzing, and communicating information on the underlying factors that lead to chronic health conditions and other risk factors that contribute to poor health (IOM, 2010a). Driven by a need for change in how healthcare is paid for, the *Affordable Care Act* was signed into law by President Obama in 2010. It is scheduled to go into effect over the span of four years beginning in 2011. Although it has the potential to change the economic landscape of healthcare, it is unclear how healthcare will be affected in the long term as the law is being challenged by several groups at the time of this book's publication.

Our healthcare system is complex, and there is no simple solution to lowering costs and improving access. The goal of this text is not to provide an overarching solution to the issues of cost, but to propose that nurses can contribute to improving the cost effectiveness and efficiency of care through the provision of evidence-based treatment guidelines to identified populations with shared needs, and by advocating for policies that address the underlying factors that impact health and healthcare. To do this, we must change the way that we deliver healthcare and become politically active. In an ideal world, healthcare policies are created based on valid and reliable evidence and population need and demand. The ideal premise is that there is equitable distribution of healthcare services and that the appropriate care is given to the right people at the right time and at a reasonable cost. The American Nurses Association (ANA) has been advocating for 20 years for healthcare reforms that would guarantee access to high-quality healthcare for all and supports the public option in the Affordable Care Act (ANA, 2009). The public option in the Affordable Care Act proposes that an insurance plan be offered by the federal government for purchase by consumers and small businesses.

Whether an individual nurse supports or does not support healthcare reform is a function of individual choice. The actions of professional organizations are driven by membership. Involvement in professional organizations as well as local, state, and national political activities (even if only minimally as a registered and active voter) is part of the professional responsibility of advanced practice nurses (APNs).

DEFINING POPULATIONS

The AACN definition of advanced practice nursing includes the importance of identifying and managing health outcomes at the population level (2004). In 2006, the AACN specified that graduates of DNP programs have competency in meeting "the needs of a panel of patients, a target population, a set of populations, or a broad community" (p. 10). A core component of DNP education is clinical prevention (health promotion and disease prevention at individual and family levels) and population health (focus of care at aggregate and community levels and examination of environmental, occupational, cultural, and socioeconomic dimensions of health) (AACN, 2006; Allan et al., 2004). Regardless of whether DNP graduates practice with a focus on clinical prevention or population health, the ability to define, identify, and analyze outcomes is imperative for improving the health status of individuals and populations (AACN, 2006).

The goal of population-based nursing is to provide evidence-based care to targeted groups of people with similar needs in order to improve outcomes. Population-based nursing uses a defined population or aggregate as the organizing unit for care. *The American Heritage Dictionary* (Population, 2002) defines a population as "all of the people inhabiting a specified area." A second definition is given as "the total number of inhabitants constituting a particular race, class, or group in a specified area" (p. 1366). Subpopulations may be referred to as *aggregates.* Many different parameters can be used to identify or categorize subpopulations or aggregates. They may be defined by ethnicity (e.g., African American or Hispanic), religion (e.g., Roman Catholic or Buddhist), or geographic location (e.g., Boston or San Diego). Aggregates can also be defined by age or occupation. People with a shared diagnosis e.g., diabetes or a shared risk factor such as smoking comprise other identifiable aggregates. Sometimes people may choose to describe themselves as members of a particular group (democrat or socialist). One person may belong to more than one such group (e.g., White, younger than 18, current smoker, etc.).

A community is comprised of multiple aggregates. The most common aggregate used in population-based nursing is the high-risk aggregate. A high-risk aggregate is a subgroup or subpopulation of a community that shares a high-risk factor among its members, such as a high-risk health condition (e.g., congestive heart failure) or a shared high-risk factor (e.g., smoking and sedentary behavior). The aggregate concept can be used to target interventions to specific aggregates or subpopulations within a community. (Porche, 2004) The implementation of standard or proven (evidence-based) strategies to prevent illness and/or improve the health of targeted groups of people can have the effect of ameliorating health problems at the population and/or aggregate level. Making change at the population level cannot only impact the health of a community in the present but for generations to come. As we learn how to approach and target populations using evidence, we improve our chance of long-term success and can strive to make lifelong changes in the health of a community.

USING DATA TO TARGET POPULATIONS AND AGGREGATES AT RISK

The collection and analysis of data provide healthcare professionals and policy makers with a starting point for identifying, selecting, and implementing interventions that target specific populations and aggregates. Many of the leading causes of death in the United States are preventable. One in three American adults has cardiovascular disease. It is the leading cause of death among both men and women in the United States, killing an average of one American every 37 seconds (AHA, 2010). In descending order, the ten leading causes of death in the United States are heart disease, malignant neoplasms, cerebrovascular diseases, chronic lower respiratory diseases, accidents, Alzheimer's disease, diabetes, influenza and pneumonia, renal diseases, and septicemia (Centers for Disease Control and Prevention [CDC], 2007b).

Several factors such as the physical environment, healthcare systems, personal behaviors, and the social environment can have a deleterious impact on individual and community health. The negative consequences of these factors are researched and well documented.

Smoking

Smoking alone has been estimated to cause 443,000 premature deaths and $96 billion in health-related costs each year in the United States. It is a leading cause of preventable morbidity and mortality. Results of the 2009 National Health Interview Survey and the 2009 Behavioral Risk Factor Surveillance System were used to estimate national and state adult smoking prevalence. In 2009, 20.6% of U.S. adults aged 18 or older were current cigarette smokers. Men (23.5%) were more likely than women (17.9%) to be current smokers. Among people below the federal poverty level, the prevalence of smoking was 31.1%, and 20.5% among persons with less than a high school diploma (while the rate was 5.6% among adults with a graduate degree). Regional differences also exist. The West has the lowest prevalence rate (16.4%), with higher prevalence in the Midwest (23.1%) and South (21.8%). The proportion of U.S. adults who were current cigarette smokers did not change substantially between 2005 (20.9%) and 2009 (20.6%) (CDC, 2010a).

A reduction in smoking by school-age children should result in reductions in tobacco-related deaths in the future; unfortunately, the downward trend in the prevalence of cigarette smoking among children has declined significantly since 2003. Smoking declined by 40% between 1997 and 2009 but only 11% between 2003 and 2009 (CDC, 2010c). There is huge potential for cost savings by preventing smoking-related illnesses. One cannot overlook the effects of secondhand smoking on the health of family members and co-workers. It is well known that secondhand smoke has long-lasting effects on the unborn fetus, infant, and child. These effects can manifest as low birth weight in newborns (Ventura et al., 2003), increased respiratory infections (U.S. Environmental Protection Agency [EPA], 2004), higher risk of asthma exacerbations (U.S. Department of Health and Human Services [DHHS], 2006), sudden infant death (Anderson & Cook, 1997), and a lower intelligence quotient (Yolton et al., 2005). Thus, it is important to recognize not only the direct effects of smoking on health but also the indirect effects on the fetus, infants, children, and family members. Not unlike in adults, the cessation of smoking early on can reverse or ameliorate the potential long-term harmful effects of secondhand smoke exposure. These data provide a starting point for targeting specific high-risk groups for intervention based on parameters such as age, education, income, and geographical location. Smoking cessation and smoking prevention programs are not the only areas that offer opportunities for improving the health of people in the United States and for saving money. Like smoking, obesity is a significant public health concern.

Obesity

As part of *Healthy People* 2010, the Unites States set a goal to reduce the percentage of obese Americans to 15% by 2010. In 1999, researchers found 20% of men were obese and 39% had abdominal obesity. By 2007, those percentages had risen to 32% and 44%, respectively. The number of obese women increased from 33% to 35% and abdominal obesity prevalence rose from 56% to 62% during the same time period (Puhl, Heuer, & Sarda, 2010). Beasley et al. (2003) used multiple databases to estimate the expected number of years of life lost (YLL) because of overweight and obesity across the life span of an adult. They concluded that obesity shortened life expectancy markedly especially among younger adults. For any given degree of overweight, younger adults generally had greater YLL than older adults. They also found that gender and ethnicity interact with obesity and YLL. Younger African Americans, for example, are more negatively impacted by YLL than older African Americans, and men are more negatively impacted than women. This is yet another example of how data can be used to identify parameters for targeting aggregates for an intervention. In this case, gender, ethnicity, and age are the targets of interest.

Jacobs et al. (2010) published a study that helps to illustrate the complexity of understanding risk factors and their relationship to the development of poor health. They studied the association between waist circumference and mortality among 48,500 men and 56,343 women 50 years or older. They determined that waist circumference as a measure of abdominal obesity is associated with higher mortality independent of body mass index (BMI). They note that waist circumference is associated with higher circulating levels of inflammatory markers, insulin resistance, type II diabetes mellitus (DM), dyslipidemia, and coronary heart disease. In recent years, the constellation of these above mentioned factors has been described as metabolic syndrome. Metabolic syndrome is a complex syndrome that encompasses many conditions and risk factors particularly abdominal obesity, high blood pressure, abnormal cholesterol and triglyceride levels, and insulin resistance and is known to be associated with an increased risk of stroke, heart disease, and type II DM (Grundy et al., 2005). The increasing prevalence of metabolic syndrome is becoming a tremendous public health concern, and more evidence is appearing in the literature to better define its treatment as well as preventive measures needed to reduce the incidence. Although it is ill defined in children and adolescents, it is clear that early interventions to reduce obesity and sedentary behavior and to improve nutrition can have long-term effects and can improve overall life expectancy. The metabolic syndrome, like many conditions, demonstrates the complexity of interactions that occurs in disease development and that no one factor in and of itself can be targeted alone. The APN needs to take into consideration the many facets of health and disease, genetics and environment, and human attitudes and behavior when determining how to implement a population-based program.

Diabetes Mellitus

The number of American adults treated for DM more than doubled between 1996 and 2007 (from about 9 million to 19 million). This includes an increase from 1.2 million to 2.4 million among people aged 18 to 44. During this time period, the treatment costs for DM climbed from $18.5 billion to $40.8 billion (Soni, 2010). The rise in both incidence and prevalence rates in DM is closely tied to rising obesity levels, which is a preventable risk factor.

The *Diabetes Data & Trends Report* (CDC, 2007a) reveals that the rate of newly diagnosed cases of DM in people aged 18 to 44 in the United States has increased from 1.7 per thousand in 1980 to 2.0 per thousand in 1990, to 2.7 per thousand in 2000, and to 3.4 per thousand in 2005. This upwards trend in the incidence rate for DM provides a clear direction for targeting prevention measures toward younger populations. There is, in fact, a huge potential for improving the health of populations by targeting children for primary health prevention measures that goes well beyond reducing diabetes rates. Implications for early interventions beginning in pregnancy and continuing through infancy and early childhood are clear. Infants are increasingly being overfed as many are using infant formula instead of or in addition to breast feeding. Evidence is increasing that early feeding patterns (Owen et al., 2005) as well as parental obesity and parental eating patterns are linked to the increased likelihood of developing obesity in children, which puts them at an increased risk for type II DM. There are many opportunities for APNs to apply evidence-based, primary prevention interventions to improve the long-term outcomes of children at the beginning of pregnancy and at birth. This approach may include targeting high-risk aggregates (e.g., parents with obesity and type II DM) and then expanding to communities through educational campaigns or changes in policy.

Health and the Social Environment

Most of the data discussed earlier exemplify the biologic and environmental factors that contribute to poor health in adults. However, it is becoming more apparent that social (e.g., psychological) factors starting soon after birth may play a more significant role on adult health than was once thought. Having a comprehensive understanding of the underlying causes of adult diseases (including the social, psychological, biological, and environmental) is necessary to successfully approach the problem. Without this comprehensive understanding, it may be difficult to successfully implement a primary prevention program. Studies that link adverse childhood events (ACE) with adult health help illustrate the sometimes causal relationship between the social environment and poor health. The ACE study is an ongoing, joint project of the CDC and Kaiser Permanente. This research examines the relationships between several categories of childhood trauma (e.g., physical or sexual abuse, having an incarcerated household member, or being raised with one or no parents) with adult behavioral problems (e.g., mental health issues, promiscuity, drug and alcohol problems). An ACE score based on exposure to the identified categories of adverse childhood experiences is used to determine a study participant's exposure to trauma (ACE Study, 2011). In one widely cited ACE study (Felitti et al., 1998), people who experienced a score of four or more categories of ACEs compared to those who had no history of exposure had a 4- to 12-fold increased risk for alcoholism, drug abuse, depression, and suicide attempts. They also experienced a 2- to 4-fold increase in smoking and self-reported poor health. Subsequent research provides additional evidence to support the link between childhood trauma and adverse events and poor health outcomes.

Smyth, Heron, Wonderlich, Crosby, and Thompson (2008) conducted a study of students entering college directly from high school to investigate the association between adverse events in childhood and eating disturbances. They found that childhood adverse events predicted eating disturbances in college. Childhood adverse events have also been linked to drug abuse and dependence (Messina et al., 2008) and greater use of healthcare and mental health services (Cannon, Bonomi, Anderson, Rivara, & Thompson, 2010). Building on earlier studies that linked smoking in adulthood with ACEs, Brown et al. (2010) discovered a relationship between a history of ACEs and the risk of dying from lung cancer.

Studies such as these illustrate the importance of understanding the social determinants of poor health and the potential for doing good and preventing harm to aggregates and populations by targeting problems such as child abuse and neglect for prevention and early recognition and intervention.

Population Strategies in Acute Care

Targeting evidence-based interventions toward aggregates in the acute care population also has the potential to broadly improve health outcomes. How can we improve the quality of care for our patients by taking a population-based approach? When nurses apply evidence-based interventions to identified aggregates they can improve outcomes more effectively than when interventions are designed on a case by case (individualized) basis. The following examples illustrate this point.

Several organizations including the Association for Professionals in Infection Control and Epidemiology, the Society for Healthcare Epidemiology of America, and the CDC have proposed a call to action to move toward elimination of healthcare associated infections (HAI). The key elements of the framework are data collection, evidence-based practices, and system-wide infection prevention strategies that include accurate data collection and development of credible prevention strategies including payment incentives that focus on prevention, accreditation, and public reporting (Cardo et al., 2010).

Patients in intensive care units (ICU) and who are ventilated constitute an aggregate with identifiable parameters and shared risks. Ventilator-associated pneumonia (VAP) is the most frequent nosocomial infection found in many ICUs. It occurs in 9% to 40% of intubated patients and 10% to 20% of patients who are ventilated more than 48 hours. The incidence rate is 5 to 10 episodes per 1000 hospital admissions. It is associated with prolonged length of stay, and high morbidity and mortality (Lisboa & Rello, 2008). The average cost of VAP is approximately $50,000 per person (Cocanour et al., 2006). An intervention referred to as the ventilator bundle was designed to reduce the incidence of VAP. It is composed of four protocols that provide prophylaxis against peptic ulceration and deep vein thrombosis, daily cessation of sedation, and elevation of the patient's head and chest to at least 30 degrees. Studies have shown that consistent application of the bundle results in significant changes in length of ventilation and ICU length of stay (Crunden, Boyce, Woodman, & Bray, 2005; Curtin, 2011).

Another intervention that uses protocols to improve long-term outcomes addresses the treatment of stroke in an acute care setting. It was found that stroke patients taken to hospitals that follow specific treatment protocols have a better chance of surviving than patients taken elsewhere. A study evaluated the outcomes of the first 1 million stroke patients treated at hospitals enrolled in the *Get with the Guidelines* stroke program that was started by the American Heart Association (AHA) in 2003. The American Stroke Association guidelines require that hospitals follow seven specific evidence-based steps for treating stroke patients. Between 2003 and 2009, hospitals that followed these protocols lowered the risk of death by 10% for patients with ischemic stroke (Fonarow et al., 2011).

Surveillance of poor health outcomes in acute care facilities is one way in which APNs can identify causative factors and design interventions to reduce costs and improve care. For example, recognizing the causative factors that lead to increased rehospitalization rates and super-utilization of emergency departments could be the first step in designing an intervention. Approximately 25% of all U.S. hospital patients are readmitted within one year for the same conditions that led to their original hospitalization. The Agency for Healthcare Research and Quality (AHRQ) analyzed data for 2006 to 2007 on 15 million patients in 12 states. They found that among Medicare patients, 42% were readmitted to hospitals and 30% had multiple emergency department visits. Among Medicaid patients, 23% had multiple hospital admissions and 50% had multiple emergency department visits. According to the AHRQ, better outpatient care could prevent unnecessary repeat hospital admissions (May 27, 2010). Identifying and targeting populations with specific diagnoses for which there are high readmission rates offers great return on investment. Readmissions are costly in dollars to both consumers and hospitals and negatively impact the quality of life for patients.

Chronic Conditions

In 2000, the U.S. DHHS released a report outlining a strategic framework that includes goals to foster healthcare and public health system changes to improve the health of those with multiple chronic conditions (MCC). The intention of the framework is to create change in how chronic illnesses are addressed in the United States from an individual approach to one that uses a population-focused approach. The authors of the report point out that 66% of total healthcare spending is directed toward caring for the approximately 20% of Americans with multiple concurrent chronic conditions (e.g., arthritis, heart disease, and DM). One strategy proposed by the DHHS is to define and identify populations and sub-populations with MCC broadly and to explore care models to target subgroups at high risk of poor health outcomes. Another proposed strategy addresses the need to develop systems to promote models to address common risk factors and challenges that are associated with many chronic conditions. The framework also addresses the need to create policies and interventions that identify populations and subpopulations at risk and to identify strategies and interventions that target these populations (DHHS, 2010).

The problem of chronic diseases is not restricted to the United States. The World Health Organization (WHO) has published a report that documents the global problem of noncommunicable diseases (NCD). NCDs now account for more deaths than infectious diseases even in poor countries. WHO Director General Dr. Margaret Chan is quoted as saying, "for some countries, it is no exaggeration to describe the situation is an impending disaster; a disaster for health, society, most of all for national economies" (WHO, 2011, p. v). NCDs accounted for 63% of deaths worldwide in 2008. Millions of people die each year as a result of modifiable risk factors that underlie the major NCDs. These include tobacco use, alcohol abuse, poor nutritional habits, insufficient physical activity, overweight/obesity, high blood pressure, elevated blood sugar, and high cholesterol levels. The writers of the report contend that 8% of premature heart disease, stroke, and diabetes can be prevented. Ten action points including banning smoking in public places, enforcing tobacco advertising bans, restricting access to alcohol, and reducing salt in food are listed. All of these actions require a population approach to be effective (WHO, 2011).

A survey conducted by the AHA lends an interesting perspective to this argument. They surveyed 1000 people in the United States. The AHA found that 76% of the respondents agreed that wine can be good for the heart but only 30% knew the AHA's recommended limits for daily wine consumption. Drinking too much alcohol of any kind can increase blood pressure and lead to heart failure. The survey results also found that most respondents do not know the source of sodium content in their diets and are confused by low-sodium food choices. A majority of the respondents (61%) believe that sea salt is a low-sodium alternative to table salt when in fact it is chemically the same. This survey reinforces the idea that the American public requires more understanding of nutrition and the relationship between nutrition and health. It also reinforces the argument that interventions to improve health must be addressed at the community or population level (AHA, 2011).

Interventions that are evidence-based and population appropriate can reduce the underlying causes of chronic disease. This approach has the potential to lower the mean level of risk factors and shift outcomes in a favorable direction. An example that is receiving a lot of recent attention is sodium intake. Excess sodium in the diet can put people at risk for stroke and heart disease. The CDC has reported that 9 of 10 Americans consume more salt than is recommended. Only 5.5% of adults follow the recommendation to limit sodium intake to 1500 mg a day. Most sodium does not come from salt added to foods at the table but from processed foods. These foods include grain-based frozen meals, soup, and processed meat. In this report, the IOM concludes that reducing sodium content in food requires new government standards for the acceptable level of sodium. Manufacturers and restaurants need to meet these standards so that all sources in the food supply are involved (CDC, 2010b; IOM, 2010b). A study published in the *Annals of Internal Medicine* (Smith-Spangler, Juusola, Enns, Owens, & Garber, 2010) estimates that reducing dietary salt 0.3 g per day could greatly reduce the yearly number of U.S. cases of coronary heart disease, stroke, and heart attacks with a savings of up to $24 billion in healthcare costs each year.

This discussion illustrates the need to promulgate laws and develop policies that impact health outcomes. Changing individual behavior is difficult. Using the power of legislation and regulation to make changes in the environment such as banning smoking in public places, increasing air quality, and reducing the amount of sodium in processed foods has enormous potential for improving the health of populations.

PRINCIPLES OF POPULATION-BASED APPROACH TO HEALTHCARE

The five basic principles of the population approach to care described by Ibrahim, Savitz, Carey, and Wagner (2001) provide a framework for the APN in the area of population-based care. The principles that characterize population-based care include: a community perspective, a clinical epidemiology perspective, evidence-based practice, an emphasis on prevention, and an emphasis on outcomes.

The *community perspective* refers to the collection of data related to the frequency of disease, disability, and death in an aggregate or a population and the number of people in the population of interest. The evaluation of outcome measures in populations begins with an identification of the totality of health problems, the needs of defined populations, and the differences among groups. The rates calculated from these numbers can help the APN to identify risk factors, target populations at risk and lay the foundation for designing interventions.

The *clinical epidemiology perspective* refers to the need to manage all patients with similar needs or problems—obesity, for example, or dependent elderly people being cared for at home. The care of specialized groups is the core of advanced practice. *Evidence-based practice* is defined as the conscientious integration of best research evidence with clinical expertise and patient values and needs in the delivery of quality, cost-effective healthcare (Burns & Grove, 2009). The basic sciences of public health (particularly epidemiology and biostatistics) provide tools for the APN working with specialized populations to provide evidence for effective and efficient interventions.

Prevention can also best be carried out at the population level, whether at the level of direct care or through the support and promotion of policies. For example, an evidence-based program to prevent hospital readmissions for congestive heart failure can lead to improved health and decreased health-related costs. The promulgation of policies and regulations to support primary prevention measures such as decreased sodium in prepared foods could potentially lead to decreased rates of hypertension and heart disease. Interventions that are appropriate at the individual level and applied at the population level can result in a far-reaching effect.

Outcomes measurement refers to collecting and analyzing data using predetermined outcomes indicators for the purposes of making decisions about healthcare (ANA, 2004). Outcomes research in APN practice is research that focuses on the effectiveness of nursing interventions. Outcomes measurement in population-based care begins with the identification of the population and the problem, followed by the generation of a clinical question related to outcomes. It is a measure of the process of care. An outcomes measure should be clearly quantifiable, be relatively easy to define, and lend itself to standardization.

In outcomes measurement, the APN is ultimately concerned with whether or not a population benefits from an intervention. The APN also needs to be concerned with the question of quality, efficacy (Does the intervention work under ideal conditions?), and effectiveness (Does it work under real life situations?). Other important considerations are efficiency (cost benefit), affordability, accessibility, and acceptability.

SUMMARY

The Robert Wood Johnson Foundation and the IOM have issued a report to respond to the need to transform the nursing profession. The committee developed four key messages:

1. Nurses should practice to the full extent of their education and should achieve higher levels of education training.
2. The education system for nurses should be improved so that it provides seamless academic progression.
3. Nurses should be full partners, with physicians and other healthcare professionals.
4. Healthcare in the Unites States should be re-designed for effective workforce planning and policymaking (IOM, 2010c).

To improve population health, APNs need to practice to the full extent of their education, be active in the political arena, and work collaboratively with other healthcare professionals. To promote health, APNs can use epidemiological methods to identify aggregates at risk, analyze problems of highest priority, design evidence-based interventions, and evaluate the results. An important concept in the field of population health is attention to the multiple determinants of health outcomes and the identification of their distribution throughout the population. These determinants include medical care, public health interventions, characteristics of the social environment (e.g., income, education, employment, social support, culture), physical environment (e.g., clean air, water quality), genetics, and individual behavior. These determinants can act independently but population-based care is concerned with the patterns of such determinants (Kindig & Stoddart, 2003).

A final note about the use of APN in this book: *The Consensus Model for APRN Regulation: Licensure, Accreditation, Certification & Education* was completed and published in 2008 by the APRN Consensus Work Group and the National Council of State Boards of Nursing APRN Advisory Committee. The title of advanced practice registered nurse (APRN) is used in the document to refer to certified nurse anesthetists, certified nurse midwives, clinical nurse specialists, and certified nurse practitioners. The model was created through a collaborative effort of more than 40 organizations in order to "align the interrelationships among licensure, accreditation, certification, and education to create a more uniform practice across the country" (ANCC, 2011, 1st bullet point). The goal is for implementation of the model by 2015 (ANCC, 2011; APRN Consensus Work Group, 2008). The authors of this book live and work in a state where APN is the legal title for advanced practice nursing, and we decided to use that title to refer to advanced practice nurses throughout this text. This title is inclusive of nurses who have completed a doctorate in nursing practice and advanced practice nurses educated at the master's level.

EXERCISES AND DISCUSSION QUESTIONS

Exercise 1.1 Using the table below as an example, list the parameters that describe the population(s) to whom you provide care.

POPULATION	FRAMING DEFINITIONS	PARAMETERS
Patients who have been diagnosed with congestive heart failure (CHF) and who live in the community	Adult (18 years of age and older) patients discharged from an urban medical center with a primary diagnosis of CHF	P1 = diagnosis
		P2 = age
		P3 = location/service area
Population of New Jersey	All permanent residents of New Jersey	P1 = geographical location
		P2 = permanent residency

Exercise 1.2 PolitiFact is a Web site created by the *St. Petersburg Times* and a winner of the 2009 Pulitzer Prize (http://politifact.com/truth-o-meter/). It was created to help people find the truth in American politics. Reporters and editors from the newspaper check statements by members of Congress, the White House, lobbyists and interest groups and rate them on a *Truth-O-Meter*. Find a statement that is being circulated about the Affordable Care Act, and then check the Truth-O-Meter to determine the veracity of the statement.

Exercise 1.3 Identify two or three population-based and health-related interventions at your institution or in your community. Determine if the approach has been successful in changing outcomes and/or reducing health-related costs. Identify the aggregate population and what parameters were used in this intervention. Identify any changes in policy associated with these interventions.

REFERENCES

ACE Study. (2011). *The adverse childhood experiences (ACE) study.* Retrieved from http://acestudy.org/index.html

Agency for Healthcare Research and Quality. (2010). *1 in 4 patients undergoes revolving-door hospitalizations.* (May 27, 2010). News release.

Allan, J., Barwick, T., Cashman, S., Cawley, J. F., Day, C., Douglass, ... Wood, D. (2004). Clinical prevention and population health: Curriculum framework for health professions. American Journal of Preventive Medicine, 27(5), 471–476.

American Association of Colleges of Nursing (AACN). (2006). *The essentials of doctoral education for advanced practice nursing.* Retrieved from http://www.aacn.nche.edu/DNP/pdf/Essentials.pdf

American Heart Association. (2010). Half of adults 50 and younger with low 10-year risk of CVD have high lifetime risk. Retrieved from http://www.newsroom.heart.org/index.php?s=43&item=635

American Heart Association (AHA). (2011a). *Most Americans don't understand health effects of wind and sea salt, survey finds.* Retrieved from http://www.newsroom.heart.org/index.php?s=43&item=1316

American Heart Association. (2011b). *Stroke fact sheet.* Retrieved from http://www.heart.org/idc/groups/heart-public/@wcm/@private/@hcm/@gwtg/documents/dowloadable/ucm_310976.pdf

American Nurses Association. (2004). *Nursing: Scope and standards of practice.* Washington, DC: Author.

American Nurses Association. (2009). *ANA supports public plan option for health reform, contrary to Doctors' group.* Press Release. Retrieved June 12, 2009, from http://nursingworld.org/FunctionalMenuCategories/MediaResources/PressReleases/2009-PR/ANA-Supports-Public-Plan-Option-for-Health-Reform.aspx

American Nurses Credentialing Center. (2011). *APRN fact sheet.* Retrieved from: http://www.nursecredentialing.org/Certification/APRN-Updates/APRN-Factsheet.aspx

Anderson, H. R., & Cook, D. G. (1997). Passive smoking and sudden infant death syndrome: Review of the epidemiological evidence. *Thorax, 52,* 1003–1009.

APRN Consensus Work Group & the National Council of State Boards of Nursing APRN Advisory Committee. (2008). *Consensus model for APRN regulation:* Licensure, accreditation, certification & education. Retrieved from https://www.ncsbn.org/7_23_08_Consensue_APRN_Final.pdf

Beasley, J., Kuller, L., Allison, D., Wang, C., Redden, D., Westfall, A., & Fontaine, K. (2003). Obesity and years of life lost. In K. R. Fontaine, D. T. Redden, & C. Wang, et al. (Eds.), *Years of life lost due to obesity. JAMA, 289,* 187–193; author reply. *JAMA, 289*(14), 1777–1778. Retrieved from EBSCO*host*.

Brown, D., Anda, R., Felitti, V., Edwards, V., Malarcher, A., Croft, J., & Giles, W. (2010). Adverse childhood experiences are associated with the risk of lung cancer: A prospective cohort study. *BMC Public Health, 10,* 20. Retrieved from EBSCO*host.*

Burns, N., & Grove, S. (2009). The practice of nursing research: Appraisal, synthesis, and generation of evidence (6th ed.). St Louis, MO: Saunders Elsevier.

Cannon, E., Bonomi, A., Anderson, M., Rivara, F., & Thompson, R. (2010). Adult health and relationship outcomes among women with abuse experiences during childhood. *Violence And Victims, 25*(3), 291–305. Retrieved from EBSCO*host.*

Cardo, D., Dennehy, P., Halverson, P., Fishman, N., Kohn, M., Murphy, C., & Whitley, R. (2010). Moving toward elimination of healthcare-associated infections: A call to action. *American Journal of Infection Control, 38*(9), 671–675. Retrieved from EBSCO*host.*

Centers for Disease Control. (2007a). *Diabetes data and trends.* Retrieved September 18, 2007, from http://www.cdc.gov/diabetes/statistics/incidence/fig1.htm

Centers for Disease Control and Prevention (CDC). (2007b). *Leading causes of death.* Retrieved from http://www.cdc.gov/nchs/fastats/lcod.htm

Centers for Disease Control and Prevention. (2010a). Vital signs: Current cigarette smoking among adults aged ≥ 18 years—United States, 2009. *Morbidity and Mortality Weekly Report.* Retrieved September 10, 2010, from http://www.cdc.gov/mmwr/preview/mmwrhtml/mm5935a3.htm?s_cid=mm5935a3_w

Centers for Disease Control and Prevention. (2010b). Sodium intake among adults—United States, 2005–2006. (2010). *Morbidity and mortality weekly report.* Retrieved June 25, 2010, from http://www.cdc.gov/mmwr/preview/mmwrhtml/mm5924a4.htm?s_cid=mm5924a4_w

Centers for Disease Control and Prevention. (2010c). Cigarette use among high school students—United States, 1991–2009. *Morbidity and mortality weekly report.* Retrieved July 9, 2010, from http://www.cdc.gov/mmwr/preview/mmwrhtml/mm5926a1.htm?s_cid=mm5926a1_w

Central Intelligence Agency (CIA). (2011). *The world factbook.* Retrieved from https://www.cia.gov/library/publications/the-world-factbook/rankorder/2091rank.html

Cocanour, C., Peninger, M., Domonoske, B., Li, T., Wright, B., Valdivia, A., & Luther, K. (2006). Decreasing ventilator-associated pneumonia in a trauma ICU. *Journal of Trauma, 61*(1), 122–130. Retrieved from EBSCO*host.*

Collins, S., Doty, M., Robertson, R., & Garber, T. (2010). How the recession has left millions of workers without health insurance, and how health reform will bring relief: Findings from the Commonwealth Fund Biennial Health Insurance Survey of 2010. Retrieved from http://www.commonwealthfund.org/~/media/Files/Publications/Fund%20Report/2011/Mar/1486_Collins_help_on_the_horizon_2010_biennial_survey_report_FINAL_v2.pdf

Crunden, E., Boyce, C., Woodman, H., & Bray, B. (2005). An evaluation of the impact of the ventilator care bundle. *Nursing in Critical Care, 10*(5), 242–246.

Curtin, L. J. (2011). Preventing ventilator-associated pneumonia: A nursing-intervention bundle. *American Nurse Today, 6*(3), 9–11.

Felitti, V., Anda, R., Nordenberg, D., Williamson, D., Spitz, A., Edwards, V., … Marks, J. (1998). Relationship of childhood abuse and household dysfunction to many of the leading causes of death in adults: The adverse childhood experiences (ACE) study. *American Journal of Preventative Medicine, 14,* 245–258.

Fonarow, G., Smith, E., Saver, J., Reeves, M., Bhatt, D., Grau-Sepulveda, M., … Schwamm, L. (2011). Timeliness of tissue-type plasminogen activator therapy in acute ischemic stroke: Patient characteristics, hospital factors, and outcomes associated with door-to-needle times within 60 minutes. *Circulation, 123*(7), 750–758. Retrieved from EBSCO*host.*

Garrett, B., Buettgens, M., Doan, L., Headen, J., & Holahan, J. (2010). *The cost of failure to enact health reform (2010–2020).* The Urban Institute. Retrieved from http://www.urban. org/publications/412049.html

Grundy, S. M., Cleeman, J., Daniels, S. R., Donato, K. A., Eckel, R. H., Franklin, B. A., ... Costa, F. (2005). Diagnosis and management of the metabolic syndrome: An American Heart Association/National Heart, Lung, and Blood Institute scientific statement. *Circulation, 112,* 2735.

Ibrahim, M., Savitz, L., Carey, T., & Wagner, E. (2001). Population-based health principles in medical and public health practice. *Journal of Public Health Management & Practice, 7*(3), 75–81. Retrieved from EBSCO*host.*

Institute of Medicine (IOM). (2010a). *For the public's health: The role of measurement in action and accountability.* Retrieved from http://iom.edu/~/media/Files/Report%20Files/2010/ For-the-Publics-Health-The-Role-of-Measurement-in-Action-and-Accountability/ For%20the%20Publics%20Health%202010%20Report%20Brief.pdf

Institute of Medicine. (2010b). *Strategies to reduce sodium intake in United States.* Retrieved from http://iom.edu/Reports/2010/Strategies-to-Reduce-Sodium-Intake-in-the-United-States.aspx

Institute of Medicine. (2010c, October 5). *The future of nursing: Leading change, advancing health.* Retrieved from http://iom.edu/Reports/2010/The-Future-of-Nursing-Leading-Change-Advancing-Health.aspx

Jacobs, E., Newton, C., Wang, Y., Patel, A., McCullough, M., Campbell, P., ... Gapster, S. (2010). Waist circumference and all–cause mortality in a large US cohort. *Archives of Internal Medicine, 170*(15), 1293–1301.

Kindig, D., & Stoddart, G. (2003). What is population health? *American Journal of Public Health, 93*(3), 380–383.

Lisboa, T., & Rello, J. (2008). Diagnosis of ventilator associated pneumonia: Is there a gold standard and a simple approach? *Current Opinions Infectious Disease, 21,* 174–178.

Messina, N., Marinelli-Casey, P., Hillhouse, M., Rawson, R., Hunter, J., & Ang, A. (2008). Childhood adverse events and methamphetamine use among men and women. *Journal of Psychoactive Drugs,* 399–409. Retrieved from EBSCO*host.*

National Coalition on Health Care. (2010). *Insurance.* Retrieved from http://nchc.org/ issue-areas/insurance

Obama, B. (2009, August 16). Why we need health care reform. *The New York Times,* WK9.

Orszag, P. R. (2008). Growth in health care costs. Statement before the Committee on the Budget United States Senate. Retrieved January 31, 2008, from http://www.cbo.gov/ ftpdocs/89xx/doc8948/01-31-HealthTestimony.pdf

Owen, C. G., Martin, R. M., Whincup, P. H., Smith, G. D., & Cook, D. G. (2005). Effect of infant feeding on the risk of obesity across the life course: A quantitative review of published evidence. *Pediatrics, 115*(5), 1367–77.

Population. (2002). *The American heritage dictionary of the English language* (4th ed., p. 1366). Boston, MA: Houghton Mifflin.

Porche, D. J. (2004). *Public and community health nursing practice.* Thousand Oaks, CA: Sage Publications, Inc.

Puhl, R. M., Heuer, C., & Sarda, V. (2010, September 7). Framing messages about weight discrimination: Impact on public support for legislation. *International Journal of Obesity online publication.* Retrieved September 7, 2010, from http://www.nature.com/ijo/ journal/vaop/ncurrent/pdf/ijo2010199a.pdf

Smith-Spangler, C., Juusola, J., Enns, E., Owens, D., & Garber, A. (2010). Population strategies to decrease sodium intake and the burden of cardiovascular disease: A cost-effectiveness analysis. *Annals of Internal Medicine, 152*(8), 481. Retrieved from EBSCO*host*.

Smyth, J., Heron, K., Wonderlich, S., Crosby, R., & Thompson, K. (2008). The influence of reported trauma and adverse events on eating disturbance in young adults. *International Journal of Eating Disorders, 41*(3), 195–202. Retrieved from EBSCO*host*.

Soni, A. (2010, December). Trends in use and expenditures for diabetes among adults 18 and older, *U.S. civilian noninstitutionalized population, 1996 and 2007.* Agency for Healthcare Research and Policy (AHRQ). Retrieved from http://www.meps.ahrq.gov/mepsweb/data_files/publications/st304/stat304.pdf

U.S. Department of Health and Human Services. (2006). *The health consequences of involuntary exposure to tobacco smoke: A report of the Surgeon General, U.S. Department of Health and Human Services.* Available at http://www.surgeongeneral.gov/library/secondhandsmoke/factsheets/factsheet2.html

U.S. Department of Health and Human Services (DHHS). (2010). *Multiple chronic conditions—a strategic framework: Optimum health and quality of life for individuals with multiple chronic conditions.* Washington, DC: Author.

U.S. Environmental Protection Agency. (2004). *Fact sheet: Respiratory health effects of passive smoking.* Available at http://www.epa.gov/smokefre/pdfs/survey_fact_sheet.pdf

Ventura, S.J., Hamilton, B.E., Mathews, T.J., & Chandra, A. (2003). Trends and variations in smoking during pregnancy and low birth weight: Evidence from the birth certificate, 1990–2000. *Pediatrics* 2003; 111; 1176–1180. http://pediatrics.aappublications.org/content/111/Supplement_1/1176.

World Health Organization. (2011). *Global status report on NCDs.* Retrieved from http://www.who.int/gho/ncd/en/index.html

Yolton, K., Dietrich, K., Auinger, P., Lanphear, B. P., & Hornung, R. (2005). Exposure to environmental tobacco smoke and cognitive abilities among U.S. children and adolescents. *Environ Health Perspect, 113*(1), 98–103.

TWO

Identifying Outcomes

Sonda M. Oppewal

Nurses have a long and rich history of wanting to do the most good for the most people. Today, it is imperative that advanced practice nurses (APNs) provide interventions that benefit populations in addition to providing effective interventions at community, aggregate, family, and individual levels. Identifying population level healthcare needs and healthcare disparities can help improve health outcomes at all levels.

The American Association of Colleges of Nursing's (AACN) definition of advanced practice nursing includes the importance of identifying and managing health outcomes at the population level (AACN, 2004). In 2006, the AACN specified that graduates of doctorate in nursing practice (DNP) programs have competency in meeting "the needs of a panel of patients, a target population, a set of populations, or a broad community" (p. 10). A core component of DNP education is clinical prevention (health promotion and disease prevention at individual and family levels) and population health (focus of care at aggregate and community levels and examination of environmental, occupational, cultural, and socioeconomic dimensions of health) (AACN, 2006; Allan et al., 2004). Regardless of whether DNP graduates practice with a focus on clinical prevention or population health, the ability to define, identify, and analyze outcomes is imperative for improving the health status of individuals and populations (AACN, 2006; U.S. Department of Health and Human Services [DHHS], 2000).

The purpose of this chapter is to explore how APNs can identify and define population outcomes. Specific examples from various settings such as acute care, subacute care, long-term care, and the community will be given, as well as outcomes related to health disparities and national health objectives. The identification of outcomes or key health indicators is an essential first step in planning effective interventions and is used later in the evaluation process. By comparing outcomes, APNs can advocate for needed change at local, regional, state, or national levels by identifying areas for improvement in practice, by comparing evidence needed for effective practice, and by better understanding health disparities. Health disparities are not fair or socially just; however, they are preventable. They reflect an uneven distribution of environmental, social, economic, and political factors. Health disparities are differences in incidence or prevalence of illness, mortality, injury, or violence, or differences in opportunities to reach optimal health given disadvantages because of race, ethnicity, socioeconomic status, gender, sexual orientation, geographic location, or other reasons (Centers for Disease Control and Prevention [CDC], 2008). APNs have an important collaborative role with professionals from other disciplines and community members to work toward eliminating health disparities.

IDENTIFYING AND DEFINING POPULATION OUTCOMES

Background

One of the earliest records of observed outcomes by nurses dates back to 1854 during the Crimean War at the Scutari Hospital in Turkey when Florence Nightingale, credited as the founder of modern nursing, documented a decrease in mortality among the British soldiers after providing more nutritious food, cleaning up the environment, and improving the sewage system (Fee & Garofalo, 2010). Despite the leadership and pioneer work that Nightingale provided in outcomes documentation (Hill, 1999; Lang & Marek, 1991; van Maanen, 1979), the nursing literature revealed variation in the documentation of nursing outcomes. Griffiths (1995) concluded that the literature from the mid-1960s to the mid-1990s was not very progressive in documenting nursing outcomes but showed promise of improving. Health reform efforts to improve quality and access and reduce costs spurred more work to examine outcomes while examining their relationship to indicators of structure and process. While earlier work in nursing outcomes focused on costs, it was clear that a more comprehensive model that reflected other types of outcomes was needed to advance healthcare and reflect the various outcomes that resulted from nursing interventions (Nelson, Batalden, Plume, Mihevc, & Swartz, 1995).

Defining, Categorizing, and Identifying Outcomes

Health outcomes are usually defined as an end result that follows some kind of healthcare provision, treatment, or intervention and may describe a patient's condition or health status (Hill, 1999; Kleinpell & Gawlinski, 2005; Oermann & Floyd, 2002). Classifying outcomes or categorizing outcomes can be done in several ways. For example, outcomes may be classified into categories: by describing "who" is measured such as individuals, aggregates, communities, populations, or organizations; by identifying the "what" or the type of outcome such as care-, patient-, or performance-related outcomes (Kleinpell, 2001); and by determining the "when" or the time it takes to achieve an outcome such as short-term, intermediate, or long-term outcomes (Rich, 2009). Table 2.1 provides examples of outcomes by these different classification systems and the measures by the beneficiary of the outcome, type of outcome, and time frame of the outcome.

TABLE 2.1   Examples of Outcomes and Measures by Beneficiary, Type, and Time Frame

BENEFICIARY (WHO?)	MEASURE	POTENTIAL OUTCOME
Individual outcomes	Blood pressure reading	Decreased blood pressure
Aggregate outcomes	Weekly weights of participants in an exercise class	Reduced mean weight for class members each week
Community outcomes	A town's seat belt usage per 100 drivers 20 years of age and younger computed yearly	Increased yearly rate of a town's seat belt usage per 100 drivers 20 years of age and younger
Population outcomes	Reported number of infant deaths within 1 year of birth per 1000 infants	Decreased infant mortality rate compared to previous year

TYPE (WHAT?)	MEASURE	POTENTIAL OUTCOME
Care-related outcomes	Annual rate of hospital-acquired infections determined from hospital infectious disease reports	Decreased hospital-acquired infections from previous year
Patient-related outcomes	Observation of insulin injection administration technique	Correct demonstration by patient of safe insulin administration technique
Performance-related outcomes	Chart review of protocol checklist of asthma best practices protocol	Nursing staff adherence to asthma best practices protocol

TIME FRAME (WHEN?)	MEASURE	POTENTIAL OUTCOME
Short-term outcomes	Self-report of nipple discomfort among first-time breastfeeding mothers at a regional hospital's postpartum unit	Absence of nipple discomfort among first-time breastfeeding mothers 1 week after hospital discharge from a regional hospital's postpartum unit
Intermediate outcomes	Self-report of tobacco usage by first-time outpatient clinic users during the calendar year	Smoking cessation self-reports 8 weeks after quit date by outpatient clinic users during the calendar year
Long-term outcomes	Annual communicable disease reports of HIV incidence among African Americans	Annual reduction of HIV incidence rates among African Americans

One of the early frameworks that nurses use to categorize outcomes and is still used today is based on four dimensions that correspond to points on a compass. Known as the *Clinical Value Compass*, the four dimensions or categories are: clinical (e.g., disease-specific outcomes), functional (e.g., ability to participate in activities of daily living, overall well-being), cost (e.g., number of encounters, length of stay, finances and resources), and satisfaction (e.g., patient and family satisfaction) (Nelson et al., 1995; Nelson, Mohr, Batalden, & Plume, 1996; Oermann & Floyd, 2002).

Another framework used frequently in nursing and healthcare to evaluate care relies on the examination of three components: structure, process, and outcome. Structure refers to healthcare resources such as the number and type of health and social service agencies and utilization indicators, process describes how the healthcare was delivered, and outcome refers to the change in health status based on the intervention provided (Donabedian, 1980). This framework is particularly useful in describing the health of a community (Shuster & Goeppinger, 2008). For example, the community's health can be described in terms of its structure by the number and type of health and social agencies present, its healthcare workforce, health services utilization indicators, and the community's educational and socioeconomic levels in relation to demographic measures of race, gender, and age. The community's health process measures reflect healthcare delivery methods and how well community members can work together to solve their problems, which reflects community competence (Cottrell, 1976). Community health outcomes include status measures associated with vital statistics (e.g., births, deaths, marriages, divorces, fetal deaths, and induced termination of pregnancies), morbidity or illness data and trends, social determinants of health such as housing, unemployment, and poverty rates, neighborhood safety, access to fresh fruits and vegetables, as well as physical activity venues like parks, playgrounds, and neighborhood sports fields (McDevitt & Wilbur, 2002; Shuster & Goeppinger, 2008). Other indicators of a community's health status may include the number of premature deaths, quality of life, disabilities, risk factors, and injuries. APNs can work in partnership with community members to identify what community members see as relevant and important, and then continue to work in partnership to identify strategies to intervene, monitor, and improve those outcomes (Sheilds & Lindsey, 2002).

Vital statistics provide important outcome measures that APNs can monitor and compare over time and analyze by demographic variables to detect health disparities. In the United States, the National Center for Health Statistics (NCHS) collects the official records of births, deaths, marriages, divorces, fetal deaths, and induced terminations of pregnancies (McDevitt & Wilbur, 2002) from local health departments. Personnel from local health departments analyze the data from death certificates including demographic data, the immediate cause of death, contributing factors of death, and multiple causes of death. Local data are sent to a state office for collation and then sent to the NCHS who provides this information to the public on its Web site and in an annual publication, "Vital Statistics of the United States" (Friis & Sellers, 2009).

APNs are often responsible for reviewing morbidity and mortality trends and can use this information to advocate for improved health policy, additional resources, or to develop innovative interventions. For example, if an APN notices an increase over the past year of closed head injuries in teenagers because of motor vehicle crashes (MVC), she or he may identify a plan of care that targets risk factors associated with teenage driving and MVCs. For example, the APN may review emergency department (ED) records of teenage drivers in car accidents to assess seat belt use, blood alcohol levels, prior ED visits, and age at the time of the incident (as a way of assessing characteristics of teen drivers). APNs may also approach high schools by collaborating with a school nurse and developing a peer training program whereby high school students can be trained as peer teachers to encourage classmates to wear seat belts, avoid entering a car with an impaired driver, and saying no to drug and alcohol usage. Nurse educators can encourage teachers to integrate the importance of wearing seat belts in their classes by discussing the potential for traumatic brain injury in MVCs especially in unrestrained drivers. Review of the biomechanics of accidents in a physics or science class can also provide practical knowledge for teens that may be beneficial and more easily relatable. Additionally, education regarding drug and alcohol usage and avoidance of driving under the influence could also be integrated into this type of curriculum. Finally, more advanced techniques can be employed whereby the school nurse can lead spot surveillance of seat belt usage as teenagers enter and exit the school parking lot. After developing and implementing appropriate interventions, the APN can reassess seat belt use, repeat ED visits, and blood alcohol concentrations in relation to MVCs. Collection of these data may help identify risk factors that could have significant impact on reducing teenage MVCs and ultimately lead to changes in policy and/or curriculum in schools. Policy changes for which the APN can advocate include legislation whereby any detectable blood alcohol concentration level is illegal, more stringent and enforced driving fines for unrestrained passengers and drivers, and graduated driving license laws that increase driving supervision time and/or call for limits with driving past 9 p.m. at night until the driver is older. Although this is just one example of how surveillance by an APN could lead to the development of an intervention to reduce teenage MVC's, one can see the potential value of community collaboration and the use of an intervention to improve an outcome of interest.

Morbidity data are less standardized in general than mortality data because states and local agencies decide what illnesses must be reported to the Centers for Disease Control and Prevention (CDC). Many communicable infections and diseases are required to be reported depending upon whether control measures are developed. The list of reportable or notifiable diseases is likely to change as more scientific reviews are conducted. The accuracy of morbidity data is diminished if healthcare providers fail to report a disease or illness for fear of invading the individual's privacy or because the healthcare provider misdiagnosed the illness (McDevitt & Wilbur, 2002). In some cases, many healthcare providers are not even aware of reporting requirements. Certain diseases with easy and/or rapid transmission are more likely to harm a population's health and infectious or communicable diseases such as certain sexually transmitted infections or other diseases such as rabies, rubella, plague, measles, tetanus, and food-borne illnesses (Friis & Sellers, 2009) can lead to more significant morbidity and mortality if not reported promptly.

Another way to evaluate population morbidity other than relying on the list of reportable diseases is derived from population surveys that are conducted to determine the frequency of acute and chronic illnesses and disability as well as other characteristics. The U.S. National Health Survey (NHS) is an example of a morbidity survey that was first authorized by Congress in 1956 for the purpose of informing the U.S. population about various health measures and indicators. In 1960, the NHS and the National Office of Vital Statistics merged to form the National Center for Health Statistics (NCHS), which has been part of the CDC since 1987. The NCHS works with public and private partners to collect data that provides reliable and valid evidence on a population's health status, influences on health, and health outcomes (DHHS, 2010a). APNs can review these data to identify health disparities among subgroups based on race or ethnicity, and/or socioeconomic status; monitor trends with health status and with healthcare delivery systems; support research endeavors; identify health problems; evaluate health policies; and provide important information that can be used to improve policies and health services.

The NCHS collects data in four main ways with each method yielding information that is readily available on the internet for use by healthcare providers, researchers, and educators. First, the *National Vital Statistics System* provides information about state and local vital statistics including teen birth rates, prenatal care, birth weights, risk factors related to poor pregnancy outcomes, infant mortality rates, life expectancy, and leading causes of death. Second, the *National Health Interview Survey* (NHIS) provides health information from household interviews conducted by Census Bureau personnel. Data on health status, access to care, use of health services, immunization rates, risk factors and health-related behaviors, and health insurance coverage can be gleaned from the NHIS surveys. The *National Health and Nutrition Examination Survey* (NHANES) is the third major survey source conducted through mobile examination centers held at randomly selected sites throughout the United States. Data are obtained from physical examinations, diagnostic procedures, and laboratory tests from various conditions, environmental exposures, risk factors, and indicators of growth and development including weight, diet, and nutrition. The fourth major method of data collection from the NCHS is the *National Health Care Surveys* that provides information about the patients, healthcare providers, and agency services. For example, patient safety data, clinical management of specific health conditions, disparities in healthcare utilization and health quality, patient safety indicators, and information about the use of healthcare innovations are collated and made available from these surveys (U.S. DHHS, 2010). Each of the four key methods conducted by the NCHS provides useful outcome information.

How do APNs decide what outcomes to study? There are a plethora of outcomes that exist in relation to cost, clinical and functional data, and community and environmental indicators. Often, outcomes will reflect the desired or anticipated effects of the intervention that are related to the problem or population of interest (Oermann & Floyd, 2002). Another way to select outcomes is by reviewing available epidemiological data for outcomes that may be of interest or relevance to an APN's intervention or study (Sheilds & Lindsey, 2002). Using the earlier example of designing an intervention to help identify risk factors and reduce teenage MVCs, an APN could seek out epidemiological data from the National Annenberg Risk Survey of Youth conducted by researchers at the University of Pennsylvania. This survey includes teen attitudinal risk factors and protective factors, and identifies several factors that could potentially be identified as outcomes of interest for an APN working on reducing teen MVCs (*http://www.annenbergpublicpolicycenter.org/ProjectDetails. aspx?myId=10*).

There is no shortage of available resources for identifying outcomes. The Guide to Community Preventive Services is a helpful resource available at *www. thecommunityguide.org*. It provides evidence-based recommendations about public health interventions, analyses from systematic reviews to determine program and policy effectiveness, information on whether an intervention might work in one's community, and information about the intervention's costs and benefits. A task force of nonfederal volunteers who are public health and prevention experts conduct the systematic reviews, and personnel from the CDC provide technical and administrative assistance (*http://www.thecommunityguide.org/about/ history.html*). APNs can review the topics (problems or areas of focus) for different information about outcomes. For example, adolescent health is one of the topics with systematic reviews available. By spending a few minutes exploring the posted information, one can find numerous outcomes such as number of self-reported risk behaviors including engagement in any sexual activity, frequency of sexual activity, number of partners, frequency of unprotected sexual activity, use of protection to prevent sexually transmitted infections (STIs), use of protection to prevent pregnancy, and self-reported or clinically documented STIs. Other community guide topics are listed in Table 2.2 with example outcomes adapted from the Web site.

TABLE 2.2 Community Guide Topics and Outcomes Examples

COMMUNITY GUIDE TOPICS	OUTCOME EXAMPLES
Adolescent health	Alcohol, tobacco, and drug usage; injury, violence, and suicide rates; nutrition, physical activity, and sexual behaviors
Alcohol	Daily alcohol intake (ounces per day), type of alcohol intake (beer, wine, etc.), binge drinking, underage drinking

(continued)

TABLE 2.2   Community Guide Topics and Outcomes Examples (*continued*)

COMMUNITY GUIDE TOPICS	OUTCOME EXAMPLES
Asthma	Symptom-free days, quality of life scores, school absenteeism, environmental remediation, medication usage, smoke exposure (first- or secondhand smoke)
Birth defects	Folic acid daily intake, daily alcohol consumption, medication exposures
Cancer	Cigarette smoking, physical activity, nutrition, obesity, screening test results
Diabetes	Hemoglobin A1c, incidence of skin infections, obesity, peripheral neuropathy, renal insufficiency
HIV/AIDS, STIs, and pregnancy	Abstinence, correct condom use demonstration, incidence of STIs or pregnancy
Mental health	Depression scale scores, decision making, attendance at school or work
Motor vehicle	Use of child safety seats, use of seat belts, blood alcohol concentration, use of phone while driving
Nutrition	Daily intake of fruits and vegetables, body mass index, soda intake, fat intake, fiber intake
Obesity	Daily physical activity, sedentary time in front of a TV, computer, or electronic screen, weight reduction
Oral health	Dental caries, incidence of oral or throat cancer, use of helmets, facemasks, and mouth guards in contact sports, use of chewing tobacco
Physical activity	Muscle strength and endurance activities, moderate- or vigorous-intensity aerobic physical activity
Social environment	Surroundings such as neighborhoods or workplace, involvement in church, politics or social networks
Tobacco	Out-of-pocket costs for cessation therapies, creation of smoke-free policies, retail tobacco sales to youth
Vaccines	Number of infectious cases, hospitalizations, deaths from vaccine preventable disease, immunization rates, immunization failures
Violence	Number of violence-related hospitalizations and deaths, participation in therapeutic foster care, school-based violence prevention programs, reduction of nonaccidental trauma in infants and toddlers
Worksite health promotion	Stair usage by employees, gym membership by employees, use of weight management counseling by employees

Note: Adapted from http://www.thecommunityguide.org

Outcome monitoring has become increasingly important over the years and in many cases is a necessity to justify program implementation or program funding. Electronic health records help to simplify the recording and monitoring of outcomes over time, between patient groups and populations. Outcomes are an expected part of what APNs must collect when their focus is on populations. When combined with an evidence-based practice approach, outcomes can help provide standards or parameters for developing innovative interventions, instituting approaches more likely to impact the problem, and/or develop new practice guidelines or protocols (Ibrahim, Savitz, Carey, & Wagner, 2001). For example, an APN working in a long-term care facility may gather information about falls and risk factors for falls in older adults who comprise the population of interest. An assessment can be made to determine if differences exist according to gender, comorbid conditions, race, and other variables of interest. Patients with heart disease served in a subacute setting may be closely monitored for resolution of congestive heart failure symptoms, adherence with the medication regimen, ability to perform activities of daily living, and family member satisfaction for the care provided to their loved ones. Nurses in acute care settings may establish protocols and select outcome measures such as number of patients who receive preoperative antibiotics to reduce postoperative infections, use of TeamSTEPPS communication strategies to improve a health facility's communication effectiveness within the team. (Agency for Healthcare Research and Quality [AHRQ], 2010b), and rapid response teams to improve resuscitation efforts. APNs in a mental health center who work with adolescents by providing adolescent psychotherapy and psychotropic medications may compare outcomes using a depression scale, suicide ideation rates, or subjective improvement on psychometrically tested instruments that gauge improved affective state and satisfaction with life. The following case (Case Study 2.1) highlights a community-based example of how a research team evaluated different models of healthcare delivery for women at risk of poor birth outcomes in Washington, D.C. (Palmer, Cook, & Courtot, 2010).

CASE STUDY 2.1

Background

Washington, D.C., has some of the worst pregnancy outcomes in the United States. A review of the literature by the investigators revealed studies that suggest that birth centers or midwife-run practices, group prenatal care, and provider continuity during pregnancy contribute to improved pregnancy outcomes.

Purpose

To describe three models of maternity care delivery (a hospital obstetric clinic, a safety-net clinic, and a birth center) to low-income women in Washington, D.C., and analyze how the care might be improved to better serve this population.

(continued)

Case Study (continued)

Method

The investigators used a comparative case study design with each of the three care models representing a separate case. A mix of qualitative and quantitative methods was used. Data were gathered from semistructured stakeholder interviews, structured observations, focus groups (of women receiving pregnancy care), and supplementary secondary data (such as service statistics and birth outcome data).

Results

Attention to social (such as low health literacy and transient living situations) and medical risk factors was important in this population. Providers at all sites felt they delivered high quality care. Of all of the models, the birth center seemed to address social factors in the most comprehensive fashion. As part of larger organizations, the safety-net clinic and hospital obstetric clinic were more stable financially, although the birth center was able to provide longer visits at less cost. The biggest burden to providing care was addressing both clinical needs and social risk needs, a key finding related to the timing of postpartum care. All birth center patients and first-time mothers who saw the certified nurse midwife at the safety-net clinic were seen 2 weeks postpartum. Patients at the hospital-based clinic and multifarious patients at the safety-net clinic were scheduled for postpartum visits at 6 weeks. People who were interviewed at the hospital-based clinic and safety-net clinic felt earlier postpartum visits "would better address unintended pregnancies, breastfeeding problems, and post partum depression" (Palmer, Cook, & Courtot, 2010, p. 52).

Recommendation

Components of successful models include onsite social services, patient education, peer counseling, continuity of provider care, and adequate time for providers to spend with patients. Key organizational features were breastfeeding peer counselors, group prenatal care, greater time allotted to prenatal care, continuity of provider care, and a mission that reflects a belief in holistic maternity care.

Limitations

The hospital obstetric clinic only allowed interviews with staff and the quantitative data from the hospital obstetric clinic, and the safety-net clinic were limited. The quantitative data varied in quality among all three sites of the models. Because this is primarily a qualitative study, the investigators could not make conclusions about the impact each model

Case Study (continued)
had on outcomes; however, they were able to identify key similarities and differences among the three models. They also identified factors that appear to be important components of quality care for pregnant low-income women in Washington, D.C.

Note: Adapted from Palmer L., Cook A., & Courtot, B. (2010). Comparing models of maternity care serving women at risk of poor birth outcomes in Washington, DC. *Alternative Therapies, 16*(5), pp. 48–56.

Nursing-Sensitive Quality Indicators

As documented evidence of patient safety concerns grew in the United States at a time when healthcare costs were increasing and healthcare quality was questioned, various nursing organizations started to focus on establishing a coordinated system for evaluating patient safety. In 1994, the American Nurses Association (ANA) developed Nursing's Safety and Quality Initiative (ANA, 1999) which initiated studies of patient safety with the goal of advocating for healthy change. It was clear that nurse managers and administrators needed sound data for comparing their hospital units with similar units across the nation as a means of improving quality by developing and refining quality improvement initiatives and monitoring progress. The indicators needed to be specific or sensitive to nursing care rather than ones that reflected medical care or institutional care. The indicators would have to be highly correlated with nursing quality, be measurable with a high degree of reliability and validity, and not pose undue hardships on personnel tasked with collecting the data. Donabedian's (1982) framework of focusing on structure, process, and patient-centered outcomes was used for identifying and honing the indicators. By 2003, there was a set of 10 indicators which could be placed in Donabedian's framework. *Structure* indicators included staff mix and nursing care hours per patient day; *process* indicators included maintenance of skin integrity and nurse staff satisfaction; and patient-focused *outcomes* included nosocomial infections, patient fall rates, patient satisfaction with pain management, patient education, nursing care, and overall care (Dunton, 2008; Gallagher & Rowell, 2003; Montalvo, 2007).

The National Database of Nursing Quality Indicators (NDNQI) was created in 1998 by the ANA as part of the initiative to make changes to improve safety and quality of care, to help educate nurses about measurement, and to invest in research studies that examined safe and high quality patient care. The NDNQI helped standardize information that was submitted by hospital units throughout the United States on indicators related to nursing structure (staffing level, educational level), process measures, and outcome measures (ANA, 1999). Hospitals have used these results to compare their performance to other hospitals. The database is invaluable for preparing for accreditation or certification by The Joint Commission or American Nurses Credentialing Center accreditation as nurse executives can compare staffing patterns and methods of care delivery with clinical outcomes (Quigley, 2003). The NDNQI database is housed and managed by the University of Kansas Medical Center (KUMC) School of Nursing through a contractual agreement with the ANA (Montalvo, 2007). Technical assistance and continuing education are provided by KUMC liaisons to ensure that reliable and valid data collection methods are used by hospital personnel. The database provides a wealth of information on a quarterly and annual basis of more than 1200 facilities in the United States. This allows for the comparison and evaluation of nursing care at the unit level of structure, process, and outcomes with other institutions that share similar characteristics. (Dunton, 2008; Montalvo, 2007). The NDNQI collects data on 10 of the 15 National Quality Forum (NQF) Voluntary Consensus nursing indicators (Dunton, 2008). In 2004, the NQF nursing voluntary consensus standards process endorsed 15 national standards that could be used to evaluate nursing specific care. These standards are referred to as the NQF 15 (Kurtzman & Corrigan, 2007; Montalvo, 2007).

The ANA broadened the identification of nursing-sensitive indicators from acute care hospital settings to community-based, non-acute care settings such as long-term care facilities, schools, and home healthcare settings. This work began in 1998 and by 2000, 10 indicators were named: pain management, consistency of communication, staff mix (combination and number of RNs, LPNs, nursing assistants), client satisfaction, prevention of tobacco use, cardiovascular disease prevention, caregiver activity, identification of primary caregiver, activities of daily living (ADL), and independent activities of daily living (IADL) and psychosocial interaction (Gallagher & Rowell, 2003). The ability to collect and compare data on nursing-sensitive indicators and the ability to develop new indicators over time enhances the NDNQI and provides APNs with important information to help improve the health and safety of populations and standardize the best care practices.

Standardized Language in Nursing

The use of standardized language is important in any field to ensure a level of communication that is consistent and effective in ensuring the best quality outcomes. Specifically, in nursing and other health professions, standardized language is critical for patient safety and quality. By establishing a uniform nursing language in electronic health records, research, and in the development of evidence-based practice, APNs will have a stronger foundation to build upon to improve patient outcomes and standards of care. The North American Nursing Diagnosis Association (NANDA) was developed in the 1970s as a way of classifying and standardizing nursing diagnoses. Now referred to as NANDA International or NANDA-I, the nursing diagnoses include a name or label, signs and symptoms or defining characteristics, and risk factors associated with the diagnosis. Members of NANDA worked with nursing researchers at the University of Iowa to develop the Nursing Interventions Classification (NIC) and the Nursing Outcomes Classification (NOC). NANDA, NIC, and NOC, now referred to as NNN, collectively reflect a standardized way of communicating with defined terms within and across various national and international settings (Lunney, 2006; Smith & Craft-Rosenberg, 2010). As APNs contribute to the body of evidence-based practice, and collaborate with others to generate more evidence of effective practice, their work may benefit from reviewing and using the NNN language for diagnoses, nursing interventions, and patient outcomes (Kautz & Van Horn, 2008). It is imperative that APNs use standardized language in their research and in their practice, so outcomes can be compared in similar ways with larger databases for evaluation and research purposes.

NATIONAL HEALTHCARE OBJECTIVES

Healthy People 2020

Healthy People 2020, released by the U.S. Department of Health and Human Services (DHHS) in early December of 2010, serves as a blueprint or roadmap for the United States to achieve health promotion and disease prevention objectives that are designed to ultimately improve the health of all Americans. The Healthy People initiative started in 1979 when the Surgeon General released a report that focused on promoting health and preventing disease for all Americans. It was followed by *Healthy People 2000* in 1989 and ten years later, *Healthy People 2010.* With leadership provided by the DHHS, an appointed Advisory Committee, and the collaboration of numerous public and private groups, local and state policy makers and officials, and numerous organizations (voluntary, advocacy, faith-based, and for-profit businesses), input was solicited regionally, statewide, and nationally to help craft the vision, mission, and overarching goals, as well as specific health promotion and disease prevention strategies, to help Americans live longer and healthier lives. The resulting objectives, whether on the county, state, or national level, are intended for use by broad audiences and stakeholders to help motivate, guide, and focus action for a healthier nation.

Compared to previous national health promotion blueprints, the *Healthy People 2020* framework exemplifies the importance of a variety of influences on health such as personal influences (e.g., genetic, biological, psychological), organizational or institutional, environmental (e.g., social and physical), and policy levels, and it moves beyond an individual level approach to interventions that create local policies to promote the social and physical environments that are conducive to health for all. Another change in the 2020 version is the reorganization of objectives so they can be retrieved by three broad categories: interventions, determinants, and objectives and information (with a feature for users to be able to retrieve information by local, state, or national levels). Some of the 2020 objectives have been retained from *Healthy People 2010* because they were not met, some objectives have been modified, and some are entirely new to *Healthy People 2020.* A major difference with *Healthy People 2020* is that it is intended to be web-user friendly such that users can easily retrieve, search, and interact with the database easily and effectively. Hence, APNs and other users will be able to tailor information available from *Healthy People 2020* for their specific use and according to their specific priorities in ways that were not available with earlier versions of *Healthy People*.

Table 2.3 provides a summary of the *Healthy People 2020* initiatives with the vision, mission, goals, foundation health measures, and 42 topic areas. Each topic area has a list of objectives with data sources, a baseline, and target measures to achieve. A new feature with *Healthy People 2020* is additional topic-related clinical

TABLE 2.3   Vision, Mission, Goals, Foundation Health Measures, and Topic Areas of *Healthy People 2020*

Vision	A society in which all people live long, healthy lives.
Mission	Healthy People 2020 strives to: • Identify nationwide health improvement priorities. • Increase public awareness and understanding of the determinants of health, disease, and disability and the opportunities for progress. • Provide measurable objectives and goals that can be used at the national, state, and local levels. • Engage multiple sectors to take actions to strengthen policies and improve practices that are driven by the best available evidence and knowledge. • Identify critical research, evaluation, and data collection needs.
Overarching Goals	Attain high quality, longer lives free of preventable disease, disability, injury, and premature death. • Achieve health equity, eliminate disparities, and improve the health of all groups. • Create social and physical environments that promote good health for all. • Promote quality of life, healthy development, and healthy behaviors across all life stages.
Foundation Health Measures	
CATEGORY	**MEASURES OF PROGRESS**
General health status	• Life expectancy • Healthy life expectancy • Physical and mental unhealthy days • Limitation of activity • Chronic disease prevalence • International comparison (where available)
Disparities and inequity	Disparities/inequity to be assessed by the following: • Race/ethnicity • Gender • Socioeconomic status • Disability status • Lesbian, gay, bisexual, and transgender status • Geography

(continued)

TABLE 2.3   Vision, Mission, Goals, Foundation Health Measures, and Topic Areas of *Healthy People 2020 (continued)*

Social determinants of health	Determinants can include the following: • Social and economic factors • Natural and built environments • Policies and programs
Health-related quality of life and well-being	Well-being/satisfaction • Physical, mental, and social health-related quality of life • Participation in common activitiesCategory

Healthy People 2020 Topic Areas
• Access to health services • Adolescent health • Arthritis, osteoporosis, and chronic back conditions • Blood disorders and blood safety • Cancer • Chronic kidney diseases • Dementias, including Alzheimer's disease • Diabetes • Disability and health • Early and middle childhood • Educational and community-based programs • Environmental health • Family planning • Food safety • Genomics • Global health • Healthcare-associated infections • Health communication and health information technology • Health-related quality of life and well-being • Hearing and other sensory or communication disorders • Heart disease and stroke • HIV • Immunization and infectious diseases • Injury and violence prevention • Lesbian, gay, bisexual, and transgender health • Maternal, infant, and child health • Medical product safety • Mental health and mental disorders • Nutrition and weight status • Occupational safety and health • Older adults • Oral health • Physical activity • Preparedness • Public health infrastructure • Respiratory diseases • Sexually transmitted diseases • Sleep health

(continued)

TABLE 2.3   Vision, Mission, Goals, Foundation Health Measures, and Topic Areas of *Healthy People 2020* (*continued*)

- Social determinants of health
- Substance abuse
- Tobacco use
- Vision

Note: Adapted from http://www.healthypeople.gov/2020/TopicsObjectives2020/pdfs/HP2020_brochure.pdf

recommendations, evidence-based interventions, and other resources and links with consumer health information. Information about *Healthy People 2020* can be found at *http://www.healthypeople.gov/2020/default.aspx*

The *Healthy People 2020* Web site has useful information that APNs can use to identify and monitor outcomes. Other tools referred to as indicators exist that APNs can use for determining outcomes or measures of the quality of healthcare. These tools are available from the Agency for Healthcare Research and Quality (AHRQ) Indicators Web site at *www.qualityindicators.ahrq.gov* along with software to compute the quality indicator rates, users' guides, reports, and other technical assistance and support. The inpatient quality indicators were designed to help hospitals identify possible issues and problems in need of quality improvement by using hospital administrative data to analyze mortality and mortality rates for specific conditions and procedures, hospital- and area-level procedure utilization rates, and number of procedures (for select procedures). In addition to the inpatient quality indicators, other sets of quality indicators are available including preventative quality indicators, patient safety indicators, and pediatric quality indicators (AHRQ, 2010a).

Agency for Healthcare Research and Quality's National Healthcare Quality Report

Since 2003, the AHRQ has partnered with members of the DHHS to report on healthcare quality improvement by publishing the National Healthcare Quality Report (NHQR). The intent of this report is to respond to the status of healthcare quality in the United States, identify where improvement is most needed, and describe how the quality of healthcare that is given to Americans changes over time. This report includes more than 200 health measures placed in four categories that reflect quality measures: effectiveness, patient safety, timeliness, and patient centeredness (AHRQ, 2010a).

Findings from the 2009 report (AHRQ, 2010a) revealed that healthcare for Americans is in need of improvement, specifically for those who do not have health insurance as they are at most risk for receiving healthcare of poor quality. Compared with people who have health insurance, uninsured people were less likely to receive flu vaccinations, dental care, diabetes management, preventive health services such as cancer screenings, and counseling to improve physical activity and nutrition. A second group of key findings revealed that there were more healthcare-acquired infections and suboptimal patient safety outcomes compared to the previous year and that disparities existed according to geographic region; people who lived in the Southwest and South Central parts of the country were more likely to have healthcare-acquired infections and suboptimal patient safety outcomes than people living in the Midwest or New England states. A third key finding was that the pace of improving quality was slow especially for preventive care and chronic disease management, and slower in outpatient settings than in hospital settings. Care improvements in hospitals have been evident since the Centers for Medicare and Medicaid Services (CMS) started reporting on quality measures, which can be found on the Hospital Quality Compare Web Site (*http://www.hospitalcompare.hhs.gov*). Key recommendations of the report called for removing barriers to quality care and specifically to reduce the number of Americans who lack health insurance. A second recommendation was to empower healthcare providers so they can use health technology efficiently as a tool to support health quality improvement. Another recommendation was to initiate and sustain partnerships between various community-based organizations such as public and private agencies, businesses, and leaders and healthcare providers to facilitate much-needed change to improve the overall quality of health (AHRQ, 2010).

National reports compiled by AHRQ and other researchers have revealed disparities in healthcare quality, health access, and other services. The American health system suffers from the numerous differences that exist in the quality of care among minority and vulnerable populations. APNs have numerous resources they can access to improve quality and decrease health disparities. The National Partnership for Action (NPA) to End Health Disparities (*http://minorityhealth. hhs.gov/npa/*) was started by the Office of Minority Health to mobilize individuals and groups to work to improve quality and eliminate health disparities. The National Priorities Partnership (*http://www.nationalprioritiespartnership. org*) includes key private and public stakeholders who have agreed to work on major health priorities of patients and families, palliative and end-of-life care, care coordination, patient safety, and population health. The Quality Alliance Steering Committee (*http://www.healthqualityalliance.org*) is another partnership of healthcare leaders who work to improve healthcare quality and costs (AHRQ, 2010). Various strategies to bridge the gaps in healthcare quality are available at the national level and may be applied or considered at state, regional, or local levels in collaboration with stakeholders as a means of decreasing health disparities.

Health Disparities

Healthy People 2010 maintained two overarching goals: to increase the years of healthy living and to eliminate health disparities. These goals have been retained for *Healthy People 2020* as evidence continues to mount that the United States has many problems with equity of health access, quality, and health status depending upon characteristics such as a population's color, ethnicity, gender, socioeconomic status, or residential location (Shi & Stevens, 2005). *Healthy People 2010* differed from *Healthy People 2000* in that it included a feature for monitoring objectives and subobjectives in relation to ethnicity, race, income, education, and/or gender. *Healthy People 2020* will build on these efforts and continue to monitor inequities and health disparities throughout the nation. By monitoring potential differences among groups, health professionals will have the tools to recognize why and where population disparities are occurring and ultimately can lead to creative strategies to reduce health disparities and improve equity.

There are numerous dimensions of disparities or differences related to health that can adversely affect groups of people because of specific characteristics or obstacles. It is widely recognized now that the social determinants of health such as housing, education, access to public transportation, access to safe water, access to fresh food, and residential neighborhood are all related to a population's health. If some populations have a health outcome that is greater or lesser than another population, this is an example of a disparity. In addition to race and ethnicity, other characteristics also contribute to the presence of disparities or the achievement of good health such as gender, sexual orientation, geographic location, cognitive, sensory or physical disability, and socioeconomic status. The outcomes identified in the objectives of *Healthy People 2020* are intended to improve the health of all groups of people and bridge those gaps. *Healthy People 2020* will assess health disparities in U.S. populations in future years by tracking morbidity and mortality outcomes in relation to specific factors such as race and ethnicity, gender, sexual identity and orientation, presence of special healthcare needs or disability status, and geographic location based on urban or rural living.

CDC Office of Minority Health and Health Disparities

Established in 1988, the Office of Minority Health and Health Disparities (OMHD) within the CDC monitors health disparities such as race, ethnicity, socioeconomic status, gender, and geographic area. Resources available from this office may be used by APNs to obtain data that demonstrate how minority populations compare with the U.S. population as a whole. For example, Blacks or African Americans, Hispanics or Latinos, American Indians and Alaska Natives, and Native Hawaiian and Pacific Islanders face different challenges with health status, quality, and services in comparison with the majority population. Such disparities are complicated to analyze and explain as they go beyond differences in genetics or biological characteristics. Racist and discriminatory behaviors and policies, cultural barriers, lack of access to care, and interaction of environmental, health behaviors and genetics may explain some of the disparities (DHHS, 2000). The midcourse review of *Healthy People 2010* provided evidence of substantial disparities related to health, life expectancy, and quality of life (*http://www.healthypeople.gov/2010/Data/midcourse/html/execsummary/Goal2.htm*), and numerous other reports and research studies have documented similar health disparities (AHRQ, 2009; Daniel, 2010; IOM, 2003; Kaiser Family Foundation, 2004; Koci, 2010; MacMullen, Shen, & Tymkow, 2010; MacMullen, Tymkow, & Shen, 2006; Shen, Tymkow, & MacMullen, 2005).

Another resource available to APNs can be found at Quick Health Data Online (*http://www.healthstatus2010.com/owh/*). This site has several valuable components that include the Quick Health Data Online system, the Health Disparities Profile, and the Women's Health and Mortality Chartbook. The Quick Health Data Online system provides information on state- and county-level data from all 50 states, the District of Columbia, and U.S. territories and can be analyzed by stratifying into various categories including demographics, disease type, and insurance status. The Health Disparities Profile examines key health indicators by state level and by race and ethnicity. This resource is invaluable for identifying a state's health disparities. For example, North Carolina has disproportionately higher rates of diabetes and strokes among the African American population. The African American population also has higher rates of high blood pressure and obesity than the majority population (*http://www. healthstatus2010.com/owh/disparities/ChartBookData_list.asp*). Information like this is very important to APNs who wish to develop or implement interventions to target vulnerable community members and those who are most at risk of having poor health outcomes.

National Institutes of Health
Centers for Population Health and Health Disparities

The National Institutes of Health (NIH) awards grants to Centers for Population Health and Health Disparities (CPHHD) that are selected to address disparities and inequities associated with cancer and heart disease, the two leading causes of death for American adults. This program involves numerous partnerships including NIH's National Cancer Institute (NCI), the National Heart, Lung, and Blood Institute (NHLBI), and the Office of Behavioral and Social Sciences Research (OBSSR). Ten centers were awarded funds in May of 2010 to promote research collaborations among various disciplines, to train new transdisciplinary researchers to conduct collaborative research, and to increase the rigor and impact on health disparities. The Web site (*http://cancercontrol.cancer.gov/*) has different resources available, including reports on health inequalities, tool kits for research projects, and a health disparities calculator (HD*Calc). HD*Calc is statistical software that can be downloaded and used to generate and calculate eight disparity measurements (*http://seer.cancer.gov/hdcalc*).

Information about CPHHD, including information about each individual center's goals, can be easily located at the Web site noted above. APNs can contact the principal investigators or other research staff to obtain information, to explore collaborative endeavors with research, to participate with community-based participatory research, to assist with translational research studies, and to share expertise with the aim of decreasing health disparities among vulnerable populations.

Examples of Health Disparities and Outcomes

The AHRQ publishes a synopsis of minority health findings in program briefs that include summaries and citations of research studies published in various health professional journals. The studies are organized by clinical outcomes related to a disease such as cancer, cardiovascular disease, and chronic illness; by health services such as emergency care/hospitalization and preventive services; and access to healthcare including costs and insurance. Other categories include mental/behavioral health; pregnancy, childbirth, and birth outcomes; quality of care/patient safety; and reducing disparities (AHRQ, 2009).

Examples of health disparities related to chronic illness or a disease (which can be considered a clinical outcome) include findings from research studies that indicate that Mexican Americans have twice the risk of developing diabetes mellitus compared to other ethnic groups (Freeman, 2008); African Americans have a higher annual incidence of lung cancer (76.1 per 100,000 people) than Whites (69.7 per 100,00 people) with the highest incidence occurring in the South (CDC, 2010); and African Americans are more likely to have high blood pressure compared to Whites or Mexican Americans (Yoon, Ostchega, & Louis, 2010). Examples of studies that explore gender inequities include a study by an APN who explored a framework of female marginalization and found that women were more likely to die from cardiovascular disease compared with men (Koci, 2010; Vaccarino et al., 2009). Another research team explored how to tailor a diabetes self-management intervention for use by older, rural African American women (Leeman, Skelly, Burns, Carlson, & Soward, 2008), and another research team found that poor literacy was linked with poor HIV medication adherence, with this being more common among Blacks compared to Whites (Osborn, Paashe-Orlow, Davis, & Wolf, 2007).

In terms of pregnancy and childbirth, a recent report explored an ecological approach as a way of better understanding the disparities that exist in perinatal mortality for Black infants born in the United States compared to White infants. Even though the infant mortality rate in the United States has declined in recent years, and even when controlling for socioeconomic factors, Black infants compared to White infants are more than twice as likely to die in their first year of life, and the Black fetal mortality rate is more than double that of Whites (Alio et al., 2010; MacDorman, Munson, & Kirmeyer, 2007; Mathews, & MacDorman, 2007). In short, the health disparities that exist for African American infants are deplorable, and effective strategies to reverse this trend are needed urgently. While much research has been done to better understand this disparity, researchers suggest that a multidimensional approach is needed to try to understand these disparities, that contextual variables must be explored, and a history of institutionalized racism and individual racism that is embedded in every aspect of life of African American women must be recognized. More research is needed to try to improve the health of vulnerable populations. Healthcare workers need cultural competency training, communication needs to improve between providers and patients, strategies to improve community relations are needed, and adherence to nondiscriminatory health policies is also necessary to bridge the gaps in providing quality care (Alio et al., 2010).

It is critical that DNP graduates and APNs advocate for the elimination of health disparities as this work is of critical importance and urgently needed. And, from an ethical standpoint, working to eliminate health disparities is the *right thing to do*. By recognizing health disparities and developing a better understanding of how process and status impact the outcome of interest, APNs are better prepared to develop effective interventions to eliminate or reduce health disparities. Such strategies may include advocating for better health insurance coverage for poor and immigrant populations, ensuring that sufficient services exist in underserved areas, encouraging minority participation in research studies with community-based participatory research and specifically with practice-based research networks, using linguistically and culturally appropriate communication and written handouts, promoting and facilitating community partnerships, and implementing strategies to encourage people from minority populations to become healthcare professionals (Anderko, Bartz, & Lundeen, 2005; Daniel, 2010).

APNs have successfully tested interventions to decrease health disparities, and by careful and thorough review of the current literature and resources available, they have the tools to develop interventions and identify outcomes associated with less health disparities. A research team from East Carolina University tested the efficacy of having an APN provide care management and interdisciplinary group visits of rural African Americans with diabetes mellitus. The APN met with patients weekly for 12 months at the practice where the intervention was held and assisted with patient education, care management, and patient flow. An interdisciplinary team comprised of a nurse, physician, nutritionist, and pharmacist provided four group visits to patients while control patients received normal care at another practice. By the end of the 12-month period, there were significantly lower median HbA1C findings (the outcome of interest) for the intervention group compared with the control group (Bray, Thompson, Wynn, Cummings, & Whetstone, 2005).

Another research team with Home Care of Rochester (HCR) designed a theory-based outcomes improvement model based on the Sunrise Enabler approach to deliver home nursing care to Hispanic patients (Leininger, 2006). According to the 2007 National Healthcare Disparities Report published by the AHRQ, Hispanics receive a poorer quality of care than non-Hispanic Whites in 23 of the 38 core quality measures (AHRQ, 2008). In addition to paying attention to culturally and linguistically appropriate services (CLAS) and healthcare standards, the team recognized the disparity that existed for Hispanics who had difficulty accessing healthcare. By developing a model of care based on Leininger's Theory of Culture Care and Universality (2006), team members developed a plan for delivering culturally congruent care. They recruited and oriented Hispanic nurses to provide the home care and developed educational information in a way the population appreciated by using a *telenovella* or soap opera video format. HCR used the Outcome and Assessment Information Set (OASIS) to evaluate the model. They found that the acute hospitalization rate for Hispanic patients dropped almost by half following the intervention where previously it had been twice that of the overall population before the program was implemented, and there were some small gains seen in the Hispanic patients' adherence to medications and a reduction in the usage of emergency services (Woerner, Espinsoa, Bourne, O'Toole, & Ingersoll, 2009). APNs have many resources available to assist them in developing and testing innovative models of care that have the potential to decrease or eliminate health disparities while improving patient outcomes.

SUMMARY

APNs have a critical role in improving the population's health by intervening at every level from the individual to the community. Before an effective intervention can take place, it is imperative that outcomes are first identified and defined so they can later be analyzed. Outcomes may be classified by the beneficiary of the health intervention and by type such as care-, patient-, or performance-related, and also by time frame of achievement. Outcomes may also be categorized by clinical or disease-specific outcomes, and function, cost, and satisfaction outcomes. A commonly used framework to classify outcomes is Donabedian's framework (1980, 1982) of structure, process, and outcomes. This framework has been used for describing a community's health as well as for classifying nursing-sensitive indicators. Outcomes are an important part of the standardized language that nursing leaders and researchers continue to refine and operationalize as a means of improving healthcare and are particularly relevant as electronic health records grow in usage throughout the United States.

The national healthcare objectives as released in *Healthy People 2020* provide a blueprint of health promotion and disease prevention objectives that are designed to improve the health of all Americans. Building on the goal of *Healthy People 2010,* which sought to eliminate health disparities, APNs can use these web-based resources to identify outcomes and compare them with national and state data that can be further analyzed by stratifying for a population's ethnicity, race, income, education, and/or gender. Federal agencies such as the AHRQ, the CDC Office of Minority Health and Health Disparities, and the NIH Centers for Population Health and Health Disparities provide ready access to a plethora of information and resources that can be used to identify and define outcomes.

APNs have a tremendous opportunity to access and use available data to contribute to the current body of knowledge that forms the basis for evidence-based practice. By selecting and using well-defined indicators and comparing those to national norms, APNs can provide important information on trends or patterns of poor quality of care or health inequities. This information has the potential to stimulate the development of creative and innovative programs or interventions to improve health outcomes. Evidence of improved outcomes will help APNs justify and advocate for change through policy, practice, and research with the ultimate goal of eliminating health disparities and promoting health equities among all populations.

EXERCISES AND DISCUSSION QUESTIONS

Exercise 2.1 Poor infant mortality rates for African American babies in the United States are an example of a glaring health disparity in American society.

- Where would you go to find information about this problem?
- How would you obtain information regarding infant mortality rates from your local, state, or regional community?
- What interventions are designed to reduce infant mortality rates, and specifically the infant mortality rates of specific groups of infants with the highest mortality rates?
- How might an APN participate in local efforts to reduce infant mortality rates?

Exercise 2.2 An APN is interested in trying to prevent mortality from acute strokes and decides to develop an online continuing education program to teach RNs, APNs, and physician assistants about thrombolytic therapy administration of tissue plasminogen activator (tPA) and stroke protocols.

- What outcomes might the APN monitor to determine the effectiveness of this program?
- The APN takes a closer look to identify subgroups in his or her state and community with the highest risk of stroke. What ways can he or she tailor the educational intervention to better reach these groups?

Exercise 2.3 Review some of the writings of Florence Nightingale.

- What outcomes did she monitor?
- Are there similar outcomes of concern to APNs today?
- How did she measure the outcomes that she monitored?
- What impact did she have by sharing these outcomes?

Exercise 2.4 You are a psychiatric clinical nurse specialist interested in improving mental health services in your community. You decide to review the Guide to Community Preventive Services to identify a science-based intervention that will help older adults who live at home better manage depression.

■ What information is in the guide that may be relevant to your practice?
■ What other government sponsored Web sites may have useful information?
■ What types of outcomes are you interested in monitoring regarding the problem of older adults with depression?

Exercise 2.5   A recent conference you attended included a session on ways that hospitals in the Southeast are using the NDNQI. You do not know very much about nursing indicators but recognize this would be helpful to you in the new role you will have as a nurse manager.

■ Where can you obtain information about the NDNQI?
■ You later learn that the hospital where you work has just started collecting data on 5 of the 10 nursing indicators. You ask to review the data and find that the nursing care hours per patient day on your unit are low in comparison with the national data provided from the database. How can you use this information to improve patient care on your unit?

Exercise 2.6   Diabetes affects a growing number of Americans. You have been invited to join a collaborative of community agencies interested in tackling diabetes from a community perspective.

■ What resources will you use to identifydifferent outcomes related to diabetes?
■ What outcomes related to diabetes are of most interest to community members?
■ How will you compare the outcomes you select to monitor at the local level with state and national outcomes?

Exercise 2.7   APNs should not only recognize but also make it part of their practice to develop strategies to reduce or eliminate health disparities. Review information from *Healthy People 2020* and the CDC Office of Minority Health and Health Disparities Web sites.

■ What health disparities can you find that are relevant to your community?
■ How can you better advocate for minority groups who have poorer health outcomes?
■ What specific objectives in *Healthy People 2020* can help this effort?

REFERENCES

Agency for Healthcare Research and Quality (AHRQ). (2008). *2007 National healthcare disparities report*. (AHRQ Publication No. 08-0041). Retrieved from http://www.ahrq.gov/qual/nhdr07

Agency for Healthcare Research and Quality (AHRQ) (2009, August). *Minority health: Recent findings. Program Brief (AHRQ Publication No. 09-PB003).* Retrieved from http://www.ahrq.gov/research/minorfind.htm

Agency for Healthcare Research and Quality (AHRQ). (2010a, March). *2009 National healthcare quality report (AHRQ Publication No. 10-0003).* Retrieved from http://www.ahrq.gov/qual/nhqr09/nhqr09.pdf

Agency for Healthcare Research and Quality (AHRQ). (2010b). *Pocket guide: TeamSTEPPS® Strategies & tools to enhance performance and patient safety (AHRQ Publication No. 06-0020-2) Version 06.1.* Rockville, MD: Author.

Alio, A. P., Richman, A., R., Clayton, H. B., Jeffers, D. F., Wathington, D. J., & Salihu, H. M. (2010). An ecological approach to understanding black-white disparities in perinatal mortality. *Maternal Child Health Journal, 14,* 557–566. doi:10.1007/s10995-009-0495-9

Allan, J., Agar Barwick, T., Cashman, S., Cawley, J. F., Day, C., Douglass, C. W., et al. (2004). Clinical prevention and population health: Curriculum framework for health professions. *American Journal of Preventive Medicine, 27*(5), 471–476. doi:10.1016/S0749-3797(04)00206-5

American Association of Colleges of Nursing. (2004). *AACN position statement on the practice doctorate in nursing.* Washington, DC: Author.

American Association of Colleges of Nursing. (2006). *The essentials of doctoral education for advanced nursing practice.* Retrieved from http://www.aacn.nche.edu/DNP/pdf/Essentials.pdf

American Nursing Association (ANA). (1999). *Nursing facts: Nursing–sensitive quality indicators for acute care settings and ANA's safety & quality initiative.* Retrieved from www.nursingworld.org/MainMenuCategories/ThePracticeofProfessionalNursing/PatientSafetyQuality/NDNQI/Research/QIforAcuteCareSettings.aspx

Anderko, L., Bartz, C., & Lundeen, S. (2005). Practice-based research networks: Nursing centers and communities working collaboratively to reduce health disparities. *Nursing Clinics of North America, 40,* 747–758. doi:10.1016/j.cnur.2005.08.009

Bray, P., Thompson, D., Wynn, J. D., Cummings, D. M., & Whetstone, L. (2005). Confronting disparities in diabetes care: The clinical effectiveness of redesigning care management for minority patients in rural primary care practices. *The Journal of Rural Health, 21*(4), 317–321. doi:10.1111/j.1748-0361.2005.tb00101.x

CDC. (2008, April 9). *Health disparities among racial/ethnic populations.* Retrieved from http://www.cdc.gov/NCCDPHP/DACH/chaps/disparities/

CDC. (2010, November 12). Racial/ethnic disparities and geographic differences in lung cancer incidence—38 states and the District of Columbia, 1998–2006. *Morbidity and Mortality Weekly Report, 59*(44), 1434–1438. Retrieved from http://www.cdc.gov/mmwr/preview/mmwrhtml/mm5944a2.htm?s_cid=mm5944a2_w

Cottrell, L. S. (1976). The competent community. In B. H. Kaplan, R. N. Wilson, & A. H. Leighton (Eds.), *Further explorations in social psychiatry.* New York, NY: Basic Books.

Daniel, M. (2010). Strategies for targeting health care disparities among Hispanics. *Family & Community Health, 33*(4), 329–342. doi: 10.1097/FCH.0b013e3181f3b292

Donabedian, A. (1980). *Explorations in quality assessment and monitoring.* Ann Arbor, MI: Health Administration Press.

Donabedian, A. (1982). *The criteria and standards of quality.* Ann Arbor, MI: Health Administration Press.

Dunton, N. E. (2008). Take a cue from the NDNQI. *Nursing Management, 39*(4), 20–23. doi: 10.1097/01.NUMA.0000316054.35317.b

Fee, E., & Garofalo, M. E. (2010). Florence Nightingale and the Crimean war. *American Journal of Public Health, 100*(9), 1591. doi:10.2105/AJPH.2009.188607

Freeman, J. (2008). Treating Hispanic patients for type 2 diabetes mellitus: Special considerations. *Journal of the American Osteopathy Association, 108*(5), 5–13.

Friis, R. H., & Sellers, T. A. (2009). *Epidemiology for public health practice* (4th ed.). Boston, MA: Jones and Bartlett.

Gallagher, R. M., & Rowell, P. A. (2003). Claiming the future of nursing through nursing-sensitive quality indicators. *Nursing Administration Quarterly, 27*(4), 273–84.

Griffiths, P. (1995). Progress in measuring nursing outcomes. *Journal of Advanced Nursing, 21,* 1092–1100. doi:10.1046/j.1365-2648.1995.21061092.x

Hill, M. (1999). Outcomes measurement requires nursing to shift to outcome-based practice. *Nursing Administration Quarterly, 24*(1), 1–16.

Ibrahim, M. A., Savitz, L. A., Carey, T. S., & Wagner, E. H. (2001). Population-based health principles in medical and public health practice. *Journal of Public Health Management Practice, 7*(3), 75–81.

Institute of Medicine (IOM), Committee on Understanding and Eliminating Racial and Ethnic Disparities in Health Care. (2003). *Unequal treatment: Confronting racial and ethnic disparities in health care.* Washington, DC: National Academies Press.

Kaiser Family Foundation. (2004). *Racial and ethnic disparities in women's health coverage and access to care: Findings from the 2001 Kaiser women's health survey.* Menlo Park, CA: The Foundation.

Kautz, D. D., & Van Horn, E. R. (2008). An exemplar of the use of NNN language in developing evidence-based practice guidelines. *International Journal of Nursing Terminologies and Classifications.* Retrieved from http://findarticles.com/p/articles/mi_qa4065/is_200801/ai_n25138588/?tag=content;col1

Kleinpell, R. (2001). Measuring outcomes in advanced practice nursing. In R. Kleinpell (Ed.), *Outcome assessment in advanced practice nursing* (pp. 1–50). New York, NY: Springer.

Kleinpell, R., & Gawlinski, A. (2005). Assessing outcomes in advanced practice nursing practice: The use of quality indicators and evidence-based practice. *AACN Clinical Issues, 16*(1), 43–57. doi:10.1097/00044067-200501000-00006

Koci, A. (2010). Care of women and marginalized populations in the critical care setting. *Critical Care Nursing Quarterly, 33*(3), 244–247. doi: 10.1097/CNQ.0b013e3181e65fb4

Kurtzman, E. T., & Corrigan, J. M. (2007). Measuring the contribution of nursing to quality, patient safety, and health care outcomes. *Policy, Politics & Nursing Practice, 8*(1), 20–36. doi:10.1177/1527154407302115

Lang, N. M., & Marek, K. D. (1991). The policy and politics of patient outcomes. *Journal of Nursing Quality Assurance, 5*(2), 7–12.

Leeman, J., Skelly, A. H., Burns, D., Carlson, J., & Soward, A. (2008). Tailoring a diabetes self-care intervention for use with older, rural African American women. *The Diabetes Educator, 34*(2), 310–317. doi:10.1177/0145721708316623

Leininger, M. M. (2006). Culture care diversity and universality theory and evolution of the ethnonursing method. In M. M. Leininger, & M. R. McFarland (Eds.), *Cultural care diversity and universality: A worldwide nursing theory* (2nd ed., pp. 1–41). Boston, MA: Jones & Bartlett.

Lunney, M. (2006.) Helping nurses use NANDA, NOC, and NIC: Novice to expert. *Nurse Educator, 31*(1), 40–6. doi:10.1097/00006223-200601000-00011

MacDorman, M. F., Munson, M. L., & Kirmeyer, S. (2007). Fetal and perinatal mortality, United States, 2004. *National Vital Statistics Reports, 56,* 1–20.

MacMullen, N. J., Shen, J. J., & Tymkow, C. (2010). Adverse maternal outcomes in women with asthma versus women without asthma. *Applied Nursing Research, 23*(1), e9–e13. doi:10.1016/j.apnr.2009.03.004

MacMullen, N. J., Tymkow, C., & Shen, J. J., (2006). Adverse maternal outcomes in women with asthma: Differences by race. *MCN, The American Journal of Maternal/Child Nursing, 31*(4), 263–268. doi:10.1097/00005721-200607000-00012

Mathews, T. J., & MacDorman, M. F. (2007). Infant mortality statistics from the 2004 period linked birth/infant death data set. *National Vital Statistics Reports, 55*, 1–32.

McDevitt, J., & Wilbur, J. (2002). Locating sources of data. In N. E. Ervin (Ed.), *Advanced community health nursing practice: Population-focused care.* Upper Saddle River, NJ: Prentice Hall.

Montalvo, I. (2007). The national database of nursing quality indicators (NDNQI). *Online Journal of Issues in Nursing, 12*(3). Retrieved from EBSCO*host*.

Nelson, E. C., Batalden, P. B., Plume, S. K., Mihevc, N. T., & Swartz, W. G. (1995). Report cards or instrument panels: Who needs what? *The Joint Commission Journal on Quality Improvement, 21*(4), 155–166.

Nelson, E. C., Mohr, J. J., Batalden, P. B., & Plume, S. K. (1996). Improving health care, part 1: The clinical value compass. *Joint Commission Journal for Quality Improvement, 22*(4), 243–58.

Oermann, M., & Floyd, J. A. (2002). Outcomes research: An essential component of the advanced practice nurse role. *Clinical Nurse Specialist, 16*(3), 140–144. doi:10.1097/00002800-200205000-00007

Osborn, C. Y., Paasche-Orlow, M. K., Davis, T. C., & Wolf, M. S. (2007). Health literacy: An overlooked factor in understanding HIV health disparities. *American Journal of Preventive Medicine, 33*(5), 374–378. doi:10.1016/j.amepre.2007.07.022

Palmer L, Cook A, Courtot B. Comparing models of maternity care serving women at risk of poor birth outcomes in Washington, DC. *Alternative Therapies in Health & Medicine* [serial online]. September 2010; 16(5): 48–56. Available from: CINAHL Plus with Full Text, Ipswich, MA. Accessed August 5, 2011.

Quigley, E. (2003). Contributions of the professional, public, and private sectors in promoting patient safety. *Online Journal of Issues in Nursing, 8*(3, Manuscript 1). Retrieved from www.nursingworld.org/MainMenuCategories/ANAMarketplace/ANAPeriodicals/OJIN/TableofContents/Volume82003/No3Sept2003/ContributionsinPromoting.aspx

Rich, K. A. (2009). Evaluating outcomes of innovations. In N. A. Schmidt, & J. M. Brown (Eds.), *Evidence-based practice: Appraisal and application of research.* Sudbury, MA; Jones & Bartlett.

Sheilds, L. E., & Lindsey, A. E. (2002). The community. In N. E. Ervin (Ed.), *Advanced community health nursing practice: Population-focused care.* Upper Saddle River, NJ: Prentice Hall.

Shen, J. J., Tymkow, C., & MacMullen, N. (2005). Disparities in maternal outcomes among four ethnic populations. *Ethnicity & Disease, 15*(3), 492–497.

Shi, L., & Stevens, G. D. (2005). *Vulnerable populations in the United States.* San Francisco, CA: Jossey-Bass.

Shuster, G. F., & Goeppinger, J. (2008). Community as client: Assessment and analysis. In M. Stanhope, & J. Lancaster (Eds.), *Public health nursing: Population-centered health care in the community* (7th ed.), St. Louis, MO: Mosby.

Smith, K. J., & Craft-Rosenberg, M. (2010). Using NANDA, NIC, and NOC in an undergraduate nursing practicum. *Nurse Educator, 35*(4), 162–166. doi:10.1097/NNE.0b013e3181e33953

U.S. Department of Health and Human Services. (2000). *Healthy People 2010. With understanding and improving health and objectives for improving health* (2nd ed., Vol. 2). Washington, DC: U.S. Government Printing Office.

U.S. Department of Health and Human Services (U.S. DHHS), Centers for Disease Control and Prevention. (2010a). *National Center for Health Statistics, 1960–2010, celebrating 50 years.* Hyattsville, MD: Author.

U.S. Department of Health and Human Services (U.S. DHHS). (2010b, December). *Healthy People 2020.* Retrieved from http://www.healthypeople.gov

Vaccarino, V., Parsons, L., Peterson, E. D., Rogers, W. J., Kiefe, C. I., & Canto, J. (2009). Sex differences in mortality after myocardial infarction changes from 1994 to 2006. *Archives of Internal Medicine, 169*(19), 1767–1774. doi:10.1001/archinternmed.2009.332

van Maanen, H. M. T. (1979). Perspectives and problems on quality of nursing care: An overview of contributions from North America and recent developments in Europe. *Journal of Advanced Nursing, 4,* 377–389. doi.org/10.1111%2Fj.1365-2648.1979.tb00872.x

Woerner, L., Espinosa, J., Bourne, S., O'Toole, M., & Ingersoll, G. L. (2009). Project ¡ÉXITO!: Success through diversity and universality for outcomes improvement among Hispanic home care patients. *Nursing Outlook, 57,* 266–273. doi:10.1016/j.outlook.2009.02.001

Yoon, S., Ostchega, Y., & Louis, T. (2010). *Recent trends in the prevalence of high blood pressure and its treatment and control, 1999–2008.* NCHS data brief, no 48. Hyattsville, MD: National Center for Health Statistics.

THREE

Measuring Disease in Populations

Ann L. Cupp Curley

Patty A. Vitale

*E*vidence-based practice as it relates to population-based nursing combines clinical practice and public health through the use of population health sciences in clinical practice (Heller & Page, 2002). Epidemiology is the science of public health. It is concerned with the study of the factors determining and influencing the frequency and distribution of disease, injury, and other health-related events and their causes (Gordis, 2008). In addition to epidemiology, an understanding of other scientific disciplines such as biology and biostatistics are also important for understanding diseases and their causation as they relate to population health.

The focus of population-based care is on populations at risk, comparison groups, and demographic factors. It is concerned with the patterns of delivery of care and outcomes measurement at the population or sub-population level. The focus of this chapter is on understanding the natural history of disease and the approaches that are integral for the prevention of disease. It will also introduce the basic concepts that are necessary in understanding how to measure disease outcomes and design studies that are used in population-based research. Emphasis is placed on measuring disease occurrence with a fundamental discussion of how to calculate incidence, prevalence, and mortality rates. Successful advanced practice nursing in population health depends upon the ability to recognize the difference between the individual and population approaches to the collection and use of data, and the ability to assess needs and evaluate outcomes at the population level.

THE NATURAL HISTORY OF DISEASE

The natural history of disease refers to the progression of a disease from its *preclinical state* (prior to symptoms) to its *clinical state* (from onset of symptoms to cure, control, disability, or death). Disease is not something that occurs suddenly but rather it is a multifactorial process that is dynamic and occurs over time. It evolves and changes and is sometimes initiated by events that take place years, even decades, before symptoms first appear. Many diseases have a natural life history that can extend over a very long period of time. The natural history of disease is described in stages. Understanding the different stages allows for a better understanding of the approach to the prevention and control of disease.

Stage of Susceptibility

The stage of susceptibility refers to the time prior to disease development. In the presence of certain risk factors, genetics, or environment, disease may develop and the severity can vary among individuals. Risk factors are those factors that are associated with an increased likelihood that the disease will develop at a later time. The idea that individuals could modify "risk factors" tied to heart disease, stroke, and other diseases is one of the key findings of the Framingham Heart Study (NHLBI and Boston University, 2010). Started in 1948 and still in operation, the Framingham Heart Study is one of the most important population studies ever carried out in the United States. Before Framingham, for example, most healthcare providers believed that atherosclerosis was an inevitable part of the aging process. Although not all risk factors are amenable to change (e.g., genetic factors) the identification of risk factors is important and fundamental to disease prevention.

Preclinical Stage of Disease

During the preclinical phase, the disease process has begun but there are no obvious symptoms. Although there is no clear manifestation of disease, because of the interaction of biological factors, changes have started to occur. During this stage however the changes are not always detectable. Screening technologies have been developed to detect the presence of some diseases before clinical symptoms appear. The Papanicolaou (Pap) smear is an example of an effective screening method for detecting cancer in a premalignant state to improve mortality related to cervical cancer. The use of the Pap smear as a screening tool facilitates early detection and treatment of premalignant changes of the cervix prior to development of malignancy.

Clinical Stage of Disease

In the clinical stage of disease, sufficient physiologic and/or functional changes occur for the presence of recognizable symptoms of disease to appear. It might also be accurately referred to as the treatment stage. For some people, the disease may completely resolve (either spontaneously or with medical intervention), and for some it will lead to disability and/or death. It is for this reason that the clinical stage of disease is sometimes subdivided for better medical management. Staging systems used in malignancies to better define the extent of disease involvement is an example of a system that can help guide the type of treatment modality selected based on stage. In many cases, staging can provide an estimate of prognosis. Another example is the identification of disability as a specific subcategory of the treatment stage. Disability occurs when a clinical disease leaves a person either temporarily or permanently disabled. When people become disabled, the goal of treatment is to mitigate the effects of disease and to help people to function to their optimal abilities. This is very different than the goal for someone who can be treated and restored to the level of functioning that they enjoyed prior to their illness.

The Nonclinical Disease Stage

This nonclinical or unapparent disease stage can be broken into four subparts. The first subpart is the *preclinical stage*, which, as mentioned earlier, is the acquisition of disease prior to development of symptoms and is destined to become disease. The second subpart is the *subclinical stage* that occurs when someone has the disease but it is not destined to develop clinically. The third subpart is the *chronic or persistent stage of disease* which is disease that persists over time. And finally, there is the fourth subpart or *latent stage* in which one has disease with no active multiplication of the biologic agent (Gordis, 2008).

The Iceberg Phenomenon

For most health problems, the number of identified cases is exceeded by the number of unidentified cases. This occurrence, referred to as the "iceberg phenomenon" makes it difficult to assess the true burden of disease. Many diseases do not have obvious symptoms as stated earlier and may go unrecognized for many years. Unrecognized diseases such as diabetes, hypertension, and mental illness create a significant problem with identifying populations at risk and estimating service needs. Complications also arise when patients are not recognized or treated during an early stage of a disease when interventions are most effective. Additionally, patients who do not have symptoms or do not recognize their symptoms do not seek medical care and, in many cases, even if they do have a diagnosis, will not take their medications as they perceive that they are healthy when they are asymptomatic.

PREVENTION

Understanding the natural history of disease is as important as understanding the causal factors of disease because it provides the advanced practice nurse (APN) with the knowledge that is required to be proactive in his or her practice.

Understanding how disease develops is fundamental to the concept of prevention and provides a framework for disease prevention and control. The primary goal of prevention is to prevent a disease before it occurs. The concept of prevention has evolved to include measures taken to interrupt or slow the progression of disease or to lessen its impact. There are three levels of prevention.

Primary Prevention

Primary prevention refers to the process of altering susceptibility or reducing exposure to susceptible individuals and includes general health promotion and specific measures designed to prevent disease prior to a person getting a disease. Interventions designed for primary prevention are carried out during the stage of susceptibility and can include such things as providing immunizations to change a person's susceptibility. Actions taken to prevent tobacco usage are another example of primary prevention. Tobacco usage is one of the 10 leading health indicators used by *Healthy People 2010* to measure health. Cigarette smoking is the leading cause of preventable morbidity and mortality in the United States (Centers for Disease Control and Prevention [CDC], 2010c), and prevention or cessation of smoking can reduce the development of many smoking-related diseases. Taxes on cigarettes, education programs, and support groups to help people stop smoking and the creation of smoke-free zones are all examples of primary prevention measures. The CDC linked a series of tobacco control efforts by Minnesota to a decrease in adult smoking prevalence rates. From 1999 to 2010, Minnesota implemented a series of antismoking initiatives including a statewide smoke-free law, cigarette tax increases, media campaigns, and statewide cessation efforts. Adult smoking prevalence decreased from 22.1% in 1999 to 16.1% in 2010 (CDC 2011). This is an excellent example of a statewide primary prevention effort to reduce smoking prevalence through a variety of initiatives.

Secondary Prevention

The early detection and prompt treatment of a disease at the earliest possible stage are referred to as *secondary prevention*. The goals of secondary prevention are to either identify and cure a disease at a very early stage or slow its progression to prevent complications and limit disability. Secondary prevention measures are carried out during the preclinical or presymptomatic stage of disease. Screening programs are designed to detect specific diseases in their early stages while they are curable and also in time to prevent morbidity and mortality related to later stages of disease. The Pap smear, mentioned earlier, is such an example. Other examples include annual testing of cholesterol levels and rapid HIV testing of asymptomatic individuals.

Tertiary Prevention

Tertiary prevention strategies are implemented during the middle or late stages of clinical disease and refer to measures taken to alleviate disability and restore effective functioning. Attempts are made to slow the progression or to cure the disease. In cases where permanent changes have taken place, interventions are planned and designed to help people lead a productive and satisfying life by maximizing the use of remaining capabilities (rehabilitation). Cardiac rehabilitation programs that provide physical and occupational therapy to postoperative cardiac care patients are an example of tertiary prevention.

CAUSATION

The Epidemiological Triangle

An understanding of causation is also necessary for formulating plans to impact the health of populations. The *epidemiological triangle* is a model that has historically been used to explain causation. The model consists of three interactive factors—the causative agent (those factors for which presence or absence cause disease), a susceptible host, and the environment (includes such diverse elements as water, food, and the cultural or political environment). A change in the agent, host, and environmental balance can lead to disease (Harkness, 1995). The underlying assumptions of this model are that causative factors can be both intrinsic and extrinsic to the host and that the cause of disease is related to interaction between the three parts. This model initially was developed to explain the infectious disease process and was particularly useful when the focus of epidemiology was on infectious diseases. It is less helpful for understanding and explaining the more complicated processes associated with chronic disease. With the rise of chronic diseases as the primary cause of morbidity and mortality, a model that recognizes multiple causative factors was needed to better understand this complex interaction.

The Web of Causation

The dynamic nature of chronic diseases calls for a more sophisticated model for explaining causation than the epidemiological triangle. Introduction of the *web of causation* concept first appeared in the 1960s when chronic diseases overtook infectious diseases as the leading causes of morbidity and mortality in the United States. The foundation of the concept is that disease develops as the result of many antecedent factors and not as a result of a single, isolated cause. Each factor is itself the result of a complex pattern of events that can be best perceived as interrelated in the complex configuration of a web. The use of a web is helpful for visualizing how difficult it is to untangle the many events that can precede the onset of a chronic illness.

Critics have argued that this model places too much emphasis on epidemiological methods and too little on theories of disease causation. Newer models stress biological evolution, adaptation, and the social production of disease (Krieger, 1994).

METHODS OF ANALYSIS

Successful population-based practice depends upon the ability to recognize the difference between the individual and population approaches to the collection and use of data, and the ability to assess needs and evaluate outcomes at the population level. Several of the more recent theories of causation can be helpful in determining if an exposure is causally related to the development of disease. In particular, calculating the strength of association using statistics is one of several criteria that can be used to determine causality. However, statistics must be used with caution. Health is a multidimensional variable—factors that affect health, and that interact to affect health, are numerous. Many relationships are possible. There are problems inherent in the use of statistics to explain differences between groups. Although statistics can *describe* disparities, they cannot *explain* them. It is left to the researchers to explain the *differences*. In addition to statistics, one must also be aware of the validity and reliability of the data. There are problems associated with the categorizing and gathering of statistics during the research process that can have an effect on how the data should be interpreted. In order to be successful in research, one must do more than just collect data—one must look at the theoretical issues associated with explaining the relationship between the variables. Recognizing limitations in research and in practice is the most important step prior to making conclusions in any setting. Therefore, it is important that APNs have a commitment to higher standards with an emphasis placed on adherence to careful and thorough procedural and ethical practice.

Methods derived from epidemiology can be useful in identifying the etiology or the cause of a disease, identifying risk factors and their impact in a population, determining the extent of a disease and/or adverse events found in a population, evaluating both existing and new preventive and therapeutic measures and modes of healthcare delivery, and providing the foundation for developing public policy and making regulatory decisions.

Descriptive Epidemiology

Rates

Knowledge of the distribution of illness and injury within a population can provide valuable information on etiology and can lay the foundation for the introduction of new prevention programs. It is important to know how to measure disease in populations, and rates are a useful method for measuring attributes, illness, and injury in any population. Rates also can be used to identify trends and evaluate outcomes and can allow for comparisons within and between groups. The *Morbidity and Mortality Weekly Report* (*MMWR*) is a publication of the CDC and contains updated information on incidence and prevalence of many diseases and conditions. These rates provide healthcare providers with up to date information on the risks and burden of various diseases and conditions (CDC, 2010a). The information obtained from the *MMWR* can be used to identify trends and provide policy makers with information for designating resources. The following is an example of how such information can be used.

> In 2007, breast cancer was the second leading cause of cancer death for White women aged 45–64 and the leading cause of cancer death for Black women aged 45–64. From 1990 to 2007, the breast cancer death rate in this age group declined by 41% for White women and 24% for Black women, increasing the disparity between the two groups. In 2007, the breast cancer death rate for women aged 45–64 was 60% higher for Black women than White women (56.8 and 35.6 deaths per 100,000) [CDC, 2010a]

The above extract is from an *MMWR* published on July 30, 2010. By publishing rates and comparing two different groups of women over time, it highlights both the burden of breast cancer and the disparity between two different groups. This information can be useful to both clinicians and policy makers who make decisions about interventions and services.

When calculating rates, the numerator is the number of events that occur during a specified period of time and is divided by the denominator which is the average population at risk during that specified time period. This number is multiplied by a constant—either 100, 1000, 10,000, or 100,000—and is expressed as per that number. The purpose of expressing rates as per 100,000, for example, is to have a constant denominator, and it allows investigators to compare rates between groups with different population sizes. Simply put, the rate is calculated as follows:

Rate = Numerator/Denominator × Constant multiplier

In order to calculate rates, the APN must first have a clear and explicit definition of the patient population and of the event. An important consideration when calculating rates is that anyone represented in the denominator must have the potential to enter the group in the numerator, and all persons represented in the numerator must come from the denominator.

Rates can be either crude or specific. Crude rates apply to an entire population without any reference to any characteristics of the individuals within it. For example, to calculate the crude mortality rate, the numerator is the total number of deaths during a specific period of time divided by the denominator, which is the average number of people in the population during that specified period of time (including those that have died). Typically, the population value for a 1-year period is determined using the midyear population.

Specific rates can also be calculated for a population that has been categorized into groups. Suppose that an APN wants to calculate the number of new mothers who initiate breastfeeding in a specific hospital in 2011. The formula would be:

$$\frac{\text{Total number of new mothers who initiated breastfeeding in the hospital in 2011}}{\text{Total number of live births in the hospital in 2011}} \times 1000 = \text{Rate per 1000}$$

In order to compare rates in two or more groups, the events in the numerator must be defined in the same way, the time intervals must be the same, and the constant multiplier must be the same. Rates can be used to compare two different groups—or one group during two different time periods. Returning to the example about breastfeeding, the breastfeeding rates could be compared in the same hospital, but at two different times—before and after implementation of a planned intervention to increase breastfeeding rates.

Formulas for the rates discussed in this chapter can be found in Exhibit 3.1.

Incidence and Prevalence

Incidence rates describe the occurrence of new events in a population over a period of time relative to the size of the population at risk. Prevalence rates describe the number of all cases of a specific disease or attribute in a population at a given point in time relative to the size of the population at risk. Incidence provides information about the rate at which new cases occur and is a measure of risk. For example, the formula for the incidence rate for HIV is:

$$\frac{\text{Total number of people who are diagnosed with HIV in a community during 2011}}{\text{Population in that community at midyear of 2011}} \times 1000 = \text{Rate per 1000}$$

Period prevalence measures the number of cases of disease during a specific period of time and is a measure of burden. The formula for the period prevalence rate for HIV in 2011 is:

$$\frac{\text{Total number of people who are HIV positive in a community during 2011}}{\text{Population in that community at midyear of 2011}} \times 1000 = \text{Rate per 1000}$$

In the formula given above, all newly diagnosed cases for the year plus existing cases are included. Point prevalence is defined as the number of cases of disease at a specific point in time divided by the number of people at risk at that specific point in time multiplied by a constant multiplier. An example of the use of point prevalence would be the information gathered from a survey where an investigator asks such questions as who has diabetes, hypertension, epilepsy, or any other disease or event at that specific point in time. Prevalence, whether point or period, cannot give us an estimate of the risk of disease; it can only tell us about the burden of disease for a specified period of time. Prevalence is useful when comparing rates between populations but should be interpreted with caution. Diseases that are chronic will have a high prevalence because at any given time, those with chronic disease will always have that disease, and this can make it challenging to interpret prevalence rates for determining resources. With diseases that are short in duration, prevalence may not capture the true burden of disease for that population. Additionally, it is important to note that unidentified cases are not captured in either prevalence rates or incidence rates.

Information from the CDC revealed that in 2000, 28 states had prevalence rates of adult obesity of less than 20%, and no state had a prevalence rate greater than 30%. In 2009, the prevalence of adult obesity in the United States ranged from 18.6% in Colorado to 34.4% in Mississippi, and a total of 33 states had prevalence rates greater than 25%; nine of those states had prevalence rates of greater than or equal to 30% (CDC, 2010b). Information on the rising prevalence of adult obesity in the United States has led to increased attention to factors that cause obesity (especially in children). This has led to the development of new programs aimed at primary and secondary prevention.

Incidence rates provide us with a direct measure of how often new cases occur within a particular population and provide some basis on which to assess risk. By comparing incidence rates among population groups who vary in one or more factors, the APN can begin to get some idea of the association between a factor and the risk of developing disease. If we take the example on breastfeeding one step further and the APN discovers breastfeeding rates are significantly different among different ethnic groups the characteristics of the groups can be compared and the causes for this disparity can be hypothesized and tested.

Mortality Rates

Mortality rates, also known as death rates, can be useful when evaluating populations. As stated earlier, there are many factors that can affect the natural history of disease, and measuring mortality allows investigators to compare death rates between and within populations. The formula for *mortality rate* is:

$$\frac{\text{Number of deaths in a population}}{\text{Average population estimate}} \times \text{Constant multiplier}$$
$$\frac{\text{during a specified time}}{\text{during the specified time}}$$

Mortality rates can be specific or broad in definition and can include any qualifiers for time, age, or disease type. It is important to include those specifics in your denominator to ensure the population value used is the best estimate of the population at risk. For example, to look at the number of deaths in 2010 due to breast cancer in women aged 18–40, the denominator should *only* include the midyear population of women aged 18–40 in 2010. It is also important to include those women who died in the denominator.

Standardization of crude rates is an important consideration when comparing mortality rates between populations. Standardization is used to control for the effects of age and other characteristics in order to make valid comparisons of rates. Age adjustment is an example of rate standardization and perhaps the most important one. No other factor has a bigger affect on mortality than age. Consider the problem of comparing two communities with very different age distributions. One community has a much higher mortality rate for colon cancer than the other, leading investigators to consider a possible environmental hazard in that community, when in fact, that community's population is older which could account for the higher mortality. Direct age adjustment or standardization allows a researcher to eliminate the age disparities between two populations by using a standardized population. This allows the researcher to compare mortality or death rates between groups by eliminating age disparities between populations and comparing actual age-adjusted mortality rates to determine if age truly plays a role in the crude mortality rates.

There are two methods of age adjustment: direct, as mentioned earlier, and indirect. The direct method applies observed age-specific mortality or death rates to a standardized population. The indirect method applies the age-specific rates of a standardized population to the age distribution of an observed population and is used to determine if one population has a greater mortality because of an occupational hazard or risk compared to the general population.

The case fatality rate is a measure of the severity of disease (such as infectious diseases) and can be helpful when designing programs to reduce the rate or disparity in the population. It is a measure of the probability of death among diagnosed cases. Its usefulness for chronic diseases is limited because the length of time from diagnosis to death can be long. The case fatality rate also can be useful in determining when to use a screening test. Screening tests are useful for identifying a disease early so that an intervention or treatment can be initiated in the hopes of lessening the morbidity or mortality of that disease. Those diseases that are rapidly fatal may not necessarily be useful to screen unless the screening will allow for a cure or treatment to change the overall outcome. Case fatality rates, therefore, can be helpful for comparisons between study populations and can provide useful information that could help determine if an intervention or treatment is working. The formula for *case fatality* is as follows:

$$\% \text{ Case fatality rate} = \frac{\text{Number of deaths due to a specific disease in a specified period of time}}{\text{Number of cases of that specific disease in the same specified period of time}} \times 100.$$

The case fatality rate is usually expressed as a percentage, so in this case one would multiply this rate by a constant multiplier of 100 to obtain the percentage of disease that is fatal. It is important in all of these rates to include those that have died from the disease in the denominator. Subtracting those that have died from the denominator can change the rates significantly.

The proportionate mortality ratio is useful for determining the leading causes of death. The formula for *proportionate mortality ratio* is as follows:

$$\frac{\text{Number of deaths from a specified cause in the United States during specified time perriod}}{\text{Total deaths from all causes in the United States during the same specified time period}} \times 100$$

Again, this measure is usually reported as a percentage and reflects the burden of death due to a particular disease. This information is useful for policy makers who make decisions about the allocation of resources.

Health Impact Assessment

As mentioned previously, rates can be used to describe the distribution of disease and other health-related states and events, but sometimes the APN may be more concerned with knowing how data can be used to describe the relevancy of clinical practice. Health impact assessment is the assessment of the potential health effects, positive or negative, of a particular intervention on a population. The number needed to treat statistic (NNT), the disease impact number (DIN), and the population impact number (PIN) are formulae that are used in a health impact assessment. NNT is the number of patients needed to receive a treatment to prevent one bad outcome. DIN is the number of those with the disease in question among whom one event will be prevented by the intervention. PIN is the number of those in the whole population among whom one event will be prevented by the intervention. Years of potential life lost (YPLL) measures premature mortality, the productive years that are lost related to early death (Gordis, 2008).

Fontaine, Redden, Wang, Westfall, and Allison (2003) published a study conducted to estimate the YPLL because of overweight and obesity. They found that the risk for YPLL is greatest for the youngest age groups. They also report, "The maximum YPLL for White men aged 20 to 30 with a severe level of obesity (BMI > 45) is 13 years and is 8 years for White women. For men this would represent a 22% reduction in expected remaining life span" (p. 187). Information on YPLL helps to magnify the importance of primary prevention measures designed to address obesity and other risk factors.

More extensive information on health impact assessment formulae and standardization can be found in most advanced epidemiology texts. It is important for the APN who is involved in population-based evaluation to be aware of these concepts.

DESCRIPTIVE STUDIES

Descriptive epidemiology is used to describe the distribution of disease and other health-related states and events in terms of personal characteristics, geographical distribution, and time. There are four types of descriptive studies: case reports, case series, cross-sectional studies, and correlation or ecologic studies. The remaining portion of this chapter will focus on the use of correlation and cross-sectional studies in population analyses. The data used in descriptive studies are often readily available and can be retrieved from such sources as hospital records, census data, or vital statistics records.

Correlation Studies

Correlation studies are also referred to as ecologic studies and are used to conduct studies of group or population characteristics. In ecologic studies, rates are calculated for characteristics that describe populations and are used to compare frequencies between different groups at the same time or the same group at different times. They are useful for identifying long-term trends, seasonal patterns, and event-related clusters. Because data are collected on populations instead of individuals, an event cannot be linked to an exposure in individuals, and the investigator cannot control for the effect of other variables (confounders). Therefore, it is important to identify if the association is real or false. If the association is real, the next question that needs to be asked is: Is that association causal? A confounder is a variable that is linked to both a causative factor or exposure and the outcome. There are many examples of confounders such as age, gender, and socioeconomic status. Confounding occurs when a study is performed, and it appears from the study results that a causal relationship exists between an exposure and an outcome but that relationship is actually based on a relationship between the exposure and a confounder. An example of confounding might occur if an APN carried out a study to determine if there was a relationship between age and medication compliance without controlling for income. Younger, working patients might be more compliant not because of the age factor, but because they have the resources to buy their medications. If confounding is ignored, there can be long-term implications as the APN may implement interventions for medication compliance with education programs aimed at older patients without considering problems related to income—the intervention would ultimately not succeed because the relationship was false or not causal due to confounding. Confounders must be a known risk factor for the outcome and are associated with the exposure but cannot occur as a result of the exposure.

A study by Tresserras, Canela, Alvarez, Sentis, and Salleras (1992) provides an example of a correlational study. The authors used data from 95 countries to study the relationship between infant mortality and the prevalence of adult illiteracy. The results of these analyses indicate that adult illiteracy correlates positively with infant mortality, such that populations with a higher prevalence of illiteracy have higher infant mortality rates and populations with a lower prevalence of illiteracy have lower infant mortality rates. The authors point out, "In interpreting the results, the possible presence of some biases has to be taken into account" (p. 436). These data show that a relationship may exist between the variables, but not a causal one. There are many possible explanations for the relationship, including (but not exclusively) demographic and economic differences among the countries. Correlation studies must be interpreted with caution but important information can be obtained from the trends that could identify disparities and lead to further studies and hypothesis testing.

Cross-Sectional Studies

In cross-sectional studies, both the exposure to a factor and an outcome are determined simultaneously. These studies provide a "snap shot" at one point in time and thus exclude people who have died or who chose not to participate, which can introduce bias. Temporal relationships are difficult to determine in these studies and, therefore, the risk of developing disease cannot be estimated. Cross-sectional studies can be used to suggest possible risk factors and to identify prevalence rates but are not useful for evaluating interventions. Many cross-sectional studies are surveys that sample a population and their various characteristics. They can be inexpensive and can provide timely descriptive data about a group under study, but again they do not tell us about causality or the true risk of developing a certain outcome like disease.

Spoelstra, Given, von Eye, and Given (2010) conducted a cross-sectional study to determine if individuals with a history of cancer fall at a higher rate than those without cancer. They also examined whether or not the occurrence of falls in the elderly was influenced by individual characteristics. The study population consisted of 7,448 community-dwelling elderly who were 65 years or older living in one state in the Midwest United States. The analysis of the data revealed that having cancer was not a predictor of falls in this study. Further analysis revealed that predictors of falls in this population included race, sex, ADLs, incontinence, depression, and pain. Although cancer was not found to be a predictor of falls, the authors did find a high frequency of falls in that study population. The findings led the authors to conclude that it is important to develop a predictive model for fall risk in the community-dwelling elderly.

This study serves to illustrate both the advantages and the disadvantages of cross-sectional studies. The study was carried out at one point in time using an existing dataset (the Minimum Data Set or MDS). One limitation of the study was that it missed people whose falls were not reported. Another limitation the authors cited was they could not determine whether a specific cancer diagnosis, stage, or treatment was a risk factor for falls. Finally, they were unable to determine whether or not comorbidities may have placed individuals at a higher risk for falls. The inability to control for or identify the significance of potentially important variables is a disadvantage of using a retrospective cross-sectional study design. On the other hand, a cross-sectional study is a fairly quick method to obtain descriptive data and can be used to identify prevalence rates for specified populations.

ANALYTIC EPIDEMIOLOGY

Analytic epidemiology looks at the origins and causal factors of diseases and other health-related events. Analytic designs are often carried out to test hypotheses formulated from a descriptive study. The goal of analytic epidemiology is to identify factors that increase or decrease risk. Risk is the probability that an event will occur. For example, a patient who is obese might ask, "What is the likelihood that I will get diabetes if I do not lose weight?"

Although descriptive studies allow a basis for comparison and can provide the APN with data to identify potential risk factors and differences among groups, further studies need to be carried out in order to determine the significance of a factor. To do this, the APN can compare exposed and nonexposed groups or cases and controls—comparison is an essential component of population studies.

Comparisons can be made by following a group using treatment A compared to treatment B or treatment A can be compared to no treatment at all. There are multiple study designs but we will only focus on the most common study designs and discuss the advantages and disadvantages that each one poses in practice.

Case–Control Studies

In a case–control study, the APN must first identify a group of individuals with the attribute of interest (cases). A second group is identified without the attribute of interest (controls). The proportion of those cases who were exposed to the suspected causal factor are then compared to the proportion of the cases who were not exposed, and the proportion of the controls who were exposed are compared to the proportion of the controls who were not exposed. The measure of the effect of exposure is expressed as an odds ratio (OR), which is the ratio of the odds of having been exposed if you are a case to the odds of having been exposed if you are a not a case. If the exposure is not related to the disease or factor of interest, the odds ratio will equal 1. If the exposure is related to the disease or factor of interest, the odds ratio will be greater than 1, and if the odds ratio is less than 1 the exposure is considered protective. To calculate the odds ratio, you simply set up a 2×2 table in which you multiply the cross products to obtain your result (Table 3.1).

In a case-control study, if there is an association between an exposure and disease, the history of exposure should be higher in persons who have the disease (cases) compared to those who do not have disease (controls). It is important to keep in mind that only a subset of the population will be at risk from a particular exposure—in other words, only a proportion of those exposed will become a case as a result of their exposure. The odds ratio is not a calculation of risk and cannot predict when an exposure will become a case or disease. The fact that a person is obese may put that person at risk for diabetes, but it does not mean that that person *will* get diabetes. In case–control studies, we are dealing with prevalent cases not incident cases and as a result, we cannot conclude there is a likelihood that if you are obese you will develop diabetes but rather if you have diabetes you are more likely to be obese.

Case–control studies can be used to study the effects of an intervention. Bellman, Hambraeus, Lindback, and Lindahl (2009) studied the effects of taking part in an educational program designed for patients in Sweden who have a

TABLE 3.1   Calculation of Odds Ratio in a Case–Control Study

	CASES	CONTROLS
EXPOSURE	a	b
NO EXPOSURE	c	d
TOTALS	a + c	b + d
	Proportion of Cases Exposed = a/a + c	Proportion of Controls Exposed = b/b + d
Odds Ratio = ad/bc		

history of an acute myocardial infarction. The objective of the study was to identify the effect of the intervention on smoking habits, blood pressure, LDL, exercise, cardiac symptoms, quality of life, and hospital readmissions. Patients who participated in the program (cases) were compared to patients who did not participate in the program (controls). The analysis of the data revealed that cases stopped smoking more often than controls (OR = 2.01; 95% confidence interval (CI), 1.46–2.78). The educational program had no other effects on the other variables that were examined. One problem with this type of study is that cases and controls were not randomly assigned to either group. People who chose to participate in the program may possess certain characteristics that may make them different in some fundamental ways from those who chose not to participate. As a result, this failure to randomize can lead to selection bias which could cause researchers to believe their program was successful when in reality it was the participants selected in the program who were more likely to succeed.

Selection of the sample is an important step in case–control studies. Definite criteria should be used so that there is no ambiguity about how to distinguish between a case and a control. Exposure is not always all or nothing. Controls should resemble the cases as closely as possible except for exposure to the factor under study. If the cases are drawn from a particular clinic, then ideally the controls should be drawn from the same clinic population. Matching is one method that can be used to select a sample so that potential confounders are distributed equally between the cases and controls. For example, if an APN planned to evaluate an intervention to reduce burden among caregivers of dependent elderly in the home it would be important to recognize the characteristics of the population studied prior to implementing the intervention. It is known that men and women have differing characteristics that affect their role as caregiver (e.g., women find the physical demands of caregiving more burdensome than men). By matching for gender in the study, the APN can eliminate this potentially confounding factor (gender). The problem with matching is that the investigator is not always aware of all of the potential confounding factors, and it can be difficult to match each subject in a study and in some cases investigators can over-match. When an investigator over-matches one loses the ability to look at the matched variables as outcomes of interest.

Cohort Studies

Cohort designs can be either prospective or retrospective. In a prospective cohort design, the investigator begins with a defined population and then follows a group of individuals who were either exposed or nonexposed to a factor of interest and then follows both groups to compare the incidence of an outcome or disease. Multiple exposures can be followed, and the incidence of multiple diseases can also be determined. In a retrospective cohort design, exposure is ascertained from past records and outcome is ascertained at the time the study is begun. If an association exists between the exposure and the outcome, then the incidence rate in the exposed group will be greater than the incidence rate in the nonexposed group. The ratio of these is the relative risk (RR), which is the incidence rate in the exposed group divided by the incidence rate in the nonexposed group. RR is the measure of the strength of an association between an exposure and an outcome or disease (Table 3.2).

If the RR is equal to 1 (the numerator equals the denominator), then the risk to the two groups is equal. If the RR is greater than 1 (the numerator is greater than the denominator), the risk in the exposed group is greater than the risk in the non-exposed group and can be considered possibly causal. If the RR is less than 1 (the denominator is greater than the numerator), the risk in the exposed group is less than the risk in the nonexposed group and can be considered protective.

Attributable risk (AR) or absolute risk is the amount of risk that can be attributed to an exposure. For example, it is well known that smoking can cause lung cancer but lung cancer can also occur in nonsmokers. The amount of disease that is associated with risks/exposures other than smoking is called the *background risk*. In order to calculate the risk attributable to a particular exposure, subtract the incidence of disease (lung cancer) in the exposed group (smokers) minus the incidence of disease (lung cancer) in the nonexposed group (background risk). This value is considered the attributable risk due to exposure (Table 3.2). The AR can also be calculated as a proportion of the exposed population or a proportion of the total population. For example, to determine the amount of lung cancer attributable to smoking in the total population (AR Proportion), one would have to know the incidence in the total population, (to review how to calculate the incidence in the total population, please refer to an advanced epidemiology textbook). APNs should be familiar with how to calculate and interpret RR and AR, as these values are reported commonly in the literature and reports such as the *MMWR*.

A cohort study was carried out in Norway to ascertain characteristics that would predict the risk of fibromyalgia. The authors examined the association between leisure time, physical exercise, body mass index (BMI), and risk of fibromyalgia (FM) (Mork, Vasseljen, & Nilsen, 2010). A longitudinal study followed

TABLE 3.2   Calculation of Relative Risk and Attributable Risk in a Cohort Study

	DISEASE	NO DISEASE	TOTALS	
EXPOSURE	a	b	a + b	Incidence in Exposed (Inc Exp) = a/a + b
NO EXPOSURE	c	d	c + d	Incidence in Nonexposed (Inc NonExp) = c/c + d
Relative Risk (RR) = Incidence in the Exposed/Incidence in the Nonexposed				
Attributable Risk (AR) = Incidence in the Exposed − Incidence in the Nonexposed				
AR Proportion in the Exposed Population = $\dfrac{Inc\,Exp - Inc\,NonExp}{Inc\,Exp}$				
AR Proportion in the Total Population = $\dfrac{Incidence\,in\,Total\,Population - Inc\,NonExp}{Incidence\,in\,Total\,Population}$				

15,900 women without FM or physical impairment at baseline for 11 years. At the end of the study period, there were 380 reported cases of FM and relative risks were calculated for each of the study variables (exposures). Women who reported the highest exercise level had a RR of 0.77 (95% CI 0.55–1.07). In looking at exercise, the authors controlled for the potential confounding factor of BMI. Overweight or obese women (BMI > 25.0 kg/m²) had a 60–70% higher risk compared with women with normal weight (BMI 18.5–24.9 kg/m²). Overweight or obese women who exercised >1 hour per week had an RR of 1.72 (95% CI 1.07–2.76) compared with normal-weight women with a similar activity level. The risk for overweight or obese women who were inactive (RR 2.09, 95% CI 1.36–3.21) or exercised <1 hour per week (RR 2.19, 95% CI 1.39–3.46) showed an association between risk of developing FM and low levels of exercise. The authors concluded that being overweight or obese was associated with an increased risk of FM, especially among women who also reported low levels of physical exercise, and recommended that community-based measures aimed at reducing the incidence of FM should emphasize maintaining a normal weight and regular exercise.

Cohort studies are best carried out when the investigator has good evidence that links an exposure to an outcome, when the time interval between exposure and the outcome is short, and when the outcome occurs relatively often. One of the major problems with cohort studies is that they can be time consuming and expensive, especially if the cohort needs to be followed for any length of time. Diseases that are rare or that take many years to develop may be better suited for a case–control study as it can be difficult to follow participants for many years especially if the outcome of interest is rare. The longer the time period, the more likely participants will be lost to follow-up, and multiple exposures can confound the relationship. Finally, cohort studies are not feasible if there is difficulty involved in identifying exposed versus nonexposed populations, or when data for the subjects are incomplete or lacking.

It is important to understand that the difference between case–control and cohort studies is not a function of calendar time. In case–control studies, the investigator begins with cases and controls and goes back retrospectively to look for exposures. In cohort studies, the investigator begins with exposed and nonexposed individuals and follows individuals over time to see who develops or does not develop an outcome or disease. Case–control studies allow the APN to look at cases and the probability of having an exposure to a specified variable. Cohort studies allow an APN to follow a cohort over time to determine if exposure to a variable impacts the likelihood of developing a disease—or improves outcomes (as in an intervention). If associations are found, further studies are necessary to determine causal links and to prevent ecologic fallacy. When examining the results of case–control and cohort studies, it is important for the APN to consider whether or not all other explanations for an identified association have been eliminated. No single epidemiological study can satisfy all criteria for causality. The APN needs to look at the accumulation of evidence, as well as the strength of individual studies.

Randomized Controlled Trials

Randomized controlled trials (RCTs) or clinical trials are useful for evaluating treatments (including technology) and for assessing new ways of organizing and delivering health services. In population-based studies, the issue is often health promotion and disease prevention, rather than treatment of an existing disease. The intervention is undertaken on a large scale—with the target involving defined populations rather than individuals and often involving educational, program, or policy interventions. When carefully designed, RCTs can provide the strongest evidence for a cause-and-effect relationship.

The basic design of a RCT is to assign the sample randomly to either receive the new treatment/intervention or not to receive the new treatment/intervention. The difference between a RCT and a cohort study is that in a randomized trial, the subjects are randomly assigned to either an exposed or nonexposed group. Inclusion and exclusion criteria for the participants must be precise and written in advance to eliminate any errors within the study or any future comparison studies. As with cohort studies, RCTs can compare more than two groups. Analysis is carried out to compare outcomes between the randomized groups. As mentioned earlier, comparisons can be made between different interventions, different treatments, or to a control group that has received no intervention or treatment.

A randomized trial of a fall prevention strategy was carried out by Dykes et al. (2010). The objective of the study was, "To investigate whether a fall prevention tool kit (FPTK) using health information technology (HIT) decreases patient falls in hospitals" (1912). The design was a cluster randomized study. In a clustered design, study groups of subjects (instead of individuals) are randomized to each intervention. In this case, medical units that met the inclusion criteria for the study were matched for unit census, length of stay, and fall rates. Matched units were then randomly assigned to either the intervention group or the control group. Eight units in four hospitals met the inclusion criteria and were entered into the study. The four units in the control group received an educational program on fall risk assessment and prevention and provided usual care. The four units in the intervention group received the FPTK software integrated into an existing HIT application. The FPTK tailors fall prevention interventions to the identified risk factors of each patient. The software also produces alerts such as bed posters, educational handouts for patients, and individualized plans of care. The primary outcome measure was falls per 1000 patient days. As part of the data analysis, the researchers adjusted for possible confounders such as age and fall risk scores. The intervention and control groups had similar lengths of stay and no differences in gender composition. The researchers also monitored adherence to the protocol. Analysis revealed that the intervention group had a significantly lower adjusted fall rate (3.15, 95% CI 2.54–3.90) per 1000 patient days as compared to the control group (4.18, 95% CI 3.45–5.06). The researchers hypothesized, after completion of the study, that the intervention effect was greater in older patients than younger patients. Further analysis revealed that patients aged 65 and older benefited the most from the FPTK.

This study illustrates how useful the randomized trial design is for testing a new intervention. An advantage of the cluster randomized design is the ability to study interventions that cannot be directed toward selected individuals. In this case, the design simplified the ability of the researchers to control confounders and to prevent *contamination bias* (discussed further in Chapter 4) which occurs when patients in the control group inadvertently receive the intervention.

Sample Size

Sample selection and sample size determination are critical steps in the research process. Sample size determination is necessary to identify a minimum number needed to enroll in the study to identify true differences and associations between groups, and thus has implications for the investigators as they need to allocate ample resources based on sample size to carry out the study. Power analysis is used to determine sample size. There are several factors that influence the size of the sample: power, effect size, and significance. Significance is the probability that an observed difference or relationship exists. Power is the capacity of the study to detect differences or relationships that actually exist in the population or the capacity to correctly reject a null hypothesis; that is, prevent a type II error. The larger the power required, the larger the necessary sample size. The smaller the sample size, the smaller the power of the study. Effect size is the actual differences between groups and treatments that you hope to see in your study. One way to identify effect size is to review previous studies, and a second method is to conduct a pilot study. The smaller the effect size, the more stringent the significance level, the greater the necessary sample size. The significance level that is used in most nursing studies is 0.05, and the most frequently used power is 80%. Effect sizes occur along a range of values. For example, if you want to see a 5% change in results of an outcome you will need many more participants than if you want to see a 30% change.

Power analysis can be calculated using computer programs. There are many free software programs available on the Internet to assist with power analysis. Typing sample size calculation in a search engine such as Yahoo or Google will lead the investigator to many sites (Burns, 2000; Duffy, 2006).

Screening

Screening is a tool used to detect disease in groups of asymptomatic individuals with the goal of reducing and/or preventing morbidity and mortality. Screening tests can be applied to groups of individuals or to high-risk populations and as a result can lead to variances in test results. There are multiple examples of screening tests including the Pap smear, prostate-specific antigen test, the mammogram, etc.

Determining if a screening test is appropriate requires the APN to address several aspects of the disease of interest. Screening is neither available nor appropriate for all diseases. In order for a screening program to be effective, certain criteria should be met. The target population needs to be identifiable and accessible and the disease should affect a sufficient number of people to make screening cost effective. The preclinical period should be sufficient to allow treatment before symptoms appear so that early diagnosis and treatment make a difference in terms of outcome.

Finally, it is necessary for the screening test to be sensitive enough to detect most cases of the disease and to be specific enough to limit the number of false-positive tests. Screening tests should also be relatively inexpensive, easy to administer, and have minimal side effects.

The validity of a screening test refers to its ability to accurately identify those who have the disease. Sensitivity and specificity are measures of a screening test's validity. Sensitivity is a measure of a screening test's ability to accurately identify disease when it is present. Specificity is a measure of screening test's ability to correctly identify a person without disease with a negative test. The positive predictive value (PPV) is a measure of the probability of a positive test result when the disease is present. The negative predictive value (NPV) of a test is a measure of the probability that the disease is absent when there is a negative test (Table 3.3).

Directing screening tests toward high-risk populations has many advantages. By screening populations with a higher disease prevalence, we can actually increase the positive predictive value of that test. Screening low prevalence populations can lead to more false positives, which can be costly and harmful to the patients. Thus, selection of the disease to be tested and the patient population to be screened are both important to consider when designing a new test.

The APN can evaluate the success of screening programs by looking at a variety of outcomes. For example, some of the outcomes that can be followed include: reduction in overall mortality in screened individuals, a reduction in the case fatality rate in screened individuals, an increase in percent of cases detected at earlier stages, a reduction in complications, and improvement of quality of life in screened individuals.

In 2009, the U.S. Preventive Services Task Force (USPSTF) released their recommendations for breast cancer screening (USPSTF, 2009). One of the recommendations is that biennial screening with mammography begin at age 50 for most women. The recommendation is based on the findings that the highest

TABLE 3.3 Computing Sensitivity, Specificity, and Predictive Values in Screening Tests

	DISEASE	NO DISEASE	TOTALS	
+TEST	a	b	a + b	PPV = a/a + b
−TEST	c	d	c + d	NPV = d/c + d
TOTALS	a + c	b + d		
	Sensitivity = a/a + c	Specificity = d/b + d		b = false positives c = false negatives

false-positive test rate and the most unnecessary biopsies occur in the 40- to 50-year age group. The recommendation also takes into consideration the belief that the cumulative effect of exposure to multiple mammographies over time is not benign. There is ample evidence that the most benefit for breast screening using mammography is derived from screening women aged 50 to 74 every 2 years (Lefevre, Calonge, Dietrich, & Melnikow, 2010; USPSTF, 2009). These guidelines provide an example of how evidence on the specificity and sensitivity of a screening test can be used to design clinical guidelines. Therefore, screening tests need to be tailored to the disease under investigation, and many factors need to be taken into consideration (e.g., How many false negatives can be missed? How many false positives are acceptable? Can screening and early detection really make a difference in the outcome of the disease?). Understanding these factors and balancing them with targeted screening in high-risk populations are important considerations in screening implementation.

SUMMARY

The natural history of disease refers to the progression of a disease from its preclinical state to its clinical state, and these stages provide a framework for understanding approaches to the prevention and control of disease. Primary prevention refers to the process of altering susceptibility or reducing exposure to susceptible individuals and includes general health promotion and specific measures designed to prevent disease prior to a person getting a disease. Primary prevention measures are generally carried out during the stage of susceptibility. With secondary prevention, it is sometimes possible to either cure a disease at a very early stage or slow its progression to prevent complications and limit disability. Secondary prevention measures are carried out during the preclinical or presymptomatic stage of disease. Tertiary prevention takes place during the middle or later stages of a disease (the clinical stage of disease) and refers to measures taken to alleviate disability and restore effective functioning.

The dynamic nature of disease calls for a sophisticated model for explaining causation. When designing interventions for populations, the APN needs to keep in mind that disease develops as the result of many antecedent factors and not as a result of a single, isolated cause.

Descriptive epidemiology is used to describe the distribution of disease and other health-related states and events in terms of personal characteristics, geographical distribution, and time. Analytic epidemiology looks at the origins and causal factors of diseases and other health-related events. Epidemiologic methods can be used to identify populations at risk and to evaluate interventions provided to patient populations. Population-based evaluation and planning depend upon understanding the many and varied factors that influence health and disease. APNs can use their understanding of epidemiological methods in concert with their clinical expertise in order to develop policies and implement and evaluate new programs and interventions to improve population outcomes.

EXHIBIT 3.1

Calculating Rates

Incidence rates describe the occurrence of *new* disease cases in a community over a period of time relative to the size of the population at risk.

$$\text{Incidence rate} = \frac{\text{Number of } new \text{ cases during a specified period}}{\text{Population at risk during the same specified period}} \times \text{Constant multiplier}$$

Prevalence rates are the number of *all* existing cases of a specific disease in a population *at a given point in time* relative to the population at risk.

$$\text{Prevalence rate} = \frac{\text{Number of } existing \text{ cases at a specified time}}{\text{Population at risk at the same specified time}} \times \text{Constant multiplier}$$

Crude rates summarize the occurrence of births (crude birth rate) or deaths (crude death rate). The numerator is the number of events, and the denominator is the average population size.

$$\text{Crude death rate} = \frac{\text{Number of deaths in a population during a specified time}}{\text{Average population estimate during the same specified time}} \times \text{Constant multiplier}$$

Specific rates are used to overcome some of the biases seen with crude rates. They are used to control for variables such as age, race, gender, and disease.

$$\text{Age–Specific death rate} = \frac{\text{Number of deaths for a specified age group during a specified time}}{\text{Population estimate for the specified age group}} \times \text{Constant multiplier}$$

Case fatality rate is used to measure the percentage of people who die from a certain disease and within a certain time after diagnosis. This rate tells you how fatal or severe a disease is compared to other diseases.

$$\text{Case fatality rate} = \frac{\text{Number of individuals dying during a specified period of time after disease onset or diagnosis}}{\text{Number of individuals wiith the specified disease}} \times \text{Constant multiplier}$$

(*continued*)

(continued)

Proportionate mortality ratio is useful for determining the leading causes of death.

$$\text{Proportionate mortality ratio} = \frac{\begin{array}{c}\text{Number of deaths from}\\\text{a specified cause in the United}\\\text{States during specified time period}\end{array}}{\begin{array}{c}\text{Total deaths in the United States}\\\text{during the same time period}\end{array}} \times 100$$

Calculations Used in Health Impact Assessment

Number Needed to Treat (NNT) is the number of patients needed to receive a treatment to prevent one bad outcome. Before the NNT can be calculated, the absolute risk reduction (ARR) must be identified.

$$\text{ARR} = \text{Risk in exposed} - \text{Risk in un-exposed}$$

$$\text{NNT} = 1/\text{ARR}$$

Disease Impact Number (DIN) is the number of those with the disease in question among whom one event will be prevented by the intervention.

Population Impact Number (PIN) is the number of those in the whole population among whom one event will be prevented by the intervention.

Years of Potential Life Lost (YPLL) is used for setting heath priorities. Predetermined standard age at death in the United States is 65 years.

$$\text{YPLL (65)} = 65 - \text{age at death from a specific cause}$$

Add the years of life lost for each individual for specific cause of death = YPLL

Calculations used in Screening Programs

Sensitivity: the ability of a screening test to identify accurately those persons with the disease

$$\text{Sensitivity} = \text{TP}/(\text{TP} + \text{FN})$$

TP = True positives

FN = False negatives

Specificity: reflects the extent to which it excludes the persons who do not have the disease

$$\text{Specificity} = \text{TN}/(\text{TP} + \text{FP})$$

TN = True negatives

FP = False positives

Note. Adapted from Fulton, J. S., Lyon, B. L., & Goudreau, K. A, (2010). *Foundations of Clinical Nurse Specialist Practice.* New York: Springer.

EXERCISES AND DISCUSSION QUESTIONS

Exercise 3.1 A study was conducted surveying men and women for high blood pressure. The results showed that there were 50 men and 75 women per 100,000 who had high blood pressure. The male and female population totals were 230,000 and 189,000, respectively.

- What is the absolute number of men and women affected (i.e., how many men and women were identified with high blood pressure in this study)?
- Is this incidence or prevalence? Why?

Exercise 3.2 You are working in a community hospital in a small town in Tennessee. The town's population is 23,000. There were 6 new cases of Rocky Mountain spotted fever diagnosed in the past year.

- Calculate the incidence of Rocky Mountain spotted fever per 100,000.

Exercise 3.3 A rapid screening test for women with HPV is being evaluated for its effectiveness and sensitivity as a screening test in college health-care clinics. In order to determine the effectiveness of the HPV test, it was administered to 2000 female college students. Tests were confirmed by comparisons to the gold standard testing (Pap smears). Prevalence of HPV was 12% in the college population; 443 students tested positive for HPV. The HPV test was found to be 92% specific. Create a 2 × 2 table which accurately describes this test.

	HPV	NO HPV	TOTALS
+TEST			
−TEST			
TOTALS			

- What is the sensitivity of this test?
- What is the positive predictive value of this test?
- What is the negative predictive value of this test?
- If everything else remained the same, what would happen to the predictive value of a positive test if the disease prevalence increased in the population?
- How many false negatives are there with this test?
- How many false positives are there with this test?
- If the gold standard test (Pap smear) has a sensitivity of 94% and a specificity of 88%, which test—HPV or Pap test—would you prefer to use in your healthcare clinic *if you want to reduce the number of false negative test results* in your clinic? Explain your answer using results from above.

Exercise 3.4 An investigator samples a group of clients from a clinic based on their disease status—in particular, whether or not they have high blood pressure (HTN). Of the 250 people sampled, 40% were found to have HTN. Knowing their disease status, a questionnaire is administered to the people in the study to determine how many have a family history (FHx) of stroke (in a first-degree relative). Of the people without HTN, 8% had a FHx of stroke. Of the people with HTN, 37% had a FHx of stroke. Generate the 2×2 table to describe this relationship.

	HTN	NO HTN	TOTALS
+FHX STROKE			
−FHX STROKE			
TOTALS			

- What type of study design is this?
- Can you calculate relative risk using the above data? Why or why not?
- Can you calculate odds ratio?
- Calculate the correct descriptive statistic for this study (either RR or OR).
- What are possible errors that could be made in this type of study?
- What is the correct interpretation of the statistic used?
  a. Patients with a family history of stroke are 6.75 times more likely to develop high blood pressure than patients with no family history of stroke.
  b. Patients with high blood pressure are 6.75 times more likely to have a family history of stroke than those with normal blood pressure

Exercise 3.5 A study is conducted at your hospital to learn about the relationship between HIV and IV drug usage. You identify patients from your emergency department who are IV drug users and those that are not and follow them for 1 year. You find there are 69 cases of HIV out of 253 who are IV drug users, and there are 17 cases of HIV out of 450 who are not IV drug users. (The overall rate in both groups combined = 86 cases of HIV out of 703.) You are interested in developing an intervention to reduce the incidence of HIV and you would like to target a prevention program addressing risk factors. Use this information to answer the following questions.

	+HIV	−HIV
+IV DRUG USE		
−IV DRUG USE		
TOTALS		

■ Calculate the incidence rate of HIV in the IV drug users (R_1), in the non-IV drug users (R_0), and overall (R). Express all rates "per 1000."
■ Calculate the relative risk for this exposure.
■ Calculate the attributable risk for this exposure.
■ Calculate the attributable risk proportion for this exposure.
■ What are some problems that may be associated with this kind of study design?
■ What are possible confounders?

Exercise 3.6 For the following scenarios, describe the type of study design: Answer a, b, c or d.

a. cross-sectional study,
b. case–control study,
c. cohort study, or
d. ecologic study.

_____ A study was done to look at melanoma and sun exposure in a population in Arizona. Prevalence rates in Arizona were compared to prevalence rates of melanoma and sun exposure in Alaska. The researchers found people in Arizona had a higher prevalence of melanoma and sun exposure than those in Alaska.

_____ Over a 3-month period, 12,000 patients with hepatitis will be categorized as alcoholic or nonalcoholic. Then over the next 20 years, new cases of liver cancer will be classified of the 12,000.

_____ Over a 6-month period, all incoming residents into a nursing home over 55 years of age were asked if they currently have diabetes and whether they have a history of skin infections.

_____ Over a 1-year period, all new cases of hepatitis and a similar number of persons without hepatitis were asked if they have a history of alcohol usage.

_____ All school children in five schools are given a physical fitness test during May and June of 2010. At the time the test results are collected, current risk factors for obesity were ascertained.

Exercise 3.7 During the course of the spring semester at the School of Nursing (SON), 13 students developed colds. There are 22 students who enrolled in the SON for the first time at the start of the spring semester (new to school), and 88 students are continuing at the school from the previous fall semester. Thirty-two students had a cold at some point during the spring semester. According to a survey done by students at the SON on the last day of the spring semester, three students claimed to have a cold at the time of the survey.

■ What was the *point prevalence* per 1000 of colds at the time of the survey?
■ What was the *incidence* per 1000 of colds during the spring semester?
■ What was the *period prevalence* per 1000 of colds during the spring semester?

Exercise 3.8   You are asked to assess the state of health after a natural disaster. Your community has a population of 90,150. You have obtained some statistics 1 year after the disaster, and your hospital administrator would like you to assess the impact of the disaster on the community. You are asked to look at illnesses due to *Escherichia coli*, which have peaked since the disaster. You determined there were 2905 total deaths during the year ending December 31, 2009. This includes 128 deaths from *E. coli*; 274 people were sick with *E. coli* during 2009.

■   What was the cause-specific mortality rate per 100,000 from *E. coli* in 2009?
■   What was the case-fatality rate from *E. coli*?
■   What is the crude mortality rate per 100,000 in this community?

REFERENCES

Bellman, C., Hambraeus, K., Lindback, J., & Lindahl, B. (2009). Achievement of secondary preventive goals after acute myocardial infarction: A comparison between participants and nonparticipants in a routine patient education program in Sweden. *Journal of Cardiovascular Nursing, 24*(5), 362–368.

Burns, K. (2000). Power and effect size: Research considerations for the clinical nurse specialist. *Clinical Nurse Specialist, 14*(2), 61–68.

Centers for Disease Control and Prevention. (2010a). *Morbidity and mortality weekly report (MMWR).* Retrieved from http://www.cdc.gov/mmwr/about.html

Centers for Disease Control and Prevention. (2010b). *Vital signs: State specific obesity prevalence among adults, 2009 (MMWR Morbidity and Mortality Weekly Report Vol. 59 Early release August 3, 2010).* Retrieved from http://www.cdc.gov/mmwr/preview/mmwrhtml/mm59e0803a1.htm

Centers for Disease Control and Prevention. (2010c). *Vital signs: Nonsmokers' exposure to secondhand smoke—United States, 1999–2008 (MMWR Morbidity and Mortality Weekly Report Vol. 59 September 7, 2010).* Retrieved from http://www.cdc.gov/mmwr/pdf/wk/mm59e0907.pdf

Centers for Disease Control and Prevention. (2011). Decrease in smoking prevalence—Minnesota 1999–2010. *Morbidity and Mortality Weekly Report (MMWR), 60*(5), 138–141, Retrieved from http://www.cdc.gov/mmwr/preview/mmwrhtml/mm6005a2.htm?s_cid=mm6005a2_w

Duffy, M. (2006). Resources for determining or evaluating sample size in quantitative research reports. *Clinical Nurse Specialist, 20*(1), 9–12.

Dykes, P., Carroll, D., Hurley, A., Lipsatz, S., Benoit, A., Chang, F., . . . Middleton, B. (2010). Fall prevention in acute care hospitals: A randomized trial. *JAMA, 304*(17), 1912–1918.

Fontaine, K., Redden, D., Wang, C., Westfall, A., & Allison, D. (2003). Years of life lost due to obesity. *JAMA, 289*(2), 187–193.

Gordis, L. (2008). *Epidemiology* (4th ed.). Philadelphia, PA: Elsevier Saunders.

Harkness, G. (1995). *Epidemiology in nursing practice.* New York, NY: Mosby.

Healthy People, (2010). *What are the leading health indicators?* Retrieved November 18, 2010, from http://www.healthypeople.gov/LHI/lhiwhat.htm

Heller, R., & Page J. (2002). A population perspective to evidence based medicine: "Evidence for population health." *Journal of Epidemiology and Community Health, 56,* 45–47.

Krieger, N. (1994). Epidemiology and the web of causation: Has anyone seen the spider? *Social Science and Medicine, 39*(7), 887–903.

Lefevre, M., Calonge, N., Dietrich, A., & Melnikow, J. (2010). Mammography screening for breast cancer: Recommendatiuon of the U.S. Preventative Services Task Force. [Editorial]. *American Academy of Family Physicians, 304,* (17). Retrieved from www.aafp.org/afp

Mork, P. J., Vasseljen, O. and Nilsen, T. I. L. (2010), Association between physical exercise, body mass index, and risk of fibromyalgia: Longitudinal data from the Norwegian Nord-Trøndelag Health Study. *Arthritis Care & Research,* 62: 611–617. doi:10.1002/acr.20118

National Heart, Lung and Blood Institute and Boston University. (2010). *The framingham study.* Retrieved November 20, 2010 from http://www.framinghamheartstudy.org/about/history.html

Spoelstra, S., Given, B., von Eye, A., & Given, C. (2010). Falls in the community-dwelling elderly with a history of cancer. *Cancer Nursing, 33*(2), 149–155.

Tresserras, R., Canela, J., Alvarez, J., Sentis, J., & Salleras, L. (1992). Infant mortality, per capita income, and adult illiteracy: An ecological approach. *American Journal Of Public Health, 82*(3), 435–438.

U.S. Preventative Services Task Force (USPSTF). (2009). *Screening for breast cancer.* Retrieved from http://www.uspreventiveservicestaskforce.org/uspstf/uspsbrca.htm

FOUR

Applying Epidemiological Methods in Population-Based Nursing Practice

Ann L. Cupp Curley

Patty A. Vitale

In order to provide leadership in evidence-based practice, advanced practice nurses (APNs) require skills in the analytic methods that are used to identify population trends and evaluate outcomes and systems of care (American Association of Colleges of Nursing [AACN], 2006). APNs need to be able to carry out studies with strong designs and solid methodology, taking into account the factors that can affect study results. This chapter will discuss the complexities of data collection, the strengths and weaknesses of study designs used in population research, and the fundamentals of developing a database. Critical components of data analysis will be discussed including bias, causality, confounding, and interaction.

ERRORS IN MEASUREMENT

A dilemma that can be faced with population research is the difficulty of controlling for variables that are not being studied but that may have an impact on the results. Finding a statistical association between an intervention and an outcome or an exposure and a particular disease is meaningful only if variables are correctly controlled, tested, and measured. The purpose of a well-designed study is to properly identify the impact of the variable (or variables) under study, and to avoid design flaws caused by another, unmeasured variable.

Statistics are used to analyze population characteristics by inference from sampling (Statistics, 2000). It helps us to translate and understand data. Before we can begin to understand a measured difference between groups, we have to identify the variation. But statistical analysis cannot overcome problems caused by a flawed study. When a researcher draws the wrong conclusion because of a problem with the research methodology, the result is a type I or type II error, also referred to as *errors of inference*. A type I error occurs when a null hypothesis is rejected when in fact it is true. A type II error occurs when a null hypothesis is accepted when in fact it is false. Take, for example, an APN who carries out a study to determine if a particular intervention improves medication compliance in hypertensive patients. To keep the example simple, the intervention will simply be referred to as "Intervention A." A null hypothesis proposes no difference or relationship between interventions or treatments. In this case, the null hypothesis is: There is no difference in medication compliance in hypertensive patients who receive Intervention A compared to no intervention. Let us assume that the APN completes the study and carries out the statistical analysis of the data. The following conclusions are possible.

1. There is no difference in medication compliance between the two groups.
2. There is a difference in medication compliance between the two groups.

Now let us assume that the correct conclusion is number 1, but the APN concludes that there is a difference in medication compliance between the two groups (rejects the null hypothesis when it is true). The APN has committed a type I error. If the correct conclusion is number 2 but the APN concludes that there is no difference in medication compliance between the two groups (accepts the null hypothesis when it is false), then a type II error has occurred.

When using data or working with datasets, it is critical to understand that mistakes can occur where measurements are involved. There are two basic forms of error of measurement: random error (also known as nondifferential error) and systematic error (also known as bias). Random error occurs when there are fluctuations around a true value because of sampling variability. Systematic error is any difference between the true value and the value actually obtained because of all causes other than sampling variability. Systematic error is generally considered the more critical of the two. It can be the result of either a weak study design or a deliberate distortion of the truth.

Random Error

Random error measurements tend to be either too high or too low in about equal amounts because of random factors. Although all errors in measurement are serious, random errors are considered to be less serious than bias because they are less likely to distort findings. Random errors do, however, reduce the statistical power of a study and can occur because of unpredictable changes in an instrument used for collecting data or because of changes in the environment. For example, if the temperature in one of three rooms being used to interview subjects became overheated occasionally during data collection, making the subjects uncomfortable, it could affect some of their responses. This effect in their responses is an example of a random error of measurement.

Systematic Error

There are several different types of systematic error or bias and all of them can impact the validity of study results. Bias can occur because of the study design selected, how subjects are selected, how information is collected, how the study is carried out (the conduct), or how the study is interpreted by investigators. These problems can result in a deviation from the truth which can lead to false conclusions.

Selection Bias

Selection bias occurs when the selected subjects in a sample are not representative of the population of interest or representative of the comparison group and as a result, this selection of subjects makes it appear there is an association between an exposure and an outcome when in fact there is no real association. Selection bias is not simply an error in selection of subjects for a study, but rather the systematic error that occurs with "selecting subjects in one or more of the study groups" (Gordis, 2008). This can occur with studies using convenience samples and volunteers. People who volunteer to participate in a study may have characteristics that are different from people who do not volunteer, and this can impact the outcome of the results and is simply referred to as *volunteer bias*. Similarly, people who do not respond to surveys may possess different characteristics than those who do respond to surveys. Thus, it is important to characterize nonresponders as much as possible as the characteristics of responders may be very different from nonresponders and can lead to errors in survey interpretation. The best way to avoid this type of bias is to keep it at a minimum unless the characteristics of nonresponders can be identified and addressed. Another form of selection bias is *exclusion bias* and that can occur when one establishes different eligibility criteria to the cases and controls (Gordis, 2008). Finally, *withdrawal bias* can occur when people of certain characteristics drop out of a group at a different rate than those in another group or are lost to follow-up at a different rate. This can also lead to systematic error in the interpretation of data. All of these types of systematic error can have an impact on how data are interpreted; therefore, APNs must be aware of these types of error early in their study design. Minimizing these types of error through randomization, careful assessment of subject selection and eligibility criteria, and monitoring of characteristics in the populations of interest are critical for successful research and program implementation.

Information Bias

Information bias deals with how information or data are collected for a study. This includes the source of data that is collected such as hospital records, outpatient charts, or national databases. Many of these types of data are not collected for research purposes, so they may be incomplete, inaccurate, or contain information that is misleading. This can complicate data analysis as the information abstracted from these sources may be incorrect and can lead to invalid conclusions. *Measurement bias* is a form of *information bias* and occurs during data collection. It can be an error in collecting information for an exposure or an outcome. Calibration errors can occur when using instruments to measure outcomes. This type of bias can also occur when an instrument is not sensitive enough to measure small differences between groups or when interventions are not applied equally (e.g., some nurses in an hourly rounding study round every 2 hours instead of every hour). Information bias also includes how the data are recorded and classified. This leads to *misclassification bias* where a control may be recorded as a case or a case is classified as having an exposure or exposures that they did not actually have. Misclassification bias can be subdivided into differential and nondifferential. For example, *differential misclassification* occurs when a case is misclassified as having more exposures more often than controls. In this case, this type of bias usually leads to the appearance of a greater association between exposure and outcome than one would find if this bias was not present (Gordis, 2008). Whereas in *nondifferential misclassification*, the misclassification occurs as a result of the data collection methods such that a case is entered as a control or vice versa. In this situation, the association between exposure and outcome may be "diluted," and one may conclude there is not an association when one really exists (Gordis, 2008). Another example of misclassification bias occurs when members of a control group are exposed to an intervention. This results in *contamination bias*. An example would be a nurse who floats from the floor where hourly rounding is being carried out to a control floor where no rounding is supposed to occur—but the nurse carries out hourly rounding on the control floor. In this case, contamination bias minimizes the true differences that would have been seen between groups. However, these cases should not be reassigned; in fact, any unexpected or unplanned crossover that occurs should be analyzed in the original group it was assigned from the investigator.

If information is obtained from interviews, there can be bias introduced based on how the question is asked or there may be variance between interviewers in how questions are prompted to the subject. *Recall bias* happens when subjects are asked to remember or recall events from the past. For example, women who experience a traumatic event in their lives may recall events of that day more accurately and with more detail than someone asked to recall events from a day without significance. *Reporting bias* occurs when a subject may not report a certain exposure as they may be embarrassed or not want to disclose certain personal information, or they may report certain things to gain approval from the investigator (Gordis, 2008). The effects of bias can impact a study in two ways. It can make it appear that there is a significant effect when one does not exist (type I error) or there is an effect but the results suggest there is none (type II error).

Finally, an APN needs to be aware of *publication bias*, particularly when carrying out systematic reviews or meta-analyses. Publication bias refers to the tendency of peer-reviewed journals to publish a higher percentage of studies with significant results than those studies with nonsignificant or negative statistical results. Song et al. (2009) completed a meta-analysis to determine the odds of publication by study results. Although they identified many problems that were inherent in studying publication bias (for example, they pointed out that studies of publication bias may be as vulnerable as other studies to selective publication), they concluded that, "There is consistent empirical evidence that the publication of a study that exhibits significant or 'important' results is more likely to occur than the publication of a study that does not show such results" (p. 11). Among their recommendations was that all funded or approved studies should be registered and publicly available. The publication of both categories of research provides a more balanced and objective view of current evidence.

In summary, bias must be recognized and addressed early in the study design. Ultimately, bias should be avoided when possible, but if it is recognized it should be acknowledged in the interpretation of results and addressed in the study discussion.

Confounding

Confounding occurs when it appears that a true association exists between an exposure and an outcome, but in reality, this association is confounded by another variable or exposure. An interesting study by Matsumoto et al. raised questions about the potential confounding effect of weather on differences found among communities in Japan. They investigated the rural–urban gap in stroke incidence and mortality by conducting a cohort study that included 4,849 men and 7,529 women in 12 communities. On average, subjects were followed for 10.7 years. Information on geographic (such as population density and altitude), demographic (including risk factors for stroke), and weather information (such as rainfall and temperature) were obtained and analyzed using logistic regression. The researchers discovered a significant association between living in a rural community and stroke, independent of risk factors. However, further analyses revealed that the actual link may be between weather and stroke. They proposed that the difference seen in incidence of stroke in these communities may be related not to living in a rural versus an urban community, but by the weather differences between communities. Low temperatures are known to cause an increase in coagulation factors and plasma lipids, and therefore differences in weather could have an impact on the incidence of stroke. They cite the small number of communities as a limitation of the study, and for this reason they did not generalize their findings. But they did raise an important point: It is important to be aware of the many variables (e.g., biologic, environmental, etc.) that may confound a relationship in population studies (Matsumoto, Ishikawa, & Kajii, 2010).

Confounding variables can result in the observation of differences seen between study groups when they really do not exist or it can result in the observation that no differences exist between study groups when in fact they do exist. Another example of confounding occurs when two variables are closely associated but only one is measured in a study. For example, if an investigator studied education but not income levels in a study of caregiver burden, conclusions may be drawn, which do not take into account the potential effect of income level. If the study demonstrates that caregivers who have higher educational levels experience less burden, what the researcher might not recognize is that caregivers may experience less burden because of the material resources that are available to them because of their income level. In this case, education level and socioeconomic status (SES) may be closely related, and as a result may affect the final interpretation of the study if not acknowledged early in the process.

There are some techniques that the APN can use to reduce the effects of confounding variables. Random assignment to treatment and nontreatment groups can reduce confounding by ensuring each group has similar shared characteristics that otherwise might lead to confounding. For example, using the earlier example, if you were concerned about SES and education level, you may stratify early on for those characteristics and randomly assign from those groups so they are equally represented in your intervention and nonintervention groups. When random assignment is not possible, the matching of cases and controls for possible confounding variables can improve equal representation of subjects and can minimize the effect of confounding. Investigators can match groups or individuals. Group matching allows groups with similar characteristics of interest to be matched to each other. Each group should share a similar proportion of the characteristics of interest. Usually, cases should be selected first, and the control group should be selected with similar proportions of the characteristics of interest (Gordis, 2008). In individual matching, each individual case is matched to a control with similar characteristics of interest. This is referred to as matched pairs. One has to be careful not to match cases and controls for too many characteristics, as it can be difficult to find a control or the control may be too similar to the case and true differences may not be able to be demonstrated in the analysis phase. Using strict inclusion and exclusion criteria also can be helpful and should be applied similarly for comparison groups. There are limitations to the latter two methods. Although it is possible to match for known confounding variables, there may be other unknown confounding variables that cannot be controlled for and if not recognized, this can impact study conclusions. If the study groups are matched for gender, then gender cannot be evaluated in the final analysis. Additionally, if the study is matched for too many variables, this can also limit the study as all of those variables cannot be studied, and this may limit the ability to make valid conclusions. There is a similar problem with inclusion and exclusion criteria. If men are excluded from a study, then that variable also should be excluded from the analysis phase.

The method for analyzing data can also help reduce problems related to confounding. Multivariable regression, for example, can measure the effects of multiple confounding variables. This method is only useful when the variables are recognized and acknowledged. Recognition of confounders requires a basic understanding of the relationship between an exposure and a disease or an outcome, and also can be determined by performing a stratified analysis first. Once confounders are determined, then these variables can be introduced into the model one at a time. Interaction needs to be assessed, and evaluation of the exposure disease relationship is determined. These inferential methods estimate the contribution of each variable to the outcome while holding all other variables constant in the model. The objective is to include a set of variables that are theoretically or actually correlated with both the intervention and the outcome to reduce the bias of treatment effect. The goal of regression analysis is to select the best set of confounding variables; that is, to include the most important factors likely to account for differences between intervention and comparison groups (Munro, 2005; Starks, Diehr, & Curtis, 2009).

Interaction

Whenever two or more factors or exposures are being studied simultaneously, the possibility of *interaction* exists. Interaction occurs when one factor impacts another factor such that one sees a greater or lesser effect than would be expected by one factor alone. *Synergism* occurs when the combined effect of two or more factors is greater than the sum of the individual effects of each factor. And conversely, the opposite or negative impact can be seen with *antagonism* of factors. One example of antagonism is seen with the interaction of exercise and diet. The combination of these two factors can actually reduce the risk of heart disease more than each factor alone. Synergistic models can have an additive effect in which the effect of one factor or exposure is added to another or can have a multiplicative effect in which the effect of one factor multiples the effect of another factor. For example, epidemiologists identified an interactive effect between cigarettes and alcohol; these two factors together have a multiplicative effect on the risk of developing digestive cancers (Sjödahl et al., 2007). There are many synergistic effects that can be found in clinical practice, especially as they pertain to drugs. First generation antihistamines such as chlorpheniramine, for example, have a synergistic effect on opioids such as codeine. Patients are warned not to take them in combination as the sedative effects are more significant when taken together. APNs who carry out investigations need to be aware of the potential interactions when examining the effects of multiple exposures on an outcome. A discussion on how to determine whether a model is multiplicative or additive can be found in more detail in an advanced epidemiologic textbook, but a basic understanding is necessary for interpreting the different outcomes that can occur from multiple exposures.

There are clearly many sources of error that can occur while conducting a study. The informed APN needs to identify and acknowledge these types of errors and work to minimize them. Therefore, it is essential that APNs are aware of when errors occur and how they can impact a study, and should be familiar with measures that can be taken to avoid or minimize erros.

Randomization

Randomized controlled trials (RCTs) are considered inherently strong because of their rigorous design. Random selection of a sample and random assignment to groups are objective methods that can be used to prevent bias and produce comparable groups. Random assignment helps to minimize bias by ensuring that every subject has an equal chance of being selected, and that results can more likely be attributed to the intervention being tested and not to some other extraneous factor such as how subjects were assigned to the treatment or control group. It is impossible to know all of the characteristics that could influence results. The random assignment of subjects to case and control groups helps to ensure that study groups are similar in the characteristics that might affect results such as age, gender, ethnicity, and general health. As a general rule, the greater the number of subjects that are chosen and assigned into the treatment or nontreatment groups, the more likely that the groups will be similar for important characteristics (Shott, 1990).

Blinding

Another problem encountered in research occurs when investigators or subjects themselves have an effect on study results. This can happen when a researcher's personal beliefs or expectations of subjects can influence their interpretation of the outcome. Sometimes observers can err in measuring data toward what is expected. If subjects know or believe that they are given a placebo or the nonexperimental treatment, it may cause them to exaggerate symptoms that they would dismiss if given the experimental treatment. These actions by both investigators and subjects are not necessarily intentional—they can occur subconsciously.

The best way to eliminate or minimize this type of bias is to use a single blind study design or a double blind study design. In a double blind study, both the subjects and the data collectors are blinded, that is, unaware of which group is receiving the experimental treatment or intervention. Sometimes it is impossible to blind the investigator because of the nature of the treatment, in which case a single blind design—where the subjects are unaware of which group they are in—can be used. If blinding cannot be used, measures need to be taken that ensure that study groups are followed with strict objectivity.

DATA COLLECTION

As mentioned earlier, how data are collected and analyzed can lead to bias when conducting a study. The training of investigators to ensure that data are collected uniformly from all subjects and the use of a strict methodology for data collection and analysis contribute to a strong study design. Objective criteria should be used for the collection of all data. Strict inclusion and exclusion criteria should be developed in writing so that there are no questions as to what criteria are to be applied to the study. Avoiding subjective criteria is important as it can lead to inconsistent application of criteria. For example, if you chose "ill appearance" as an exclusion criterion it may be difficult to apply this criterion uniformly as each APN may have different levels of experience making this assessment. Objective criteria such as heart rate >120, respiratory rate >24, or oxygen saturations <90% are easy to apply uniformly. Of course, even those criteria can be incorrectly assessed by someone who is inexperienced; however, one can see that these types of data are more easily reproducible within and between studies. One way to assess reliability between raters in a study is by using the *kappa statistic*. This statistic tests how

reliable different investigators or data collectors are in their assessment or interpretation of data beyond what one would expect by chance alone.

$$\text{Kappa} = \frac{(\text{Percent agreement observed}) - (\text{Percent agreement expected by chance alone})}{100\% - (\text{Percent agreement expected by chance alone})}$$

If you were to evaluate two observers without any training you would expect
them to agree a certain percent of the time and that percent represents the chance
of agreement, usually around 50%. Using the kappa statistic, you can estimate how
reliable this agreement is by subtracting out the percent expected by chance alone.
Kappa values that are greater than 0.75 represent excellent agreement, and those
values less than 0.40 represent poor agreement. These values, although not perfect,
can give an investigator an assessment of how well their observers are agreeing
in their data interpretation (Landis & Koch, 1977). The kappa statistic appears frequently in the literature, and the APN should be familiar with its use and limitations (Maclure & Willett, 1987).

The type of analysis that is used should match the level of data that are
collected and answer the research question. One of the first steps in data analysis is to compare the demographic information of cases and controls to ensure
that they are matched for important characteristics and that they represent the
population of interest. Frequencies of data can be generated and compared for
similarities and differences. This should be done early on so that any imbal-
ance between groups is addressed before it becomes a problem in the analysis
stage. This reiterates the importance of generating strict inclusion and exclusion
criteria that can be followed with minimal error. Randomization can eliminate
this problem early on if stratification is made prior to grouping of the potential
confounders.

CAUSALITY

Ernst Mach, an Austrian professor of physics and mathematics and a philosopher,
argued that all knowledge is based on sensation and that all scientific measurements are dependent upon the observer's perception. He proposed that "in nature
there is no cause and effect" (Mach, 2011). This is a relevant quote to begin a discussion of causality, because causality is a complex issue faced by all investigators.
A single clinical disease can have many different "causes," and one cause can have
several clinical consequences. Causality becomes even more complex when we
begin to look at chronic diseases. Chronic diseases can have multiple etiologies.
Cardiac disease, for example, has multiple causes such as genetic predisposition,
obesity, smoking, lack of exercise, poor diet, or any combination of these factors.

A useful definition of causation for population research is that an increase in the
causal factor or exposure causes an increase in the outcome of interest (e.g., disease).
This is an example of a dose–response relationship. There are many theories of causation, some of which have been addressed in Chapter 3, but no one theory can
explain entirely the complex interactions of an exposure with the development of
disease or an event. Several guidelines have been introduced by the United States

Department of Health, Education and Welfare in 1964 in reference to smoking and health. These guidelines have been modified over the years (2009). They are not absolute but rather an aid to help investigators evaluate their data and consider alternative explanations, that may help defend or refute their theory of causation.

There are three basic steps in determining causality. The first is the determination of a statistical association: Statistics are used to test hypotheses: Is an exposure or risk factor present significantly more often in a population with the disease? If a new intervention is put into place, is there a significant improvement in the targeted outcome? The second is the confirmation of a temporal relationship: The suspected exposure or risk factor needs to occur before the disease or outcome. The third is the elimination of all known alternative explanations: One of the best ways to ensure this is by using a well-designed study (Jekel, Katz, & Elmore, 2001).

Causes can be both direct and indirect. An example of a direct cause would be an infectious agent that causes a disease. Pertussis (whooping cough) is caused by *Bordetella pertussis* (a bacterial infection). The organism is a direct cause of the disease. Toxic shock syndrome is an example of an indirect cause. Although the staphylococcal organism and its toxins are the direct cause of the syndrome, the indirect cause (and the first factor that was identified) is tampons. Even the infectious disease process is not simple. Both the host and the environment can have an impact on the infectious disease process. Characteristics of the host (e.g., age, previous exposures, general health, and immune status) can influence the development of the disease. Environmental conditions also play a role. A good example is influenza, which is most prevalent during certain times of the year. Infectious disease departments document these trends during the year, and they are available for hospitals to review. Such information can assist in antibiotic selection, hospital staffing, and educational campaigns to insure immunizations or prevention programs are put into place.

It is important for an APN to be aware of seasonal fluctuations in certain diseases, trends in drug resistance, or changes in the community that affect the overall management of a patient. By following these trends, the APN can better assess the needs of the community and ensure that appropriate resources are available to address the fluctuations that occur naturally in all communities.

Deliberate Distortions of the Truth (Fraud)

No one wants to believe that there are investigators who commit fraud by deliberately distorting research findings, but it does happen. Unfortunately, in some cases, the fraud is intentional; in other cases it occurs via a series of missteps from methodology to analysis. As mentioned earlier, multiple forms of bias or confounding can be introduced into a study, and if ignored can lead to spurious results. Intentionally ignoring these issues, especially without addressing them as a limitation, can be fraudulent. Acceptance for publication in a prominent peer-reviewed journal and/or evidence that the protocol was approved by an Institutional Review Board (IRB) does not ensure the accuracy and/or ethical conduct of that research.

Perhaps, one of the most infamous cases of fraud involved a well-respected peer-reviewed journal. In 1998, the *Lancet* published an article written by Andrew

Wakefield and 12 others that implied a link between the measles, mumps, and rubella vaccine (MMR) with autism and Crohn's disease. Although epidemiologists pointed out several study weaknesses including a small number of cases, no controls, and reliance on parental recall, it received wide notice in the popular press. It was 7 years before a journalist uncovered the fact that Wakefield altered facts to support his claim and exploited the MMR scare for financial gain. The *Lancet* retracted the paper in 2010 (Editorial, 2011). A series of articles in the *British Medical Journal* (Deer, 2011) revealed how Wakefield and his associates distorted data for financial gain. Before this paper was retracted, it caused widespread fear among parents and accelerated an antivaccine movement that many blame for the resurgence of infectious diseases among children. In 2010, 10 children in California died from whooping cough, the most since 1958. Although no one can prove a direct cause-and-effect relationship between those 10 deaths and Wakefield's article, it can certainly be posited that his article has had an impact on vaccination rates.

In 2006, a writer for *The New York Times* (Interlandi, 2006) wrote an article that described a case of fraud that involved a formerly tenured professor at the University of Vermont. Dr. Eric Poehlman was tried in a federal court and found guilty. He was sentenced to 1 year and 1 day in jail for fraudulent actions that spanned 10 years. His misconduct included using fraudulent data in lectures and in published papers, and using these same data to obtain millions of dollars in federal grants from the National Institutes of Health (NIH). He pleaded guilty to fabricating data on obesity, menopause, and aging. Interlandi's article, which includes a very detailed account of Dr. Poehlman's actions and his downfall, documents how a "committed cheater can elude detection for years by playing on the trust—and self-interest—of his or her junior colleagues" (p.3).

It is safe to say that the majority of researchers carry out their research with scrupulous attention to detail and with integrity, but APNs need to be aware that instances such as those mentioned earlier do happen. As stated in Chapter 3, it is important that when an APN is making decisions related to population-based evaluation, the decisions need to be based on a sound methodological framework that includes ethical considerations of the effect of the research on the population as a whole. It is also important that APNs are aware that fraud occurs in research and that they should be vigilant not only in how they carry out research, but also in how they critically review the results of studies by other investigators.

STUDY DESIGNS

There is no perfect study design; however, there are strategies that can be used to decrease the threat of bias and increase the likelihood that hypotheses are answered accurately. The awareness that bias and confounding can cause a threat to the validity of study results is important and may be unavoidable; however, recognizing these limitations and addressing them within your study is even more critical. The design of high quality and transparent studies are a good foundation for evidence-based practice. Table 4.1 outlines the strengths and weaknesses of study designs used in population research.

TABLE 4.1   **Strengths and Weaknesses of Study Designs**

TYPE OF STUDY	STRENGTHS	WEAKNESSES
Randomized controlled trials	• Lowers likelihood of confounding variables • Minimizes bias in treatment assignment • Able to control intervention or exposure	• Labor intensive • Costly • Lengthy • Sometimes impractical or unethical to conduct
Cohort designs	• Able to measure confounding and address in design • Able to control intervention or exposure • Able to calculate relative risk and incidence rates • Can study multiple exposures and multiple outcomes	• Labor intensive • Costly • Lengthy
Case control	• Inexpensive • Shorter time to completion • Able to study variables with long latency or impact periods • Provides a means to compare groups • Able to calculate odds ratios • Able to study fatal diseases or assess smaller populations • Can study multiple exposures	• Risk of bias and confounding variables • Sometimes unable to measure or determine exposure • Selection bias • Measurement error • Recall bias • Not able to assess risk
Cross-sectional	• Able to calculate prevalence • Provides a snapshot of study population • Inexpensive	• Risk of confounding variables • Selection bias • Inability to control for or identify the significance of potentially important variables • Not able to assess risk

Randomized Controlled Trials

When carefully designed, randomized controlled trials (RCTs) can provide the strongest evidence for a cause-and-effect relationship. Subjects are randomly assigned to the intervention group (which will receive the experimental treatment or intervention) or the control group (which will receive the nonexperimental treatment or intervention). As is true with cohort studies, more than two groups can be compared in this design. Inclusion and exclusion criteria for the participants must be precise and spelled out in advance.

RCTs are considered strong designs because of their ability to minimize bias but if the randomization is not executed in a true random manner then the design can be flawed, or if the data are not reported consistently then errors can lead to invalid conclusions. *Consolidated Standards of Reporting Trials* (CONSORT) is a method that has been developed to improve the quality and reporting of RCTs. It offers a standard way for authors to prepare reports of trial findings, facilitate their complete and transparent reporting, and aid their critical appraisal and interpretation (CONSORT, 2011). The 25-item CONSORT checklist appears in Table 4.2, and the flow diagram is presented in Figure 4.1. The checklist items focus on reporting how the trial was designed, analyzed, and interpreted; the flow diagram displays the progress of all participants through the trial (CONSORT, 2011). The CONSORT guidelines are endorsed by many professional journals and editorial organizations. It is part of an effort to improve the quality and reporting of research that is conducted to make decisions in healthcare.

TABLE 4.2   CONSORT 2010* Checklist of Information to Include When Reporting a Randomized Trial

SECTION/TOPIC	ITEM NO.	CHECKLIST ITEM	REPORTED ON PAGE NO.
Title and abstract			
	1a	Identification as a randomized trial in the title	
	1b	Structured summary of trial design, methods, results, and conclusions (for specific guidance, see CONSORT for abstracts)	
Introduction			
Background and objectives	2a	Scientific background and explanation of rationale	
	2b	Specific objectives or hypotheses	
Methods			
Trial design	3a	Description of trial design (such as parallel, factorial) including allocation ratio	
	3b	Important changes to methods after trial commencement (such as eligibility criteria), with reasons	
Participants	4a	Eligibility criteria for participants	
	4b	Settings and locations where the data were collected	
Interventions	5	The interventions for each group with sufficient details to allow replication, including how and when they were actually administered	

(continued)

**TABLE 4.2 CONSORT 2010 Checklist of Information to Include
When Reporting a Randomized Trial (*continued*)**

SECTION/TOPIC	ITEM NO.	CHECKLIST ITEM	REPORTED ON PAGE NO.
Outcomes	6a	Completely defined pre-specified primary and secondary outcome measures, including how and when they were assessed	
	6b	Any changes to trial outcomes after the trial commenced, with reasons	
Sample size	7a	How sample size was determined	
	7b	When applicable, explanation of any interim analyses and stopping guidelines	
Randomization			
Sequence generation	8a	Method used to generate the random allocation sequence	
	8b	Type of randomization; details of any restriction (such as blocking and block size)	
Allocation concealment mechanism	9	Mechanism used to implement the random allocation sequence (such as sequentially numbered containers), describing any steps taken to conceal the sequence until interventions were assigned	
Implementation	10	Who generated the random allocation sequence, who enrolled participants, and who assigned participants to interventions	
Blinding	11a	If done, who was blinded after assignment to interventions (for example, participants, care providers, those assessing outcomes) and how	
	11b	If relevant, description of the similarity of interventions	
Statistical methods	12a	Statistical methods used to compare groups for primary and secondary outcomes	
	12b	Methods for additional analyses, such as subgroup analyses and adjusted analyses	
Results			
Participant flow (a diagram is strongly recommended)	13a	For each group, the numbers of participants who were randomly assigned, received intended treatment, and were analyzed for the primary outcome	
	13b	For each group, losses and exclusions after randomization, together with reasons	
Recruitment	14a	Dates defining the periods of recruitment and follow-up	
	14b	Why the trial ended or was stopped	

(*continued*)

**TABLE 4.2   CONSORT 2010 Checklist of Information to Include
When Reporting a Randomized Trial (*continued*)**

SECTION/TOPIC	ITEM NO.	CHECKLIST ITEM	REPORTED ON PAGE NO.
Baseline data	15	A table showing baseline demographic and clinical characteristics for each group	
Numbers analyzed	16	For each group, the number of participants (denominator) included in each analysis and whether the analysis was by original assigned groups	
Outcomes and estimation	17a	For each primary and secondary outcome, results for each group, and the estimated effect size and its precision (such as 95% confidence interval)	
	17b	For binary outcomes, presentation of both absolute and relative effect sizes is recommended	
Ancillary analyses	18	Results of any other analyses performed, including subgroup analyses and adjusted analyses, distinguishing pre-specified from exploratory	
Harms	19	All important harms or unintended effects in each group (for specific guidance see CONSORT for harms)	
Discussion			
Limitations	20	Trial limitations, addressing sources of potential bias, imprecision, and, if relevant, multiplicity of analyses	
Generalizability	21	Generalizability (external validity, applicability) of the trial findings	
Interpretation	22	Interpretation consistent with results, balancing benefits and harms, and considering other relevant evidence	
Other information			
Registration	23	Registration number and name of trial registry	
Protocol	24	Where the full trial protocol can be accessed, if available	
Funding	25	Sources of funding and other support (such as supply of drugs), role of funders	

*We strongly recommend reading this statement in conjunction with the CONSORT 2010 Explanation and Elaboration for important clarifications on all the items. If relevant, we also recommend reading CONSORT extensions for cluster randomized trials, non-inferiority and equivalence trials, non-pharmacological treatments, herbal interventions, and pragmatic trials. Additional extensions are forthcoming: For those and for up to date references relevant to this checklist, see www.consort-statement.org.

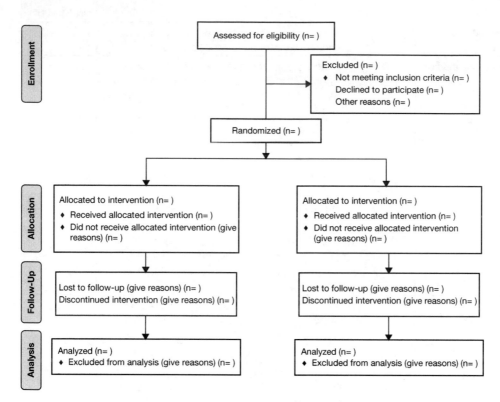

FIGURE 4.1 CONSORT statement 2010 flow diagram.

Source: From Schulz, K.F., Altman, D.G., Moher, D., for the CONSORT Group. CONSORT 2010 Statement: updated guidelines for reporting parallel group randomised trials. *BMJ* 2010;340:c332. For more information, visit www.consort-statement.org

RCTs are believed to provide the most reliable scientific evidence but they can be expensive, time consuming, and sometimes difficult to conduct for ethical reasons. There are general guidelines that APNs can follow when conducting a study to provide a framework for a quality design. They are as follows:

■ Formulate an answerable research question.
■ Complete an extensive review of the literature to determine what is currently known about the problem and to provide a sound theoretical background.
■ Select a design that will answer the research question.
■ Choose a design that is feasible in terms of both time and money.
■ Once a design is chosen, plan every step of the research process before beginning the study.

- Ensure that comparison groups are as similar as possible; stratify for possible confounders early on to avoid differences between groups.
- Determine sufficient sample size to ensure the study has adequate power for result interpretation.
- Use objective criteria for the collection of all data.
- Train all investigators to ensure that data are collected uniformly.
- Choose the appropriate method of data analysis.
- Provide sufficient and clear details of the study in papers and presentations to allow others to understand how the study was carried out and to allow them to assess for possible biases (e.g., provide an audit trail).

Cohort Studies

Cohort designs can be either prospective or retrospective. In a prospective cohort design, the investigator selects a group of individuals who were exposed to a factor of interest and compares it to a group of nonexposed individuals and follows both groups to determine the incidence of an outcome (e.g., disease). This type of design should be carried out when the APN has good evidence (a sound theoretical base) that links an exposure to an outcome. A well-designed, prospective cohort study has the potential to provide better evidence than a poorly designed RCT. One of the major problems with cohort studies is that they can be time consuming and expensive if the sample needs to be followed for a prolonged period of time, and the longer the time period involved, the more likely that participants can and will be lost to follow-up. This potential loss of subjects can result in *withdrawal bias* particularly when people with certain characteristics drop out of one group at a different rate than those in another group or are lost to follow-up at different rates. Both of these occurrences can cause changes in important characteristics between groups. For example, subjects who participate for the duration of a study may be healthier than those who drop out, leading to potential characteristic differences between groups that may affect the final analysis. These types of differences can falsely dilute observed differences between groups or falsely strengthen results and should be avoided when possible.

Descriptive reports on cohort studies should provide detailed information on the following: subjects' data that are lost or incomplete, subjects' rates of withdrawal or loss to follow-up, characteristics of subjects that are lost to follow-up or who have withdrawn from the study, and, when possible, reasons for the drop outs. They should also include detailed descriptions of the groups who are included in the analysis of outcomes such as age, gender, family history, and severity of disease.

Case–Control Studies

In a case–control study, the investigator first identifies a group of individuals with the attribute of interest (cases), and a second group is identified without the attribute of interest (controls). Cases and controls can be matched for variables that might cause confounding (e.g., age, gender, and ethnicity) or they can be unmatched. If unmatched, then each group should have similar characteristics. As mentioned earlier in the chapter, matching can be on an individual level or group level. The odds ratio is calculated to determine the odds of an event occurring in one group compared to the odds of it occurring in the other group. Calculation of an odds ratio in a matched pair study is different than an unmatched pair study and can be calculated as follows: odds ratio = b/c (Table 4.3).

TABLE 4.3   2 × 2 Table for Calculating Odds Ratio in a Case–Control Study

	Cases	Controls
EXPOSURE	a	b
NON EXPOSURE	c	d
OR = ad/bc (unmatched pairs) OR = b/c (matched pairs)		

Case–control studies tend to be inexpensive and relatively quick to complete, but there are several weaknesses. Because subjects in the groups are not randomly assigned, associations found in the analysis may be the result of exposure to another, unknown variable. To decrease the likelihood of bias, definite criteria should be used so that there is no ambiguity about how to distinguish between a case and a control. Controls should resemble the cases as closely as possible except for exposure to the factor under study. If the cases are drawn from a medical surgical unit in an acute care hospital, then ideally the controls should be drawn from the same population. Matching, as previously described, is one method that can be used so that potential confounders are distributed equally between the cases and controls. A problem with this study design is that data are usually abstracted from medical records that are not designed for collection of research material, so data obtained from medical records may be limited and may not provide adequate or accurate information on exposures. If abstracting data from interviews, biases such as recall bias or reporting bias may play a role in how data are recorded and ultimately can affect the interpretation and final conclusions of a study.

Jarlais, Lyles, and Crepaz (2004) first presented the Transparent Reporting of Evaluations with Nonrandomized Designs (TREND) in the *American Journal of Public Health*. These guidelines provide a framework for the design and reporting of nonrandomized studies in order to facilitate research synthesis. The TREND checklist has 22 steps and was designed to be used for evaluation of intervention studies using nonrandomized designs. The TREND statement and checklist is available through the CDC Web site (*http://www.cdc.gov/trendstatement/*). These types of studies should include a defined intervention and research design that provides for an assessment of the efficacy or effectiveness of the intervention. The authors place emphasis on "description of the intervention, including the theoretical base, description of the comparison condition, full reporting of outcomes, and inclusion of information related to the design needed to assess possible biases in the outcome data" (Des Jarlais, Lyles, & Crepaz, 2004). These guidelines provide APNs with a comprehensive checklist for designing studies and writing research reports.

DATABASES

Databases have become ubiquitous in the healthcare field, and their use is growing. Many of the larger and better known databases are discussed throughout this text. There is a good reason for their frequent mention. Nurses in all fields and in all positions enter data electronically into databases of some kind. Managers use databases to assess the level of satisfaction of their patient population and nursing staff. Direct care nurses use data to assess the performance of their units on important patient care indicators (such as falls) and record patient information into electronic health records that may be linked with larger databases. Departments dedicated to quality improvement track infection rates, readmission rates, and other identified indicators of quality of care.

Some databases are for a single site (e.g., one acute care hospital or one community) but it is becoming increasingly common for databases to be linked or for databases to include information at the state, regional, and national level. State and federal regulatory agencies such as the Agency for Healthcare Research and Quality (AHRQ) and the Centers for Medicare and Medicaid Services (CMS) are requiring healthcare providers to report specific patient safety indicators. Some of these data, such as those compiled by CMS, are being posted for public view. Other organizations such as the American Nurses Credentialing Center (ANCC) are requiring data entry for accreditation by programs such as Magnet and setting performance standards using benchmarks.

Databases are being developed to meet the needs of specific populations. One such database was developed for quality improvement and service planning for palliative care and hospice facilities in North Carolina. The system was developed and implemented over a 2-year period and grew from one community-based site to four. The patient data are entered at point of care (e.g., hospital, nursing home, and hospice). The information captured by the database has strengthened the ability of providers to identify areas for improvement in quality of care and the service needs of the palliative care population (Bull et al., 2010).

Nursing care data that are captured using technology can be aggregated, analyzed, and benchmarked. The information can provide APNs with a clear picture of the population that they serve and help to guide decisions for the provision of services. Patrician, Loan, McCarthy, Brosch, and Davey (2010) described the creation of the nurse-sensitive indicators for military nursing outcomes database (MilNOD). Prospective data are collected and entered into the database each shift by nurses. Information is collected on direct staff hours by levels (RN, LPN), patient census and acuity, falls, medication errors, and other identified indicators for 56 units in 13 military hospitals. The information allows nurse leaders to track nursing and patient quality indicators and to target areas for managerial and clinical performance improvement.

There are many issues that the APN needs to be aware of when using or developing databases. Databases require a high level of technological expertise to create, maintain, and use. Trained technicians and specialized equipment are required. Unanticipated technology-related problems can happen. In North Carolina, the mountains created a barrier for wireless communication and another system had to be installed for the database to be able to communicate among sites. The authors reported that there was an identified problem with data being excluded. There was concern that if the data were not randomly excluded, that systematic bias could become a problem. They emphasized the need to focus on a standardized approach for data collection. To minimize bias in their dataset, MilNOD designers created standardized definitions and specific and detailed protocols to ensure data accuracy.

Roberts and Sewell (2011) have outlined important requirements for the development and use of databases. Among the important points that they make is that nurses must understand the basics of entering data into databases and how data must be structured. Computer systems must be able to communicate with each other. This includes systems located within one site as well as systems in other sites if it is a multisite system. They also emphasize the need to be consistent in how data are coded.

Successful databases are created collaboratively. Members of the healthcare team who will be entering and using the data need to work together with technicians who understand systems. And it is not sufficient to create a workable database. Once the data are entered, it needs to be analyzed and checked for accuracy. Posting data that are summarized and benchmarked using graphs and trend lines on shared drives that are assessable to direct care nurses as well as nurse leaders bring the information to people who directly impact care and help nurses to identify areas for improvement. Nurses at all levels should be involved in data management and analysis.

SUMMARY

APNs need to carry out studies with strong designs and understand the factors that can influence study results. One problem with population research is that it is difficult to identify and control for variables that are not part of the study but which may have an effect on the results. When a researcher analyzes data in a study and draws the wrong conclusion, the result is a type I or type II error, also referred to as *errors of inference*. A type I error occurs when a null hypothesis is rejected when in fact it is true. A type II error occurs when a null hypothesis is accepted when in fact it is false. There are two kinds of error of measurement—random error and systematic error, and it is essential that APNs are aware of when these errors can occur, how they can impact a study, and what measures can be taken to avoid or minimize them. RCTs are considered the gold standard in population research and offer the best protection for preventing bias, but they are not always feasible. Well-designed cohort and case–control studies are acceptable alternatives when RCTs are not an option.

Databases are increasing in use in healthcare. Aggregated data provide valuable information about population groups that can be used to direct care. APNs should work closely with technology experts in the planning, implementation, and use of databases in order to maximize their ability to analyze data in an accurate and systematic manner. Strong methodology and data collection with a sound research design are the foundation for an excellent study/intervention that ultimately can contribute to evidence-based practice.

EXERCISES AND DISCUSSION QUESTIONS

Exercise 4.1 Over a period of several months, you notice a significant increase in the number of pediatric patients (less than 1 year of age) who present to the emergency department (ED) with traumatic injuries. You are concerned because many of these injuries could have been prevented, and some of them appear nonaccidental. You decide to design an intervention to address risk factors for trauma in infants. There are many settings in which such an intervention can be implemented: the newborn nursery, outpatient clinics, and EDs. The target audience can be expectant parents, parents, healthcare providers, or any combination thereof.

■ Design an educational intervention to address the risk factors for traumatic injuries in infants. Decide on a site and a target audience. Identify an outcome.
■ What type of study design might you use for your proposed intervention?
■ What are the advantages and disadvantages of the design you have selected?
■ What variables could be considered confounders?
■ Describe some of the systematic errors that could occur in your study and why?

Exercise 4.2 You are an administrator in an adolescent inpatient psychiatric hospital. You are concerned about a recent increase in the use of physical restraints in the hospital. You also notice an increased use of sedating medications. You have not had any recent changes in staffing or patient mix and acuity.

■ How might you assess this situation?
■ What type of study could you perform to identify the cause(s) for the increase in both physical and chemical restraint usage?
■ How will you select your population of study?

■ How will you select a control group or comparison group?
■ What are potential errors in measurement that you may encounter?

Exercise 4.3   You are working in an ambulatory care clinic in an underserved community and are interested in improving the quality of health care that is provided in your area. You are concerned about an increase in the incidence of methacillin resistant *Staphylococcus aureus* (MRSA) in the population that you serve. Before you launch an educational campaign aimed at both your staff and the community, you need to establish the severity of the problem.

■ Identify a database at the local, state, or national level that can help you to obtain the necessary information.
   • How can you determine the incidence and prevalence of MRSA in your community?
   • What are some of the potential errors that can occur in the reporting of MRSA to a local, state, or national database?
   • How might this affect your interpretation of the data?
■ You decide to begin collecting data on MRSA-related deaths for your local hospital.
   • What are some of the problems that may occur during data collection?
   • How might you avoid these problems?
■ You determine from your investigation that there is a significant problem in your community.
   • Describe how you would address the increasing morbidity and mortality of MRSA in the population that you serve.
   • What type of study design would you use to evaluate the effectiveness of your intervention?
   • What are potential confounders?
   • Is there potential for interaction?

Exercise 4.4   Match the term with correct definition.

   a. *Decision:* Conclude treatments are not different *Reality:* Treatments are different
   b. *Decision:* Conclude treatments are different *Reality:* Treatments are different
   c. *Decision:* Conclude treatments are not different *Reality:* Treatments are not different
   d. *Decision:* Conclude treatments are different *Reality:* Treatments are not different
   ____Type I error
   ____Type II error
   ____Power

REFERENCES

American Association of Colleges of Nursing (AACN). (2006). *The essentials of doctoral education for advanced practice nursing.* Retrieved from http://www.aacn.nche.edu/DNP/pdf/Essentials.pdf

Bull, J., Zafar, Y., Wheeler, J., Harker, M., Gblokpor, A., Hanson, L., ... Abernethy, A. (2010). Establishing a regional, multisite database for quality improvement and service planning in community-based palliative care and hospice. *Journal of Palliative Medicine, 13*(8), 1013–1020.

CONSORT Group. (2011). *CONSORT: Transparent reporting of trials.* Retrieved from http://www.consort-statement.org/

Deer, B. (2011). How the case against the MMR vaccine was fixed. *BMI, 342,* 77–82.

Des Jarlais, D., Lyles, C., & Crepaz, N. (2004). Improving the reporting quality of nonrandomized evaluations of behavioral and public health interventions: The TREND statement. *American Journal of Public Health, 94*(3), 361–366.

Editorial. (2011). Wakefield's article linking MMR vaccine and autism was fraudulent. [Editorial]. *British Medical Journal (BMJ), 342,* 64–66.

Gordis, L. (2008). *Epidemiology* (4th ed.). Philadelphia, PA: Elsevier Saunders.

Interlandi, J. (2006, October 22). An unwelcome discovery. *The New York Times.* Retrieved from http://www.nytimes.com/2006/10/22/magazine/22sciencefraud.html

Jekel, J. F., Katz, D. L., & Elmore, J. G. (2001). *Epidemiology, biostatistics, and preventive medicine* (2nd ed.). Philadelphia, PA: W. B. Saunders Company.

Landis, J. R., & Koch, G. G. (1977). The measurement of observer agreement for categorical data. *Biometrics, 33,* 159.

Mach, E. (2011). in Answers.com. Retrieved from http://www.answers.com/topic/ernst-mach#ixzz1AeXJGDvd

Maclure, M., & Willett, W. C. (1987). Misinterpretation and misuse of the kappa statistic. *American Journal of Epidemiology, 126*(2), 161–169.

Matsumoto, M., Ishikawa, S., & Kajii E. (2010). Rurality of communities and incidence of stroke: a confounding effect of weather conditions? *Rural and Remote Health* 10 (online), 1493. Available from: http://www.rrh.org.au

Munro, B. (2005). *Statistical methods for health care research* (5th ed.). Philadelphia, PA: Lippincott Williams & Wlkins.

Patrician, P., Loan, L., McCarthy, M., Brosch, L., & Davey, K. (2010). Towards evidence-based management: Creating an informative database of nursing-sensitive indicators. *Journal of Nursing Scholarship, 42*(4), 358–366.

Roberts, A., & Sewell, J. (2011). Data aggregation: A case study. *Computers, Informatics, Nursing, January/February 29*(1), 3–7.

Shott, S. (1990). *Statistics for health care professionals.* New York, NY: W.B. Saunders.

Sjödahl, K., Lu, Y., Nilsen, T., Ye, W., Hveem, K., Vatten, L., & Lagergren, J. (2007). Smoking and alcohol drinking in relation to risk of gastric cancer: A population-based, prospective cohort study. *International Journal of Cancer, 120*(1), 128–132.

Song, F., Parekh-Bhurke, S., Hooper, L., Loke, Y., Ryder, J., Sutton, A., ... Harvey, I. (2009). Extent of publication bias in different categories of research cohorts: A meta-analysis of empirical studies. *BMC Medical Research Methodology, 9,* 79. Retrieved from http://web.ebscohost.com/ehost/pdfviewer/pdfviewer?hid=110&sid=01961f3d-cd2e-4770-86af-bc7107e2f85e%40sessionmgr113&vid=4

Starks, H., Diehr, P., & Curtis, J. R. (2009). The challenge of selection bias and confounding in palliative care research. *Journal of Palliative Medicine, 12*(2), 181–187.

Statistics. (2000). The *American heritage dictionary of the English language* (4th ed.). Boston, MA: Houghton Mifflin.

FIVE

Applying Evidence at the Population Level

Ann L. Cupp Curley

Nurses in advanced practice have an obligation to improve the health of the populations that they serve by providing evidence-based care. The American Association of Colleges of Nursing (AACN) has outlined eight essentials that represent the core competencies for education of advanced practice nurses (APNs). The first essential listed is Scientific Underpinnings for Practice (AACN, 2006). This competency stresses the integration of evidence-based practice into advanced nursing practice. APNs are educated at the graduate level in research and critical appraisal skills and possess specialized clinical knowledge. These specialized abilities prepare the APN to demonstrate the importance of evidence-based practice to others and to facilitate the incorporation of such evidence into practice (DeBourgh, 2001).

In this chapter, the APN will learn how to integrate and synthesize information in order to design interventions that are based on evidence to improve population outcomes. Nurses must have a sound knowledge of research methodology to support an evidence-based practice. They also require a wide array of knowledge gleaned from the sciences and the ability to translate that knowledge quickly and effectively to benefit patients (Porter-O'Grady, 2003). The goal of this chapter is to summarize the necessary skills required for an evidence-based practice and to provide specific examples of how APNs have used these skills to improve population outcomes.

The American Heritage Dictionary (Evidence, 2000) defines evidence as "A thing or things helpful in forming a conclusion or judgment" (p. 617). Burns and Grove (2007) define evidence-based practice as "the conscientious integration of best research evidence with clinical expertise and patient values and needs in delivery of quality cost-effective healthcare" (p. 539). Nurses require several skills to become practitioners of evidence-based care. They must be able to identify clinical problems, recognize patient safety issues, compose clinical questions that provide a clear direction for study, conduct a search of the literature, appraise and synthesize the available evidence, and successfully integrate new knowledge into practice. The APN plays an important role in this complex process of incorporating evidence-based practice into policies and standards of care to improve population outcomes. In population-based care, there is additional complexity in determining the values and needs of groups of people. Making decisions related to population-based health requires considerations of the effect of the intervention on the population as a whole. Balancing the overall needs of groups of people with the rights of individuals requires careful and thoughtful consideration. A sound evidence-based practice provides a foundation to better assess those needs based on evidence.

ASKING THE CLINICAL QUESTION

There are many situations that drive clinical questions. Clinical practice and observation as well as information obtained by reading the professional literature can lead nurses to ask questions such as "Why is this happening?"; "Would this approach to care work in my clinical practice?"; or "What can we do to improve this outcome?" An APN who reads an article about an innovation in practice that leads to an improvement in a population outcome might wonder if such an intervention would work in another setting. The observation that the readmission rates for a particular diagnosis are increasing, or that rates for a particular disease are higher in one population than another, or that patient satisfaction scores for a particular group of patients are lower can all lead to a search of the literature for evidence to change and improve outcomes. It may also lead to further research to improve outcomes or design interventions to change outcomes. But before the search can begin, it is important that clinical questions are defined clearly and in a way that can be answered and applied to practice.

Clinical questions need to be written in a format that provides a clear direction for examination. The PICO format provides a clear-cut method for developing clinical questions and is also one of the most popular methods used for this purpose. PICO is an acronym that stands for population studied (P), intervention (I), comparison (C), and outcome (O). As you are formulating your PICO question, it is helpful to describe the type of question you are asking to better define your research method. Is this an intervention, diagnosis, etiology, or prognosis type of question? (Camden University Library, 2010) In PICO once you have decided the type of question you wish to ask, the next step is to describe the patient population to be studied. When retrieving information, it must be relevant to the targeted population. Think about how to describe the population that you are interested in learning more about. What are its most important characteristics? For example, an APN employed in a state correctional facility may observe both high rates of diabetes in the prison population and low rates of compliance with diabetes self-management. To accurately define the patient population, an APN needs to identify any important characteristics of the population that need to be addressed or examined in the proposed study or intervention. Using the same example, prison populations are known to have high rates of mental illness, and the APN decides to target this particular population for study (Conrad, 2008). Therefore, the population studied would be described as follows:

■ *Population*: Mentally ill inmates housed in state prisons diagnosed with diabetes.

The second step is to determine what intervention or process you want to study. As mentioned earlier, defining the method of study early on can help develop the PICO question more fully. In this particular example, the APN hypothesized that increasing the self-efficacy of inmates with diabetes through a self-management course might help inmates manage their diabetes better. Having read in the professional literature about self-management courses for chronic illnesses used in other settings, the APN postulates that a chronic disease self-management course might increase compliance rates with inmates through an increase in self-efficacy.

■ *Intervention*: A chronic disease self-management program (CSMP).

In this particular case, the APN planned to measure self-efficacy and diabetes management before and after the CSMP. The comparison is therefore diabetes management before and after the intervention.

■ *Comparison:* Diabetes management in mentally ill inmates housed in state prisons diagnosed with diabetes before and after implementation of the CSMP.

The last step is the outcome: What does the APN want to see improved? What does the APN expect to accomplish? The objective in this case was to increase self-efficacy and improve diabetes management in a targeted population of mentally ill inmates with diabetes after implementing a CSMP.

■ *Outcome*: Self-efficacy (measured using a validated self-efficacy scale) and hemoglobin A1c levels (as a measure of diabetes management).

Using these steps, the APN can compose the final PICO question: "Will a 6 week chronic disease self-management program increase the self-efficacy of insulin-dependent diabetic mentally ill inmates in a state prison setting?"

(Conrad, 2008). Development of the PICO question provides the APN with a better understanding of the clinical problem, allows for specific measures to be introduced, and provides the foundation for a well-designed study. The next step is to perform a thorough and comprehensive literature review.

THE LITERATURE REVIEW

The literature search should further define and clarify the clinical problem, summarize the current state of knowledge on the subject, identify relationships, contradictions, gaps, and inconsistencies in the literature, and finally, suggest the next step in solving the problem (American Psychological Association [APA], 2009). The search of the literature can be conducted by the APN, or the APN can engage the assistance of a research librarian if available. Librarians are educated to find and access information and are excellent resources for assisting with literature reviews. Navigating databases in order to find relevant information can be a complex process. The searcher needs to use the correct terms, search the correct databases, and use a well-designed and methodical search strategy. The searcher should also document each step of the process in order to provide an audit trail and avoid duplication of work (Hallyburton & St. John, 2010). An audit trail provides clarity to the method used to find the evidence and allows others to follow the decision-making process (Houde, 2009). In the absence of a librarian, there are steps that the APN can take to increase the likelihood of a successful search.

In order to find the most relevant literature to inform decision making, the searcher should use key terms from the PICO question (i.e., population studied, intervention, comparison, and outcomes of interest). The first step is to search each key term separately and then to take steps to refine the search.

The APN should use at least two databases for the literature search. Access to some databases requires a subscription while others are free. The Cochrane Library which can be accessed through the Cochrane Collaboration web site (*www.cochrane.org*) and PubMed are both free resources. The Cochrane Collaboration is an international organization that provides up-to-date systematic reviews (currently more than 4000) (The Cochrane Collaboration, 2010). PubMed (which includes MEDLINE) is the National Library of Medicine (NLM) journal literature search system. It includes more than 20 million citations for biomedical literature from MEDLINE, journals, and online books, and includes citations from full-text content (NLM, 2010). A free tutorial for searching PubMed is available at *http://www.nlm.nih.gov/bsd/pubmed_tutorial/m1001.html*.

The Joanna Briggs Institute (*www.joannabriggs.edu*) and the Cumulative Index to Nursing and Allied Health Literature (CINAHL) are excellent databases that both require a subscription. The Joanna Briggs Institute (JBI) includes The JBI Library of Systematic Reviews, which is an international, not-for-profit, membership-based organization located within the University of Adelaide (Australia) (JBI, 2010). There are discounted rates for students to join. CINAHL is a comprehensive resource for nursing and allied health literature that is made up of four databases. Two of them offer full texts. It is owned and operated by EBSCO Publishing (EBSCO Publishing, 2010).

Searches of a single key word can result in a very large number of articles. For example, a CINAHL search for full-text articles using the key word "diabetes" yielded a list of 97,956 articles. Including more than one concept in the search is more likely to provide relevant and useful articles. Boolean logic is the term used to describe certain logical operations that are used to combine search terms in many databases. Using the Boolean connector AND narrows a search by combining terms; it will retrieve documents that use two key words. Combining words with a Boolean connector such as AND (prisoner and diabetes) can narrow the search. In CINHAL, using prisoners AND diabetes yielded 13 articles. Using OR, on the other hand, broadens a search to include results that contain either of the words that are typed in the search. OR is a good tool to use when there are several common spellings or synonyms of a word. An example in this case would be inmate OR prisoner. Using NOT will narrow a search by excluding certain search terms. NOT retrieves documents that contain one but not the other of the search terms entered. It is appropriate to use when a word is used in different contexts. An example would be prisoners NOT captives. Parentheses indicate relationships between search terms. When they are used, the computer will process the search terms in a specified order and also combine them in the correct manner. (Inmate OR prisoner) AND diabetes combines inmate or prisoner and diabetes to get the results that are needed. A search conducted in the full-text database of CINAHL using these words and connectors yielded 232 articles.

There are other methods that can be used to make searches more relevant and useful. Specifying limits such as English language only, peer-reviewed journals only, randomized controlled trials only, and a date range can be used to narrow a search and increase the relevance of the information retrieved. Keep in mind that the more limits that are placed on the search, the fewer the results. A search using (inmate OR prisoner) AND diabetes, full text only, English only, limited to articles published in the last 5 years yielded 31 articles.

For the PICO question mentioned earlier, the following key words were used both alone and in combinations: Chronic Disease, Chronic Disease Management Program, Diabetes, Incarcerated, Mentally ill, Mental Illness, Prison, Self-Efficacy and Self-Management (Conrad, 2008).

A search for the most current known evidence about a topic is not complete after the search of electronic databases. A hand search of current and relevant journals can reveal information that has not yet been entered into an electronic database. Studies can also appear in publications other than journals such as books, working papers, and unpublished doctoral dissertations. Projects and reports that are completed by specialized organizations such as foundations and professional membership groups may only appear on Web sites. Internet searching can help locate such resources and can scan organizational Web sites of professional and specialized organizations such as the American Diabetes Association, the American Nurses Association, and the Robert Wood Johnson Foundation. The APN should also consider contacting experts who may be aware of important findings and recent discoveries in a particular field. A technique known as snowballing (citation tracking using the citation databases such as Science Citation Index, Social Sciences Citation Index, and Arts and Humanities Citation Index) might also be helpful (CRD, 2010). Finally, after reviewing the literature, many references can be found that may not have been yielded in an internet search by simply reviewing the references of collected literature.

ASSESSING THE EVIDENCE

Once a list of articles is obtained, the next step is to assess and synthesize the evidence. Appraising evidence for its usefulness can be a challenge. While reviewing the evidence, the APN needs to ask some fundamental questions that address the relevance of information such as "How confident am I that the relationships and knowledge in this particular study will apply to the situation in question?" Shapiro and Donaldson (2008) have identified some important questions related to evidence-based practice changes. They are as follows: "When is the evidence strong enough to use the results? Are the findings applicable to my setting? If I adopt the practice, what will it mean to the target population?" Another important question relates to the "efficacy" (evidence of an effect under ideal conditions, such as double-blind, randomized controlled trials) and "effectiveness" (evidence of what actually works in practice) of the findings or study. In summary, during the process of determining which studies to include in a synthesis, the APN needs to ask not only "Does this intervention work?" and "For whom does this intervention work?" but also "When, why, and how does it work?"

All published evidence is not completed with equal rigor and, therefore, the value of the published articles varies on a continuum from lowest highest value. A search can potentially find an enormous number of articles, but not all articles may be useful. Because there is often a limited amount of time that is available to assess and synthesize the evidence, it is helpful to have a method that provides guidance as to which articles might be the most valid and useful. In addition to conducting an extensive search of sources, the APN must establish criteria for inclusion and exclusion of studies (Melnyk & Fineout-Overholt, 2005).

There are several organizations that provide guidelines for the conduct of systematic reviews and help healthcare professionals keep pace with the professional literature by providing completed systematic reviews. Information on five of them is listed in Table 5.1. According to Polit and Beck (2008), "a systematic review is a state-of-the art summary of what is best evidence at the time the review was written" (p. 32). Reviews are completed using strict inclusion and exclusion criteria, and the aim is to include as much as possible of the research relevant to the research question. The overall objective of an appraisal is to assess the general strength of the evidence in relation to the particular issue. The Evidence for Policy and Practice Information Coordinating Centre at the Institute of Education, University of London (EPPI-Centre) has identified four key elements of a systematic review:

1. It uses explicit and transparent methods.
2. It is research that follows standard stages.
3. It is accountable, replicable, and able to be updated.
4. There is a requirement of user population studies: Who benefited and who did not? (EPPI, 2010)

TABLE 5.1 Online Resources for Evidence-Based Practice

ORGANIZATION	DESCRIPTION	WEB LINK
The Cochrane Collaboration	The Cochrane Collaboration is an independent, not-for-profit organization	http://www. cochrane.org/
	Systematic Reviews are published in *The Cochrane Library*—summaries and abstracts are free of charge. A subscription is required for full use of the resources	
	Publishes the *Cochrane Handbook for Systematic Reviews*	
The Joanna Briggs Institute, Australia (JBI)	JBI is a professional, peer review organization	http://connect. jbiconnectplus. org/
	The *JBI Library of Systematic Reviews* is a refereed library that publishes systematic reviews of literature. Subscription is required; student rates are available	
Centre for Reviews and Dissemination (CRD), University of York, UK	The CRD is part of the National Institute for Health Research (NIHR)	http://www.york. ac.uk/inst/crd/
	The CRD makes available systematic reviews on health and public health questions	
	Produces the DARE, NHS EED, and HTA databases and guidelines for undertaking systematic reviews	
The Evidence for Policy and Practice Information Coordinating Centre at the Institute of Education, University of London (EPPI-Centre)	The EPPI-Centre is part of the Social Science Research Unit at the Institute of Education, University of London	http://eppi.ioe. ac.uk/cms/
	Provides the main findings, technical summary, or full technical report of individual EPPI-Centre Systematic Reviews	
	Available online: Methods for a Systematic Review	

(continued)

TABLE 5.1   Online Resources for Evidence-Based Practice (*continued*)

ORGANIZATION	DESCRIPTION	WEB LINK
United States National Library of Medicine (NLM)	PubMed (which includes MEDLINE) is the National Library of Medicine (NLM) literature search system. It includes more than 20 million citations for biomedical literature from MEDLINE, journals, and online books. It includes citations from full-text content	http://www.nlm.nih.gov/
	PubMed Central (PMC) is a web-based repository of biomedical journal literature providing free, unrestricted access to more than 1.5 million full-text articles	
	Publishes and provides the following: systematic reviews, meta-analyses, reviews of clinical trials, evidence-based medicine, consensus development conferences, and guidelines	

To begin, it is helpful to use a table to group and summarize information according to key areas. Table 5.2 is an example of a tool that can be used to document the critical elements of the evidence such as the design of the study, the study population, and the outcomes. It provides the APN with a standard method for evaluating the important points gleaned from a literature search and can also act as an audit trail, so that others can judge how well the review was carried out.

One step in the research review process is the organization and grading of the evidence using a hierarchy. The level of evidence approach is a useful method of ranking evidence and helps to remove subjectivity from the assessment of the evidence. In hierarchies, levels of evidence are ranked according to the strengths of the evidence. The strength of the evidence is based on the design of the study used by investigators to minimize bias. Most hierarchies classify the best evidence (studies that provide the most reliable evidence) at the top of the list and the least reliable evidence at the bottom of the list. "Grading systems allow practitioners a tool for determining the best evidence for a given practice or management strategy for a particular disease or condition" (Armola et al., 2009, p. 406).

Many groups have established hierarchies of evidence based upon scientific merit. An example of some of the groups that have established hierarchies of evidence are as follows: The American Academy of Pediatrics, the Oncology Nursing Association, the Oxford Centre for Evidence-based Medicine, The Cochrane Institute, and the Joanna Briggs Institute.

The AACN's evidence-leveling system in Table 5.3 is an example of this type of system and is a useful tool in the appraisal of research evidence. As with most hierarchal systems, the AACN system classifies the levels of evidence in descending order, with the highest level of evidence in Level A and the lowest in Level M

TABLE 5.2 Literature Review and Synthesis for Evidence-Based Practice

CLINICAL QUESTION

TITLE OF ARTICLE	AUTHORS WITH CREDENTIALS	RESEARCH QUESTION	STUDY DESIGN	LEVEL OF EVIDENCE	DESCRIPTION OF SAMPLE	OUTCOME MEASURES	RESULTS

TABLE 5.3   AACN's Evidence-Leveling System

	DESCRIPTION
Level A	Meta-analysis of multiple controlled studies or metasynthesis of qualitative studies with results that consistently support a specific action, intervention, or treatment
Level B	Well-designed controlled studies, both randomized and nonrandomized, with results that consistently support a specific action, intervention of treatment
Level C	Qualitative studies, descriptive or correlational studies, integrative reviews, systematic reviews, or randomized controlled trials with inconsistent results
Level D	Peer-reviewed professional organizational standards, with clinical studies to support recommendations
Level E	Theory-based evidence from expert opinion or multiple case reports
Level M	Manufacturer's recommendation only

Source: Armola, R., Bourgault, A., Halm, M., Board, R., Bucher, L., Harrington, L., ... Medina, J. (2009). Upgrading the American association of critical-care nurses' evidence-leveling system. American Journal of Critical Care, *18*(5), 405–409. Used with permission from American Association of Critical-Care Nurses (AACN).

(Armola et al., 2009). An evidence-leveling system that includes study designs used in population research (such as case-control and cohort studies) appears in Exhibit 5.1. This system is used by the Centre for Reviews and Dissemination at the University of York (CRD). Like the AACN system, it classifies levels of evidence in descending order, with well-designed randomized controlled trials at the top and case studies at the bottom.

The incorporation of many designs into a systematic review can provide valuable insight as it has a direct impact on the complexity of the information. For example, although qualitative studies are not classified as high levels of evidence, they can still provide an APN with important information for understanding phenomena. The purpose of qualitative studies is to increase the understanding and meaning of a phenomenon when the goal is to describe or understand an experience. A classic example is the qualitative study that was carried out by Beck (1993) using grounded theory to develop an understanding of postpartum depression. Because of the nature of qualitative studies, the results cannot be generalized to the population of all women with postpartum depression; however, the publication of her results does provide the reader with a vivid description of the women in her study and insight into how the researcher arrived at the theme of "teetering on the edge" to describe the phenomena.

Validity

Once the APN has completed collecting evidence, each individual study needs to be appraised for the internal and external validity of the design. A hallmark of

EXHIBIT 5.1

Hierarchy of Study Designs to Assess the Effects of Interventions

Centre for Reviews and Dissemination, University of York, UK

This list is not exhaustive, but covers the main study designs.

Randomized Controlled Trials (RCT)

The simplest form of RCT is known as the parallel group trial which randomizes eligible participants to two or more groups, treats according to assignment, and compares the groups with respect to outcomes of interest. Participants are allocated to groups using both randomization (allocation involves the play of chance) and concealment (ensures that the intervention that will be allocated cannot be known in advance). There are different types of randomized study designs, such as:

Randomized Crossover Trials

All participants receive all the interventions; for example in a two-arm crossover trial, one group receives intervention A before intervention B, and the other group receive intervention B before intervention A. It is the sequence of interventions that is randomized.

Cluster Randomized Trials

A cluster randomized trial is a trial where clusters of people rather than single individuals are randomized to different interventions. For example, whole clinics or geographical locations may be randomized to receive particular interventions, rather than individuals.

Quasi-Experimental Studies

The main distinction between randomized and quasi-experimental studies is the way in which participants are allocated to the intervention and control groups; quasi-experimental studies do not use random assignment to create the comparison groups.

Nonrandomized Controlled Studies

Individuals are allocated to a concurrent comparison group, using methods other than randomization. The lack of concealed randomized allocation increases the risk of selection bias.

(continued)

(continued)

Before and After Study

Comparison of outcomes in study participants before and after the introduction of an intervention. The before and after comparisons may be in the same sample of participants or in different samples.

Interrupted Time Series

Interrupted time series designs are multiple observations over time that are "interrupted," usually by an intervention or treatment.

Observational Studies

A study in which natural variation in interventions or exposure among participants (i.e., not allocated by an investigator) is investigated to explore the effect of the interventions or exposure on health outcomes.

Cohort Study

A defined group of participants is followed over time and comparison is made between those who did and did not receive an intervention.

Case–Control Study

Groups from the same population with (cases) and without (controls) a specific outcome of interest are compared to evaluate the association between exposure to an intervention and the outcome.

Case Series

Description of a number of cases of an intervention and the outcome (without comparison with a control group). These are not comparative studies.

Used with permission from Centre for Reviews and Dissemination, University of York, UK.

good research is that it is carried out by researchers who are aware of the existence of error and who design studies in such a way that errors are minimized. Table 5.2 is a useful tool that facilitates the appraisal of evidence by providing a method to organize the individual aspects or components of the study design. The APN needs to use this information to conduct an analysis of the information. Interpreting the findings of a study depends upon the design, conduct, and analyses (internal validity), as well the populations, interventions, and outcome measures (external validity) (CRD, 2010).

When appraising the quality of a study, the APN should attempt to assess how accurate the findings are and whether they are of relevance in the particular setting or population of interest. The appraisal should include the appropriateness of study design to the research question, the risk of bias, the overall quality of the methods used to carry out the study, the outcome measure, the quality of the intervention, appropriateness of the analysis, the quality of the research report, and the generalizability of the results.

Blegen (2009) makes an excellent point that "Persons in training to conduct or apply research must understand the basis for making judgments about the strength of the evidence. It is not about qualitative or quantitative data, but whether the evidence was produced using procedures that promote certainty and to groups whose care we wish to improve" (p. 381). When assessing a qualitative study, the APN should take into account the theory that was used in the design of the research, analysis, and interpretation of the data. The APN also needs to decide in advance how qualitative evidence will be used. Qualitative evidence can be used in the discussion and interpretation of the results of the quantitative studies to help gain a better understanding of the overall findings from a review or can be included in the review along with the quantitative findings. This is sometimes referred to as "parallel synthesis." (Beck, 2009).

Nurses are often intimidated when faced with evaluating the data analysis section in a research article. An important fact to keep in mind is that statistical significance is not synonymous with proof and that sometimes overemphasis is placed on statistically significant findings. It is important to understand the significance of the results and how they apply to clinical practice. According to Hayat (2010), "Statistical significance is not an objective measure and does not provide an escape from the requirement for the researcher to think carefully and judge the clinical and practical importance of a study's results" (p. 219). The APN should review the results section of a research report carefully to determine whether or not the method of analysis used by the researcher answers the research question(s) or hypothesis, and provides enough information to support the interpretation of the results.

Transparency

Transparency is another important concept for consideration during the appraisal of a research report. Transparency in research is a reflection of both the accountability and the integrity of the investigator(s). It also takes into account the clarity and completeness of the research report. It should be possible, for example, for the study and results to be replicated by others. There should also be disclosure of relationships that have the potential to cause a conflict of interest. A conflict of interest may occur when a researcher's objectivity is impacted by economic (ownership of stocks or shares), commercial (payouts by companies), or personal interests (when a researcher's status may be impacted by the results of the research) (APA, 2009). For example, an investigator with ties to a company that is closely related to the area of research may stand to profit from steering the results in a particular direction. Even when investigators disclose their conflicts of interest, the APN must still critically review the research for potential bias.

Research Synthesis

The literature review not only provides a historical account of past work in the area of interest but also supports or refutes the necessity for ongoing study. The background for any study is founded upon a thorough and comprehensive literature review. It serves as a justification for current research goals and introduces the reader to important past studies that have similar outcomes of comparison. Although not all studies will have an array of historical evidence in the literature, review of similar study designs or interventions can still provide a strong justification if the background is well researched.

The overall purpose of the example described earlier was to determine if a 6-week chronic disease self-management program (CSMP) would increase self-efficacy of mentally ill inmates with diabetes in a state prison setting. According to Conrad (2008), people with diabetes should all receive care that meets national standards, and this standard should apply to those who are incarcerated as well as those who are not. Conrad found few evidence-based models of self-management support delivered to prison populations but did find evidence that this model worked well with other diabetic populations. The literature review provided evidence of potential benefit for a disease self-management program for people with diabetes, and also evidence of the relationship between self-efficacy and health behavior. The literature review completed by Conrad (2008) is provided in Table 5.4.

Upon completion of a systematic review, Conrad wrote a proposal to pilot study a 6 week self-efficacy course for mentally ill inmates with diabetes. The literature review provided sufficient information such that she was able to justify the pilot study of the program to corrections officials. The outcome measures were self-efficacy and hemoglobin A1c levels. Preliminary results have shown an improvement in both outcomes after the implementation of the CSMP. The project is ongoing at the time of this writing (M. Conrad, personal communication, March 22, 2010). The summation of this work by Conrad (2008) from literature review, to research synthesis, to pilot project is an excellent example of how APNs can use this approach to design interventions to improve population outcomes.

TABLE 5.4 Tool to Assess Literature Review: Interventions, Purpose, Populations, and Outcomes

	TITLE/AUTHOR	DESCRIPTION OF INTERVENTION	PURPOSE AND POPULATIONS	OUTCOMES ACHIEVED
1.	American Diabetes Association. (2008). *Diabetes management in correctional institutions.* Retrieved November 1, 2008, from http://www.guideline. gov/summary/summary. aspx?doc_id=12189&nbr=00 6286&string=dabetes	N/A	Not a study A guideline for diabetes management in prisons	N/A
2.	American Diabetes Association. (2008). Standards of Medical Care in Diabetes 2008. *Diabetes Care, 31*(S12–S54).	N/A	Not a study 2008 standards for diabetes care	N/A
3.	Chiverton, P. (2007). Well balanced: 8 steps to wellness for adults with mental illness and diabetes. [Journal Article, Pictorial, Research, Tables/Charts]. *Journal of Psychosocial Nursing and Mental Health Services, 45*(11), 46–55.	A well-balanced program incorporated health promotion, disease management, and evidence-based practice guideline into a16-week, 8-steps-to-wellness program for a community-based mental health population	Seventy-four adults with both serious mental illness and diabetes were evaluated using nursing wellness 8-step model	Improvements of health risk status, decreased A1C levels, and an increase satisfaction with the program were noted

(continued)

TABLE 5.4 Tool to Assess Literature Review: Interventions, Purpose, Populations, and Outcomes *(continued)*

	TITLE/AUTHOR	DESCRIPTION OF INTERVENTION	PURPOSE AND POPULATIONS	OUTCOMES ACHIEVED
4.	Chodosh, J., Morton, S. C., Mojica, W., Maglione, M., Suttorp, M. J., Hilton, L., et al. (2005). Meta-analysis: chronic disease self-management programs for older adults. [Meta-Analysis Research Support, U.S. Gov't, Non-P.H.S.]. *Annals of Internal Medicine, 143*(6), 427–438.	To determine the efficacy and important components of CSMP for older adults with diabetes Meta-analysis searched multiple sources dated through Sept 2004. Two reviewers independently indentified trials and extracted data	Meta-analysis searched multiple sources dated through Sept 2004. All RCTs were eligible for inclusion that compared outcomes of self-management interventions with a control or with usual care for diabetes mellitus	Self-management intervention led to a statistically and clinically significant decrease in hemoglobin A1c levels of about .81%
5.	Clark, B. (2006). Diabetes care in the San Francisco County Jail. [Journal Article, Research, Tables/Charts]. *American Journal of Public Health, 96*(9), 1571–1574.	Retrospective chart review of the electronic medical record for 200 inmates identified as diabetic in the San Francisco County Jail system in 2003 The researches systematically sampled 200 inmates from all that met the criteria	To examine care guideline adherence within the correctional institute Eligible inmates for inclusion had at least one jail stay of 72 hours or greater and a diagnosis of diabetes mellitus in the medical record, or were prescribed any of the formulary medications for diabetes	Of 424 inmates having diabetes, 200 were assessed Bivariate analysis showed no evidence that adherence rates varied by race, gender, or age; longer stays were associated with greater adherence A fairly low percentage of diabetic inmates had either HbA1c or lipid profiles checked, although this increased proportionally for those incarcerated longer than 30 days

6.	Conklin, T. (2000). Self-reported health and prior health behaviors of newly admitted correctional inmates. *American Journal of Public Health, 90*(12), 1939–1941.	Interviews were conducted with 1198 inmates on day 3 of incarceration. The 15-minute interviews were conducted in a private room; 130 questions on demographic, household data, health status, health problems, medical facility use, tobacco, alcohol, drug, HIV, and other sexually transmitted infections, sexual behavior, prior jail time, and physical abuse were included	Conducted a baseline health study to better elucidate the extent of inmate pre-incarceration health problems, health facility use, and health-related risky behaviors. All inmates newly admitted to the facility over a 5-month period on the 3rd day of stay were interviewed	Data showed that newly incarcerated inmates have a high prevalence of health issues at admission, prior limited access to healthcare and very high rates of disease and unhealthy behaviors. Results of interviews confirmed the significant need for medical, mental, dental, and substance abuse healthcare, with additional prevention and education programs to modify risky health behaviors
7.	Deakin, T. (2005). Group based training for self-management strategies in people with type 2 diabetes mellitus. [Meta-Analysis Review]. *Cochrane Database of Systematic Reviews*(2), CD003417.	Randomized controlled and controlled clinical trials which evaluated group-based education programs for adults with type 2 diabetes compared with routine treatment. Studies obtained from computerized searches of electronic databases, supplemental by hand searches of reference lists of articles, conference proceedings, and consultation with experts in the field	To assess the effects of group-based, patient-centered training on clinical, lifestyle, and psychosocial outcomes in people with type 2 diabetes. Studies were only included if the length of the program included follow-up with 6 months or more, and the intervention was at least one session with a minimum of six participants	Fourteen publications describing 11 studies were included involving over 1532 participants. The results of the meta-analysis in favor of the group-based diabetes education program were reduced glycated hemoglobin. Group-based training for self-management strategies in people with type 2 diabetes is effective by improving fasting blood glucose levels, glycated hemoglobin, and diabetes knowledge and reducing systolic blood pressure levels, body weight, and the required diabetes medication

(continued)

TABLE 5.4   Tool to Assess Literature Review: Interventions, Purpose, Populations, and Outcomes (*continued*)

TITLE/AUTHOR	DESCRIPTION OF INTERVENTION	PURPOSE AND POPULATIONS	OUTCOMES ACHIEVED
8. D'Eramo. (2004). A culturally competent intervention of education and care for black women with type 2 diabetes. [Clinical Trial Controlled Clinical Trial]. *Applied Nursing Research, 17*(1), 10–20.	A 6-week cognitive behavioral culturally competent diabetes mellitus (DM) intervention program was developed and led by an APN trained in DM care and certified as a DM educator. The Cross Cultural Counseling: A guide for Nutrition and Health Counselors (1987) was used as a guide for training and intervention. By using one group, pre-test and post-test quasi-experimental design the pilot was tested for feasibility. Twenty-five women were recruited from a local urban community using multiple recruitments strategies such as numerous newspaper and radio announcements, flyers and public access television announcements, and churches	This article reports on a pilot feasibility testing of a culturally competent intervention of education and care for Black women with type 2 diabetes (T2DM). Eligible participants were between 18 and 60 years old, having a primary care provider, diagnosed with T2DM and English speaking women who were receiving insulin therapy, pregnant or breast feeding, who had comorbidities or diabetes-related complications such as visual impairment that prevented independence, end stage renal disease, or lower extremity amputations were excluded	The findings suggested that a culturally sensitive intervention of nurse practitioners diabetes care and education is beneficial for Black women with T2DM, resulting in program attendance, kept appointments, improved glycemic control and weight, and decreased diabetes-related emotional distress

| 9. | Duncan, E. (2006). A systematic review of structured group interventions with mentally disordered offenders. [Research Support, Non-U.S. Gov't Review]. *Criminal Behaviour & Mental Health, 16*(4), 217–241. | Twenty studies were retrieved that fulfilled the inclusion criteria. All included studies were of participants in hospital settings. Ten of these studies were conducted in British high security hospitals and six in British medium security hospital units. The remaining four studies were conducted in Canada or the United States of America, two of which were unclear regarding the level of security at the location where their study was undertaken | To evaluate structured group interventions with mentally disordered offenders through systematic review of the evidence for their efficacy and effectiveness
Inclusion criteria:
1. Evaluation of the efficacy or effectiveness of structured single-form group interventions applied specifically to offenders with mental disorder
2. Evaluation of the efficacy or effectiveness of structured complex group interventions applied specifically to offenders with mental disorder
Studies published in English | Twenty-two studies were retrieved that fitted the inclusion criteria. Four main themes were dominant: problem solving; anger/aggression management; self-harm; and other
Calculated effect sizes gave optimism for the efficacy of structured group interventions with mentally disordered offenders
This review confirmed that there has been some useful research into structured group therapy interventions with mentally disordered offenders |
| 10. | El-Mallakh, P. (2006). Evolving self-care in individuals with schizophrenia and diabetes mellitus. [Journal Article, Research, Tables/Charts]. *Archives of Psychiatric Nursing, 20*(2), 55–64. | Clients recruited from five sites of a regional community mental health center
The study did not go into detail on how the respondents were chosen
Twenty-six interviews were conducted among 11 respondents with varying degrees of ability to care for their coexisting illnesses | Inclusion criteria: having a comorbid diagnosis of schizophrenia and type 1 or 2 diabetes, self-reported involvement in daily diabetic self-care activities, between the age of 18–72
Exclusion criteria: having any medical problem that prevented the client from participating with the interview and being unable to understand the studies purpose and procedures | A theoretical self-care model "Evolving self-care for schizophrenia and diabetes" was developed. Findings suggested that the respondents developed realistic and informed self-care health beliefs that accurately reflected knowledge and experiences with self-care of comorbid illnesses |

(continued)

TABLE 5.4   Tool to Assess Literature Review: Interventions, Purpose, Populations, and Outcomes (*continued*)

	TITLE/AUTHOR	DESCRIPTION OF INTERVENTION	PURPOSE AND POPULATIONS	OUTCOMES ACHIEVED
11.	Enders, S. (2005). An approach to develop effective healthcare decision making for women in prison. *J Palliat Med, 8(2), 432–439.*	Female inmates were recruited through self-selection from a California women's facility to participate in a group discussion Participants were divided into 16 focus groups averaging seven participants each (113), each lasting about 2 hours, and were based on four levels of education ranging from no formal education to any college education. The focus groups were guided by a set of research questions and were facilitated by the researcher to identify informational barriers to the inmates medical care needs. All groups were audio taped	The study attempted to identify informational barriers to people making medical care and treatment decisions, especially those with low literacy. The findings were used to develop a tool to assist patients become active participants in their own care All women in this specific correctional facility were eligible. Only women detained in the reception center for evaluation or possible reassignment were excluded	The conclusion was that those who face chronic, potentially life-threatening illness cannot make meaningful decisions regarding medical care and treatment without having basic foundations of health information
12.	Foster, G. (2007). Self-management education programmes by lay leaders for people with chronic conditions. [Meta-Analysis Review]. *Cochrane Database of Systematic Reviews*(4), CD005108.	The researchers searched The Cochrane Central Registry, MEDLINE, CINHAL, and other databases, reference lists, and forward citation tracking Seventeen trials involving 7442 participants were included. The interventions shared similar structures and components but studies showed heterogeneity in conditions studied, outcomes collected, and effects	To assess systematically the effectiveness of lay-led self-management programs for people with chronic conditions Randomized controlled trials comparing structured lay-led self-management education program for chronic conditions against no intervention or clinician led programs. There were no language restrictions	Self-efficacy showed a small, statistically significant improvement in 10 studies No significant difference between groups in physicals vs general practitioner attendance. Small significance in pain reduction was noted Health behaviors also showed a small significant increase in self-reported aerobic exercise and a moderate increase in cognitive symptom management

13.	Giroux, V. A. (2000). A comparison of diabetes management in a federal prison with the National Standards of Care published by the ADA in 1998. [Masters Thesis, Research]. 59.	To measure adherence to the ADA standards, this descriptive quantitative study utilized the Diabetes Quality Assurance (DQA) Checklist to perform a chart review in a federal prison outpatient clinic The DQA Checklist major categories include referrals, blood glucose evaluation, diet and exercise, foot care, cardiovascular risk factors, and laboratory tests	The purpose of this study was to describe the medical management for inmates diagnosed with DM within the FBOP and compare this to the national standards of care published by the ADA in 1998	Cardiovascular risk factor assessment, cholesterol and triglyceride measurement, nutrition assessment, ophthalmology and ECG referrals were at greater than 87% adherence. However, the degree of adherence was significantly lower in the areas of glycohemoglobin measurement, documented foot exam, HDL and LDL cholesterol measurement
14.	Goldberg, R. (2007). Quality of diabetes care among adults with serious mental illness. [Journal Article, Research, Tables/Charts]. *Psychiatric Services, 58*(4), 536–543.	Cross-sectional analysis of medical chart data from 300 patients was used to examine indicators of the quality of care established by the diabetes quality improvement project Participants were recruited from mental health clinics and primary care clinics in urban and suburban communities Each participant met with the researcher for 2.5-hour assessment, and charts were reviewed	The study compared the quality of care for type 2 diabetes delivered to two groups with type 2 diabetes adults with serious mental illness and those with no serious mental illness in a range of community-based clinic settings All patients with a diagnosis of type 2 diabetes were identified from appointment logs. Primary care providers asked for volunteers. Any client who had received any treatment for a psychiatric disorder within the past year was excluded from the control group	The results of the investigation replicated the previous studies suggesting that people with serious mental illness and type 2 diabetes receive poorer quality of diabetes care than persons with type 2 diabetes who do not have a mental illness

(continued)

TABLE 5.4 Tool to Assess Literature Review: Interventions, Purpose, Populations, and Outcomes (*continued*)

	TITLE/AUTHOR	DESCRIPTION OF INTERVENTION	PURPOSE AND POPULATIONS	OUTCOMES ACHIEVED
15.	Harris, M., Smith, B., & Veale, A. (2005). Printed patient education interventions to facilitate shared management of chronic disease: a literature review. [Review]. *Internal Medicine Journal, 35*(12), 711–716.	The authors did not state how the studies were extracted for the review or how many reviewers there were The studies were rated on three criteria: full description of the intervention, at least 26 weeks study duration, and inclusion of process measures Databases were searched, and the reference lists of included reports were screened for further relevant studies	To evaluate the effectiveness of print-only interventions in increasing patient participation in chronic diseases management and to identify disease or intervention characteristics associated with success Controlled studies that presented baseline measures were eligible for inclusion in the review Studies reporting health outcomes and quality of life and patient disease management behaviors were included Studies of patients with the eight top nonpsychological chronic diseases cause of disability-adjusted life years in Australia including diabetes were included	The studies were combined in a narrative; seven studies were included in the review. Statically significant changes were found for a few of the measures. Knowledge improved in three studies and adherence in two. Quality of life declined in one study but a confound cause was reported
16.	MacFarlane, (1992). Diabetes in prison: can good diabetic care be achieved? *BMJ, 304*(6820), 152–155.	Survey of diabetic men serving prison sentences during a 22-month period in a large British prison Survey of 42 male diabetic prisoners of whom 23 had insulin-dependent diabetes and 19 had non-insulin-dependent diabetes	To investigate the clinical characteristics and metabolic control of diabetic patients given structured diabetic care in prison	Positive outcomes: No serious diabetic instability occurred. Between the initial assessment and a second assessment 10 weeks later, glycated hemoglobin concentration had fallen in the prisons with insulin-dependent diabetes from 10.8 to 9.8 and from 8.7 to 7.6 for non-insulin-dependent diabetic inmates Conclusions: Structured diabetic care should be offered in all prisons

17.	National Commission on Correctional Healthcare. (2008). NCCHC Clinical Guideline: Diabetes (Publication. Retrieved November 16, 2008: http:// www.ncchc.org/resources/ clinicalguides/Adult_ Diabetes.pdf	N/A	Not a study Clinical guidelines for diabetes in prison	
18.	Petit, J. (2001). Management of diabetes in French prisons: a cross-sectional study. *Diabetic Medicine, 18*(1), 47–50.	Extensive literature review	To review the literature on comorbid depression and diabetes and present a conceptual framework for integrating depression management with diabetes care in a managed care environment	A conceptual framework for the relationship between diabetes and depression was developed. Four pathways were noted: directly affecting the patients' health-related quality of life, reducing physical activity levels, limiting adherence to self-care regime, and impairing patients' ability to communicate effectively with clinicians
19.	Plugge, E. (2008) Patients, prisoners, or people? Women prisoners experiences of primary care in prison: a qualitative study	Qualitative study on-site education self-management education was provided by a certified diabetes counselor	To explore women prisoners' experience of primary healthcare provision in prison	Women prisoner perceptions of the quality of prison healthcare were mixed. The conclusions were that the prison environment presents unique challenges to providing healthcare. The study shows that there appears to be a gap between patient experiences and policy goals

(continued)

TABLE 5.4   Tool to Assess Literature Review: Interventions, Purpose, Populations, and Outcomes (*continued*)

	TITLE/AUTHOR	DESCRIPTION OF INTERVENTION	PURPOSE AND POPULATIONS	OUTCOMES ACHIEVED
20.	Shon, K. (2002). Medication and symptom management education program for the rehabilitation of psychiatric patients in Korea: the effects of promoting schedule on self-efficacy theory. [Clinical Trial Randomized Controlled Trial Research Support, Non-U.S. Gov't]. *Yonsei Medical Journal, 43*(5), 579–589.	Randomized recruitment of subjects that were diagnosed with schizophrenia, mood disorders, and delusional disorders that had been hospitalized in a psychiatric hospital and discharged Among 53 outpatients, 40 were randomized after receiving approval; 20 were classified as the experimental group and 20 were placed in the control group The study had three phases: 1. Field research using a questionnaire 2. The educational component 3. The last phase and investigation was conducted to determine efficacy of the developed medication and symptom management program Pre- and post-testing were conducted with both groups	The effectiveness of a rehabilitation program for psychiatric patients self-management of medication and symptoms	After applying the medication and symptom management education, significant differences in self-efficacy, medication compliance, and the number of relapse warning symptoms were found

21.	Siminerio, L. (2005). Implementing the chronic care model for improvements in diabetes care and education in a rural primary care practice. *The Diabetes Educator, 31*(2), 225–234.	Pilot study consisting of 104 patients with type 2 diabetes and six providers in a rural primary care practice. On-site education self-management education was provided by a certified diabetes counselor. Chart reviews were also used prior to the educational groups. Five 2-hour groups were held	To determine the impact of implementing elements of the chronic care model on provider diabetes care practices and patient outcomes in a rural practice setting Any patient over 18 with a confirmed diagnosis of diabetes or two fasting blood glucose levels over 126 seen during the calendar year of 2000	Provider adherence to standards increase. Patients gained improvements in knowledge, empowerment, A1c, and high-density lipoprotein cholesterol levels
22.	Solberg, L (2006). Care quality and implementation of the chronic care model: a quantitative study. [Research Support, Non-U.S. Gov't]. *Annals of Family Medicine, 4*(4), 310–316.	The leaders of 17 primary care clinics in this medical group completed the Assessing Chronic Illness Care (ACIC) survey measure of chronic care model (CCM) implementation before and after care system changes were made The changes involved in the group's care transformation efforts addressed all six elements of the CCM to a varying extent, although the main focus was on delivery system design	To test whether improvements in care quality were correlated with changes in the chronic care model (CCM) in a large medical group that attempted to implement the CCM	Although all scores increased, those for delivery system design and self-management support changed the least and were not significant at $P < .05$. The overall change of 1.42 represents a 24% improvement in CCM implementation, although there was considerable variation among the clinics, and 4 clinics actually had lower scores at the follow-up time period

(continued)

TABLE 5.4   Tool to Assess Literature Review: Interventions, Purpose, Populations, and Outcomes (*continued*)

	TITLE/AUTHOR	DESCRIPTION OF INTERVENTION	PURPOSE AND POPULATIONS	OUTCOMES ACHIEVED
23.	Vermeire, E., (2005). Interventions for improving adherence to treatment recommendations in people with type 2 diabetes mellitus. [Meta-Analysis Review]. *Cochrane Database of Systematic Reviews*(2), CD003638.	Studies obtained from searches of multiple electronic databases and supplemental hand searches of references Randomized controlled and controlled clinical trails, before and after studies and epidemiological studies were included Two teams of reviewers independently assessed the trials identified for inclusion. Three teams of two reviewers assessed the trial quality and extracted data	To assess the effects of interventions for improving adherence to treatment recommendations in people with type 2 diabetes Randomized controlled and controlled clinical trials, before and after studies and epidemiological studies were included	Adaptation of dosing and frequency of medication taking showed a small effect on a variety of outcomes including HbA1c. Conclusion: Efforts to improve or to facilitate adherence of people with type 2 diabetes to treatment recommendations do not show significant benefits nor harms
24.	Wars, A. (2004). Self Management Education Programs in Chronic Disease: A systematic review and methodological critique of literature. *Archives of Internal Medicine, 164*, 1641–1649.	Searched electronic databases from 1964–1999, and then hand searched the reference sections of each article for other relevant publications Database searches were completed for studies within which self-management education interventions for a chronic disease was reported, a concurrent control group was included, and clinical outcomes were evaluated included	To evaluate the efficacy of patient self-management education programs for chronic diseases and critically reviewed their methodology Included studies if self-management education interventions for a chronic disease were reported, a concurrent control group was included, and clinical outcomes were evaluated	Conclusion: Self-management education programs resulted in small to moderate effects for selected chronic diseases

Note: The Effectiveness of a Chronic Disease Self-Management Program for Mentally Ill Inmates With Diabetes. Unpublished doctoral capstone project, University of Medicine and Dentistry of New Jersey—School of Nursing. Conrad, 2008, Newark, NJ. Used with permission of Dr. Margaret Conrad.

INTEGRATION OF EVIDENCE INTO PRACTICE

Time lags commonly occur when applying new research findings to clinical practice. This is the time period between the discovery that an intervention works and the application of new knowledge into actual practice. In 1999, the American Society of Anesthesiology (ASA) revised its practice guidelines for preoperative fasting in healthy patients undergoing elective procedures. "The newer, more liberal recommendations, based on studies showing that pulmonary aspiration occurs only rarely as a complication of modern anesthesia, allow the consumption of clear liquids up to two hours before elective surgery, a light breakfast (tea and toast, for example) six hours before the procedure, and a heavier meal eight hours beforehand" (Crenshaw & Winslow, 2002, p. 36). Crenshaw and Lewis carried out a study to determine if the guidelines were being followed. They interviewed 155 patients in one hospital about their preoperative fasting, comparing preoperative instructions for fasting, actual preoperative fasting, and ASA-recommended fasting durations for liquids and solids. They found that the majority of patients continued to receive instructions for npo after midnight for both liquids and solids, whether they were scheduled for early or late surgery. They also discovered that, on average, the patients fasted from liquids and solids for 12 hours and 14 hours, respectively, with some patients fasting as long as 20 hours from liquids and 37 hours from solids. These fasts were significantly longer than those recommended by the ASA. Clearly, in this case, the authors discovered a significant lag time between the generation of new knowledge and the implementation of that knowledge into practice. This is just one example of the time lag between research and practice.

In order to effect change, the APN needs to understand why these time intervals exist between the development of new knowledge and the incorporation of that knowledge into practice. Investigators have examined the reasons for nurses not keeping up to date in their practice. Jacobson, Ross, and Pravikoff (2005) completed a study to investigate what determines usual nursing practice. They discovered that most nurses practice what they learned in school. Because the average age of nurses at the time the study was completed was more than 40 years, this meant that the majority of nurses in the study had graduated before 1990, making much of what they learned in school out of date. Although nurses in the study acknowledged that an evidence-based practice is important, they expressed discomfort in using health-related databases; in fact, the study revealed that 76% of the respondents had apparently never searched CINAHL and 58% had never searched MEDLINE.

A qualitative study of two primary care practices was conducted by Gabbay and le May (2004). The objective of the study was to explore how primary care clinicians derive their healthcare decisions. The results revealed that clinicians rarely accessed or used current evidence but instead relied on what the authors labeled "mindlines." The authors describe mindlines as "internalized guidelines that are formed primarily from interactions with colleagues and people perceived as opinion leaders." They arise from experience and trusted personal sources.

The authors describe it as "day to day practice based on socially constituted knowledge" (p. 1015).

Depending upon the focus of their advanced degrees, APNs are educated to fill the roles of highly skilled practitioners and/or leaders and educators in their fields of expertise. They are in a position to educate other providers, work with direct care nurses to identify and remove barriers to evidence-based practice, and disseminate information. They also receive advanced education in research and because of this, they are uniquely qualified not only to implement evidence-based care but also to guide direct care nurses in developing PICO questions, searching and synthesizing the literature, and changing practice interventions to reflect current knowledge.

Models of Practice

Several models have been created to facilitate the implementation of evidence-based practice. They provide an organized approach for integrating and sustaining change. A practice model ensures that professional nursing practice is consistent and minimizes practice variations that can create risk and gaps in care. Some examples of the models in use are the Advancing Research and Clinical Practice through Close Collaboration Model (ARCC), the Johns Hopkins Nursing Model, the Chronic Care Model (CCM), and the Iowa Model of Evidence-Based Practice to Promote Quality of Care. The overriding characteristic of each is that they provide a structured method for incorporating best evidence into practice.

The focus of the ARCC Model is to bring research experts together with direct care nurses to integrate research with practice. It was developed by Bernadette Melnyk and the faculty of the School of Nursing at the University of Rochester, the School of Medicine and Dentistry, and community partners. It was originally designed to bring academic communities together with healthcare organizations that provide both acute and community-based care. The APN as mentor plays a prominent role in this model. An important component is education on evidence-based practice. Fineout-Overholt, Levin, and Melnyk (2004–2005) carried out a study to test the ARCC Model in two pediatric units at acute care facilities. The authors identified the following key strategies for implementing evidence-based practice: administrative support, creation of a clear role for nurses that includes evidence-based practice, adequate infrastructure (such as computer resources and databases), evidence-based practice mentors to work directly with direct care nurses, time and money to carry out studies, and creation of an evidence-based practice culture. Direct care nurses on the study units talked about the importance of working with APNs to bring about evidence-based practice as opposed to simply being told what to do. The authors point out that APNs can act as *information brokers* to create changes based on evidence-based practice while working closely with direct care nurses.

Like the ARCC Model, the origin of the Johns Hopkins Nursing Model can be found in a partnership with an academic institution. It was developed in collaboration with the Johns Hopkins Hospital and the Johns Hopkins University School of Nursing. "PET" is an acronym that describes the process used in this model. It stands for **P**ractice question, **E**vidence, and **T**ranslation. The essential cornerstones of the model are practice, education, and research, and the core of the model is evidence. It was developed to ensure that evidence was incorporated into practice (Newhouse, Dearholt, Poe, Pugh, & White, 2007).

The CCM (MacColl Institute, 2010) employs a holistic approach to chronic disease management through the use of evidence-based practice. It summarizes the basic elements for improving care in health systems at the community, organization, practice, and patient levels. It has six components: the healthcare delivery system, community, patient self-management support, decision support, delivery system design, and clinical information system. The emphasis in the model is on health promotion (MacColl Institute, 2010). O'Toole et al. (2010) investigated the use of this model in providing primary care to homeless veterans. They used a retrospective cohort design to compare veterans who received their primary care in a clinic that used the CCM to a matched cohort of veterans who received their primary care in "usual care" general internal medicine clinics. Veterans enrolled in the clinic using the CCM for delivery of primary care had fewer emergency department visits and greater improvements in blood pressure and low density lipoproteins than the control cohort. The authors cited the importance of the location of the clinic (the clinic was located in an urban Virginia hospital so that it was geographically convenient) and of tailoring interventions to the target population (the clinic addressed issues such as the need for housing and food). They concluded that how primary care is delivered and organized is important in chronic disease management.

The Iowa Model of Evidence-Based Practice to Promote Quality of Care was "developed to serve as a guide for nurses and other healthcare providers to use research findings for improvement of patient care" (Titler et al., 2001, p. 498). Case Study 5.1 presents an example of how one clinic used the Iowa Model to improve practice and population outcomes. Important features of the model are decision points and feedback loops that are characteristic of the ongoing process of improving care through research. Once a problem or new information is identified (Step One), a team is formed to investigate the issue (Step Two). A literature review is conducted, and the information is evaluated, critiqued, and synthesized for use in practice (Step Three). If the evidence is judged to be sufficient for a change in practice, the change is piloted and monitored. If there is not sufficient evidence to pilot a change, the team may decide to conduct a research study (Step Four). Once the evidence is deemed sufficient for a permanent adoption, the organization can move forward to institute the change in practice. The purpose of a pilot is not to test the effectiveness of the intervention but to test whether the intervention is feasible. After a determination is made to change practice, the organization continues to monitor structure, process, and outcome data. Case Study 5.1 illustrates how using a model of practice can facilitate change in a clinic setting that ultimately leads to improved patient outcomes.

CASE STUDY 5.1

Case Study: Use of the Iowa Model to Increase Breastfeeding Initiation Rates of Urban Clinic Mothers

Trigger

Nurses working in a perinatal clinic determined that the rate of breastfeeding initiation for their patients was 40 per 100 (40%). The clinic provides prenatal and maternity services to an ethnically diverse, inner city population in the northeastern United States.

Form Team

A team was created that included a clinical nurse specialist (CNS), the case managers for the perinatal clinic, and a lactation nurse specialist.

Assemble Relevant Research and Related Literature

A literature review was carried out by the CNS and the lactation nurse and more than 30 articles were retrieved and appraised.

Critique/Synthesize Information

The literature search revealed information on the benefits of breastfeeding, breastfeeding rates among inner city populations, research on effective strategies for increasing rates, and culturally appropriate materials for teaching.

Among the key findings:

- Breastfeeding can reduce the incidence of many disease states in childhood and throughout adulthood, such as diabetes, SIDS, ear infection, allergies, asthma, and obesity (American Academy of Pediatrics, 2005; Chulada, Arbes, Dunson & Zeldin, 2003).

- The opinions of healthcare providers regarding breastfeeding have enormous impact on urban women, their partners, and families (Philipp, Merewood, Gerendas & Bauchner, 2004).

- Methods to increase the rates of breastfeeding have been unsuccessful for African Americans because methods to increase rates are not culturally sensitive (African American Breastfeeding Alliance, 2005).

- The information was summarized, then shared and discussed with team members. The team created a plan to increase the breastfeeding rates of the clinic population.

Pilot Change and Carryout Study

The clinic initiated education programs for clinic staff and community providers and increased lactation services. The clinic environment was changed to include sensitive pictures of ethnically diverse Breastfeeding mothers and improvements were made in bilingual educational brochures. Each clinic counselor was given a protocol book describing specific literature, videos, and discussion to be provided to patients at each trimester. The healthcare providers documented the education that was provided to each patient, and patients completed a postpartum questionnaire that was used to evaluate interventions and factors influencing feeding choice.

Determine if the Change Is Appropriate for Adoption in Practice

Five years after the initiation of the evidence-based change, Breastfeeding initiation rates had increased to 70 per 100 (70%). Analysis of the patient evaluations revealed that counseling and reading material were cited as the most influential factors in making the choice to breastfeed. Other important factors were the opinions of family and healthcare professionals.

The nurses determined that prenatal education interventions addressing varied learning styles and delivered in defined segments may be effective in influencing the feeding decisions of new mothers. The educational programs must be culturally sensitive, and staff education is vital to ensure effective and accurate delivery of information.

Continue to Monitor Structure, Process, and Outcome Data

The team has continued to monitor lactation rates and to review new information on lactation education as it has become available. Educational materials are updated on a regular basis. Eight years after the start of the initiative, its breastfeeding rates have placed the hospital among the top ten in the state. The clinic and its associated hospital are currently working toward achieving Baby-Friendly Designation. In order to achieve this goal, the clinic will need to demonstrate that they have integrated the *"10 Steps to Successful Breastfeeding"* into their practice for healthy newborns (Baby Friendly USA, 2010).

Note: Adapted from Procaccini and Mahony (2010).

Source: Procaccini, D., & Mahony, J. (2010). *Survey of educational interventions to increase the breastfeeding initiation rates of urban clinic mothers.* Unpublished Manuscript. Used with permission.

SUMMARY

The use of research evidence to guide practice can lead to the implementation of interventions that will improve population outcomes, but this is a complex process. The ability to identify clinical problems and issues, ask clinical questions in a format that allows for study, conduct a search of the literature, appraise and synthesize the available evidence, and successfully integrate new knowledge into practice requires specialized skills and knowledge. This process can be challenging and time consuming. Researchers have identified many barriers to evidence-based practice, including the lack of belief by practicing nurses that research can make a real difference. APNs are uniquely situated to influence care through their roles as leaders, educators, and clinical experts. This chapter has described some of the basic skills that are needed to integrate and synthesize information in order to design interventions that are based on evidence to improve population outcomes. APNs need to use their specialized knowledge and advanced practice roles to identify the barriers to evidence-based practice in order to build the capacity to adopt change. They also require the ability to involve individuals, teams, and organizations in the process. By adopting a culture of evidence-based practice in the work environment, APNs have the opportunity to facilitate change that can lead to improved quality of care.

EXERCISES AND DISCUSSION QUESTIONS

Exercise 5.1   Write a clinical question using the PICO format.

Exercise 5.2   Carry out a literature review for the PICO question.

■ Establish criteria for inclusion and exclusion of studies.
■ Synthesize and appraise the information using Table 5.2.

Exercise 5.3   Determine whether or not you have enough evidence to change current practice.

■ Will you need to conduct a study in order to test the effectiveness of the intervention? Provide your rationale.
■ If you need to conduct a study, describe the method that you will use to evaluate the effectiveness of the intervention.
■ Describe what outcomes of interest you will identify in your study.

Exercise 5.4   Describe how you will incorporate this change into practice.

REFERENCES

African American Breastfeeding Alliance (AABA). (2004). *An Easy Guide to Breastfeeding for African American Women.* Retrieved November 21, 2005, from http://www.aabaonline.com

American Academy of Pediatrics (AAP). (1999). 10 Steps to supporting a parents' choice to breastfeed their baby. In *AAP Task Force on Breastfeeding* (pp. 1–5). Author.

American Association of Colleges of Nursing (AACN). (2006). *The essentials of doctoral education for advanced practice nursing.* Retrieved from http://www.aacn.nche.edu/DNP/pdf/Essentials.pdf

American Psychological Association (APA). (2009). *Publication manual of the American psychological association* (6th ed.). Washington, DC: Author.

Armola, R., Bourgault, A., Halm, M., Board, R., Bucher, L., Harrington, L., … Medina, J. (2009). Upgrading the American association of critical-care nurses' evidence-leveling system. *American Journal of Critical Care, 18*(5), 405–409.

Baby Friendly USA. (2010). Retrieved from http://babyfriendlyusa.org/

Beck, C. T. (1993). Teetering on the edge: A substantive theory of post partum depression. *Nursing Research, 42*(1), 42–48.

Beck, C. T. (2009). Metasynthesis: A goldmine for evidence-based practice. *AORN, 90*(5), 701–710.

Blegen, M. (2009). Qualitative or quantitative is beside the point. *Nursing Research, 58*(6), 381.

Burns, N., & Grove, S. K. (2007). *Understanding nursing research: Building an evidence-based practice* (4th ed.). St. Louis, MO: Saunders/Elsevier.

Camden University Library, University of Medicine and Dentistry of NJ. (2010). Real time *EBP: the PICO model.* Retrieved from http://libraries.umdnj.edu/camlbweb/EBM/picomodel.htm

Centre for Reviews and Dissemination (CRD). (2010). *Systematic reviews: CRD's guidance for undertaking reviews in health care [Internet].* York: University of York; 2009 [accessed 12/9/2010]. Retrieved from: http://www.york.ac.uk/inst/crd/systematic_reviews_book.htm

Chulada, P.C., Arbes, S.J., Dunson, D. & Zeldin, D.C. (2003). Breast-feeding and the prevalence of asthma and wheeze in children: analyses the Third National Health and Nutrition Examination Survey, 1988-1994. *J Allergy Clin Immunol, 111*(2), 328–36.

The Cochrane Collaboration. (2010). *About us.* Retrieved from http://www.cochrane.org/about-us

Conrad, M. (2008). *The effectiveness of a chronic disease self-management program for mentally ill inmates with diabetes.* Unpublished doctoral capstone project, University of Medicine and Dentistry of New Jersey – School of Nursing, Newark, N.J.

Crenshaw, J. T., & Winslow, E. H. (2002). Preoperative fasting: Old habits die hard. *American Journal of Nursing, 102*(5), 36–44.

DeBourgh, G. (2001). Champions for evidence-based practice: A critical role for advanced practice nurses. *AACN Clinical Issues, 12*(4), 491–508.

EBSCO Publishing. (2010). *CINAHL Databases.* Retrieved from: http://www.ebscohost.com/cinahl/

Evidence. (2000). *The American Heritage Dictionary of the English Language* (4th ed.). Boston, MA: Houghton Mifflin Company.

Evidence for Policy and Practice Information Coordinating Centre (EPPI). (2010). *Quality and relevance appraisal.* Retrieved from http://eppi.ioe.ac.uk/cms/Default.aspx?tabid=177&language=en-US

Fineout-Overholt, E., Levin, R., & Melnyk, B. (2004–2005). Strategies for advancing evidence-based practice in clinical settings. *Journal of the New York Nurses Association. Fall/Winter, 35*(2) 8–32.

Gabbay, J., & le May, A. (2004). Evidence based guidelines or collectively constructed "mindlines?" Ethnographic study of knowledge management in primary care. *BMJ. 329,* 1013–1017.

Hallyburton, A., & St. John, B. (2010). Partnering with your library to strengthen nursing research. *Journal of Nursing Education, 49*(3), 164–167.

Hayat, M. (2010). Understanding statistical significance. *Nursing Research, 59*(3), 219–223.

Jacobson, A., Ross, J., & Pravikoff, D. (2005). Evidence-based nursing... "Readiness of U.S. nurses for evidence-based practice" (Original research, September). *American Journal of Nursing, 105*(12), 15, 40–51.

The Joanna Briggs Institute. (2010). *About us.* Retrieved from http://www.joannabriggs.edu.au/about/about.php

Houde, S. C. (2009). The systematic review of the literature: A tool for evidence-based policy. *Journal of Gerontological Nursing, 35*(9), 9–12.

MacColl Institute. (2010). *The Chronic care Model.* Retrieved from http://www.improvingchroniccare.org/index.php?p=The_Chronic_Care_Model&s=2

Melnyk, B., & Fineout-Overholt, E. (2005). Evidence-based practice. Rapid critical appraisal of randomized controlled trials (RCTs): an essential skill for evidence-based practice (EBP). *Pediatric Nursing, 31*(1), 50–52.

Newhouse, R. P., Dearholt, S. L., Poe, S. S., Pugh, L. C., & White, K. M. (2007). *Johns Hopkins* nursing evidence-based practice model and guidelines. Indianapolis, IN: Sigma Theta Tau International.

O'Toole, T., Buckel, L., Bourgault, C., Redihan, S., Jiang, L., & Friedman, P. (2010) Applying the chronic care model to homeless veterans: Effect of a population approach to primary care on utilization and clinical outcomes. *American Journal of Public Health, 100*(12), 2493–2499.

Philipp, B.L., Merewood, A., Gerendas, E.J., & Bauchner, H. (2004). Breastfeeding information in pediatric textbooks needs improvement. *J Hum Lact. 20*(2), 206–10.

Polit, D., & Beck, C. T. (2008). *Nursing Research: Generating and Assessing Evidence for Nursing Practice* (8th ed.). Philadelphia, PA: Lippencott Williams & Wilkins.

Porter-O'Grady, T. (2003). Nurses as knowledge workers. *Creative Nursing, 9*(2), 6–9.

Procaccini, D., & Mahony, J. (2010). *Survey of educational interventions to increase the breastfeeding initiation rates of urban clinic mothers.* Unpublished Manuscript.

Shapiro, S., & Donaldson, N. (2008). Evidence-based practice for advanced practice emergency nurses, part II Critically appraising the literature. *Advanced Emergency Nursing Journal, 30*(2), 139–150.

Titler, M., Kleiber, C., Steelman, V., Rakel, B., Budreau, G., Everett, C., Buckwalter K.C., Tripp-Reimer T., & Goode C.J. (2001). The Iowa Model of Evidence-Based Practice to Promote Quality Care. *Critical Care Nursing Clinics of North America, 13*(4), 497–509.

U.S. National Library of Medicine. (2010). *About the National Library of Medicine.* Retrieved from http://www.nlm.nih.gov/about/index.html

SIX

Using Information Systems to Improve Population Outcomes

Ann L. Cupp Curley

People access the World Wide Web everyday to obtain health information. It is an increasingly popular source of information for both healthcare providers and consumers. The most common sources of information for U.S. adults remains health professionals (86%), friends or family members (68%), and the Internet places third (57%), just ahead of printed material (54%) (Pew Research Center, 2008). All of the chapters in this text describe Internet resources and/or online references that are useful for advanced practice nurses (APNs). From online databases that can be used for literature reviews to support evidence-based practice to integrated electronic health care records, modern technology provides the APN with valuable and useful resources. The fourth competency for the doctor of nursing practice (DNP) degree as outlined by the American Association of Colleges of Nursing (AACN, 2006) states, "DNP graduates are distinguished by their abilities to use information systems/technology to support and improve patient care and healthcare systems, and provide leadership within healthcare systems and/or academic settings" (p. 12). This chapter will describe resources that can be found on the Internet and how to evaluate them for quality. It will also describe how technology can be used to enhance population-based nursing.

USE OF THE INTERNET TO OBTAIN HEALTH INFORMATION

There are a variety of means to access information on the Internet. Once available almost exclusively on personal computers, people can now also use smart phones and tablet computers to access health information. According to Internet World

Stats (2010) in 2010, more than 200 million people in North America (77%) have access to the Internet. This represents an increase of 146% since 2000. And there is ample evidence that people around the world use the Internet to obtain health-related information and that this trend is growing. Schwartz et al. (2006) sampled patients from several family medicine practices in the United States to determine the extent of access to the Internet, the types of information sought, and how patients determined accuracy of the information. They found that 65% of the patients reported having access to the Internet, and 74% of those with access used it to search for health information. The most commonly sought information was disease-specific information, information on medications, and information on nutrition and exercise. The patients in this study reported that they assessed the accuracy of the information by checking for endorsements by government or professional organizations or by checking the credentials of authors. They also checked information across Web sites and discussed information that they found with their physicians.

In the United Kingdom, Schembri and Schober (2009) conducted a study "to determine how frequently patients attending a genitourinary (GU) medicine clinic use the Internet to diagnose their own symptoms, and to assess the accuracy of their diagnoses" (p. 231). Of the 223 symptomatic patients enrolled in this study, 45% looked up their symptoms on the Internet, and 14% of the individuals who looked up their symptoms on the Internet made the correct diagnosis. The authors noted that 90% of the patients who used the Internet to access information chose the Google search engine to start their search. Although the Internet can be a rich source of information, the ability to interpret and assess that information accurately can be a challenge. APNs should be aware of the resources available to their patients so they can answer questions or anticipate potential misguidance from Internet resources.

Underhill and McKeown (2008) used the findings from the 2005 Canadian Internet Use Survey to examine how Canadian adults use the Internet for health information. They found that 68% of adult Canadians used the Internet for nonbusiness reasons during 2005 and that 35% went online to search for health information. The most commonly sought information was information on specific diseases, lifestyle factors, symptoms, medications, and alternative therapies. In the Canadian survey when respondents were asked if they had discussed information that they found on the Internet with a physician, only 38% reported that they had. This reinforces the necessity for APNs to familiarize themselves with Internet resources and the importance of asking patients how they obtain health-related information. By anticipating needs, the APN can serve as a reference for reliable and quality Internet resources for patients. This can lead to better communication between patients and their healthcare providers as it allows patients to be involved and proactive in their own care.

An international survey commissioned by researchers at the London School of Economics determined that 81% of people with access to the Internet use it to search for advice about health, medicine, and medical conditions but only about 25% of these users check where the information comes from. The countries that were surveyed for this study included Australia, Brazil, China, France, Germany, India, Italy, Mexico, Russia, Spain, the United Kingdom, and the United States (McDaid & Park, 2010).

There is evidence to suggest that certain groups of people are more likely to access the Internet for health information than others. "Digital divide" is the term used to describe disparities in the use of the Internet and other forms of technology. The Pew Internet Project tracks Internet use in many fields including healthcare. Findings from a U.S. survey completed in 2008 reveal that Whites (65%) access health information on the Internet more often than African Americans (51%) and Latinos (44%). More women (64%) access health information online than do men (57%) and families with an annual income of less than $30,000 a year (44%) access the Internet for health information less often than families with annual incomes of $75,000 or more (82%). It is not surprising that 93% of teens aged 12 to 17 access the Internet for information and of these 73% use social networking, 31% use the Internet for health information, and 17% of these teens use the Internet to search for sensitive information such as sexual health, depression, and drug use. Three quarters of teens report that they own cell phones and 88% use text messaging. The same report reveals that Latinos and African Americans tend to access health information from smart phones and other mobile devices more so than personal computers. As the number of these devices increases, the authors of the report speculate that the number of Latinos and African Americans who access health information online may increase (Pew Research Center, 2008, 2011). APNs need to know the patterns of Internet use among different aggregates and the types of technology favored by different groups in order to be proactive in educating patients on using the Internet safely and to design effective and innovative interventions using technology.

The Internet has revolutionized the way that consumers access information and communicate with each other. This is important, because it provides APNs with fundamental information on who uses the Internet, what types of information they are looking for, and what types of devices and methods they use to search for information. Advances in technology have made it faster and easier than ever before to find information. It is disingenuous to believe that people rely solely on healthcare providers for information regarding their health or that they will always confirm the accuracy of what they have found on the Internet with their healthcare provider. Although there is a lot of information on the Internet that is valuable and of high quality, some of the information is dubious at best. It is clear that a "digital divide" exists and that APNs need to be aware of this disparity. APNs also need to acquire the skills to improve access to health technology for those who will benefit the most from it. It is for these reasons that APNs need to be proactive in talking to patients about their use of the Internet and other new technologies to better serve and manage their healthcare needs.

Accuracy of Internet Sites

APNs need to be confident that when they direct patients to Web sites for health information those sites are current and maintained by a reliable source. They also need to educate patients on how to evaluate Internet resources. An interesting additional finding of the Pew Internet Project is that 42% of all adults report that they or someone they know has been helped by following medical advice or health information found on the Internet, while 3% of all adults say they or someone they know has been harmed by following medical advice or health information found on the Internet (Pew Research Center, 2008). In fact, studies show that the Internet provides both accurate and inaccurate information. It is equally important to note that a benefit of obtaining health information on the Internet is that it is more readily accessible, especially for some patients, than access to a physician. They can also use various social networking sites and communication methods such as e-mail, chat rooms, and texting to exchange information with other people with similar health conditions (Stone & Jumper, 2001).

A second report by the Pew Research Center, *Peer to Peer Healthcare* (2011) describes the results of a survey to determine how people use technology to talk to people with similar problems. One of the revealing findings is that 1 in 4 Internet users with chronic conditions such as high blood pressure and cancer go online to find people with similar conditions. Only 15% of Internet users who do not have a chronic health condition have sought similar help online. Other people who the survey identified as going online to share health concerns are people who have suffered a recent medical crisis or people who have had a significant change in health status (Pew Research Center, 2011).

There are many studies that illustrate the importance of being vigilant in knowing the patterns of Internet use by consumers. Stone and Jumper (2001) conducted a study to identify what type of information people find when looking for information about age-related macular degeneration (ARMD) on the Internet and how the information compares to what is found in the peer-reviewed literature. These authors found that 1 in 5 sites that they reviewed discussed "some form of nonconventional treatment..." (p. 24). Two thirds of these nonconventional sites provided information that lacked scientific evidence, and one third offered information that the authors labeled "experimental." The authors stressed the importance of physicians educating patients about "the often inaccurate information nature of Internet medical information" (p. 25).

England and Nicholls (2004) used an evaluation tool to determine if the Internet is a useful source of information for people with celiac disease and whether or not transparency criteria can be used to identify accurate online sites. The authors searched the Internet for 2 months in 2002. They excluded Web sites and pages that were designed for healthcare professionals. The remaining sites were evaluated for accuracy of information, transparency, and the use of *kitemarks* (the Kitemark is a registered certification mark owned and operated by British Standards Institution [BSI] and is used to designate a quality product). The researchers concluded that most of the Web sites that they reviewed contained only basic information that is most useful to newly diagnosed patients and they found inaccurate or potentially harmful information on approximately 15% of the Web sites. The authors also reported that "No correlation was found between sites that scored highly for accuracy and those that scored highly for transparency" (p. 547). They recommended that patients who access the Internet for information on celiac disease be encouraged to discuss the information with healthcare professionals and furthermore, healthcare professionals should recommend credible sites to patients.

Holland and Fagnano (2008) completed a systematic review of Web sites to determine the accuracy of information on antibiotic use for otitis media. Only 31% of the sites that they visited mentioned the new 'wait and watch' guidelines, and only 41% mentioned the importance of finishing a complete course of antibiotics.

Ten diabetes-focused social media sites were evaluated for quality of information and privacy protection of users (Weitzman, Cole, Kaci, & Mandl, 2010). The authors note that only 50% of the sites presented evidence-based information, and inaccurate information about diabetes and ads for unfounded "cures" were found on three sites. In fact, of nine sites with advertising, transparency was missing on five. They also found that privacy protection was poor "with almost no use of procedures for secure data storage and transmission; only three sites supported member controls over personal information" (p. 5).

Clearly, people use the Internet to seek out information on health-related matters and, just as clearly, the Internet is used as a source of both good and bad information. It is critical that APNs and the patients to whom they provide care understand how to evaluate Web sites for current and accurate information as is evidenced by studies that show that most Internet consumers do not confirm the validity of the Internet resources that they use. APNs have an opportunity to better serve their population by helping consumers use the Internet wisely.

Evaluating Online Information

The Medical Library Association (MLA), the National Cancer Institute, the Health on the Net Foundation, and the U.S. National Library of Medicine (NLM) provide guidelines for evaluating online information. Links to these sites can be found in Table 6.1. The NLM has partnered with MEDLINEPlus to create the tutorial *Evaluating Internet Health Information: A Tutorial from the National Library of Medicine* that is accessible through the NLM Website. The tutorial is useful for both APNs and consumers.

TABLE 6.1   Links for Evaluating Online Information

RESOURCE	INTERNET ADDRESS	INFORMATION AVAILABLE
Medical Library Association (MLA)	http://www.mlanet.org/	Use the "For Health Consumers" link to find: MLA user's guide to finding and evaluating health information on the Web, MLA's top 10 Web sites, and Deciphering Medspeak
U.S. National Library of Medicine (NLM)	http://www.nlm.nih.gov/hinfo.html	Use the health information site to find: the guide to healthy Web surfing, medical information on the Internet tutorial (from MEDLINE), Health Library Directory, dozens of links for safe health resources for consumers
National Cancer Institute	http://www.cancer.gov/cancertopics/factsheet/Information/internet	Among its many other useful fact sheets for consumers, this site includes information on how to evaluate health information on the Internet
Health on the Net Foundation	http://www.hon.ch/HONcode/Patients/visitor_safeUse2.html	Includes guidelines for evaluating Web sites and the criteria for HONcode accreditation

There are commonalities present in all of the guidelines. The following questions can be used to evaluate Internet sites for healthcare information.

Questions to ask when evaluating a site:

1.   Who runs the site?

Check the address (*Uniform Resource Locator* or URL) of the Web site. Government sites have *.gov* in the address, educational institutions have *.edu*, and professional sites have *.org*. Commercial sites have *.com* in the address. Commercial sites may exist for commercial reasons—to sell products—but many provide useful and balanced information. Go to the *"About Us"* page. The sponsor and the credentials of the people who run the site should be clearly identified. The site should also include a method for contacting the Webmaster or the people responsible for maintaining the site.

2.   Why have they created the site?

Identify the intended audience. Some sites have separate sections for both consumers and for health professionals, while other sites are designed exclusively for either health professionals or consumers.

3. Who is sponsoring the site? Does the information favor the sponsor?

   The Web site should disclose all financial relationships such as the source of funding for the site. Advertisements should be clearly labeled as such. Users should examine sites for balanced information that does not favor a sponsor.

4. Where did the information come from? Is the information reviewed by experts?

   Web sites should provide the credentials of contributors and the process for selecting information that is posted. Look for information on an editorial board, this can usually be found on the "About Us" page. Look for a statement that indicates that it is a peer-reviewed site. The information on the site should be presented clearly and should be factual not opinion.

5. Is it up to date?

   Web sites, especially those that provide health-related information, should be current and updated on a regular basis. Dates should be clearly posted.

6. What is the privacy policy?

   There should be a privacy policy posted on the site. Check the policy to see if information is shared. Do not provide personal information unless the privacy policy clearly states what information is and is not shared and you are comfortable with the policy (MLA, 2011; MEDLINEPlus, 2011).

The Health on the Net (HON) Foundation is a private organization that has created a code of conduct for medical and health Web sites (HONcode). It does not rate the quality of information but holds Web site developers to basic ethical standards in the presentation of information. Both APNs and patients can look for HONcode certification when searching for reliable Web sites. Certification is free of charge. All HONcode certified sites are reviewed annually. In addition to the annual review, the HON Foundation relies on users to report noncompliance with the HONcode and investigates complaints (HON Foundation, 2010). The HON Foundation code of conduct for medical and health Web sites can be found at *http://www.hon.ch/HONcode/Webmasters/Conduct.html*.

The Internet can be a very helpful tool for APNs and their patients to track and monitor progress or to explore alternative practices for the common goal of improving overall health. But both groups need to be vigilant when using the World Wide Web. APNs should provide their patients with a list of reliable health Web sites to visit, and patients should be encouraged to visit more than one site to check information. Patients can be taught to look for the seal of certification from an accrediting organization like the HON Foundation, and they need to be warned "to be careful not to believe claims or promises of miraculous cures, wonder drugs, and other extreme statements unless there is proof to these claims" (HON Foundation, 2010, para 8.). It is critical that APNs encourage patients to discuss anything they learn on the Internet with their healthcare provider and that they confirm that patients know how to evaluate medical and health Web sites.

USING TECHNOLOGY TO IMPROVE POPULATION HEALTH

New technologies are creating revolutionary changes in healthcare delivery and how healthcare information is communicated. Although new technologies are not universally available or put into practice, there is evidence that technology offers many possibilities for designing unique interventions to impact population outcomes. Published research provides examples of such technological interventions. One promising use of new technology is telehealth, which is being used by some healthcare providers who serve hard-to-reach populations. Preliminary evidence suggests that telehealth is promising as a way to increase access to populations in rural and underserved areas.

In an article by Wendel, Brossart, Elliot, McCord, and Diaz (2011), the authors describe a program to increase access to mental health services in a rural Texas community. They cite the many obstacles to rural health including limited healthcare resources and services and a shortage of healthcare professionals. They also recognized that travel time to medical clinics or hospitals was one barrier to accessing healthcare services for rural residents. Rural settings have significant health disparities compared to urban communities and one of the contributing factors is limited access to healthcare resources. They designed a program to counteract one such disparity by increasing access to mental health services in a rural community. The researchers used a collaborative effort to improve transportation to services and combined this with a telehealth-based counseling program staffed by doctoral students under the supervision of experienced faculty. After 18 months, the authors reported that 43 clients with a variety of mental health issues were provided with telehealth services for a total of 278 sessions. Their experience led them to conclude that telehealth is a promising method for providing care to hard-to-reach patients. The authors note that it is imperative that there is a mechanism for secure transmissions when technology is used to transmit communications between providers and patients. They also reported that technical difficulties during the study caused some interruption in services.

Protecting patient confidentiality and providing reliable services are hallmarks of good care. When planning services using advanced technologies, APNs need to be aware of both the benefits and the barriers. It is essential that experts in the use of technology are included as team members to help design new interventions that incorporate the use of technology.

In an article by Avdal, Kizilci, and Demirel (2011), the authors acknowledged transportation as a barrier to access to care in rural communities and in urban areas with poor public transportation. They explain that in Turkey, people with diabetes are monitored and treated in polyclinics, which provide outpatient services for a wide range of health conditions. Polyclinics can be problematic as they can be crowded and diabetic patients often cannot reach healthcare providers in a timely manner. In addition, people in Turkey frequently have to travel long distances to get to polyclinics, also causing problems with access. The result is that people with diabetes are frequently poorly monitored.

They designed a study to evaluate the use of telehealth in improving the outcomes of diabetic patients in Turkey. Approximately 25% of people in Turkey have access to the Internet. The researchers selected 122 people with type 2 diabetes who had access to the Internet and who had completed basic diabetes education and shared common situational characteristics. Of these, 61 were randomly assigned to the experimental group and 61 were randomly assigned to the control group. The control group received "usual care," that is, they could continue to use the polyclinic whenever they needed it. They were encouraged to participate in weekly group training classes and to get checkups every 3 months. The experimental group received the same instructions but in addition received Web-based diabetes education from the researcher. Frequently asked questions were posted on the Web site, and daily blood sugar monitoring could be viewed by both the researcher and the individual patients. Six months after the study began, checkups were statistically higher for the experimental group, while no changes were found in the control group. At the beginning of the study, hemoglobin A1c levels were similar in both groups. Six months after the study began, hemoglobin A1c levels were significantly lower in the experimental group, while no changes were detected in the control group. The authors were encouraged by the results and concluded that Web-based education is effective as a complementary tool to help patients manage their chronic health conditions (Avdal, Kizilci, & Demirel, 2011).

Access is not always a function of the physical distance between aggregates and healthcare providers. In some cases, patients can become socially isolated because of their physical or financial limitations. The following two studies provide examples of how Web-based technology has the potential to alleviate problems with access to services and to improve population outcomes.

Researchers have investigated the use of technology to enrich the environment of people who live in long-term care facilities. Tak, Beck, and McMahon (2007) describe the results of a study to examine the extent of computer use and Internet access of residents in a national chain of long-term care facilities. A second goal of the authors was to identify the benefits of and barriers to Internet access in nursing homes. A total of 64 nursing homes constituted the sample. In this study, 14% of the nursing homes provided computers for residents to use and 11% had Internet access. An average of one resident per nursing home owned a personal computer. On average, five residents per facility used the computers offered by the nursing homes, and most computers were located in a common area. The most popular computer applications were games (89%) and e-mail (67%). A small percentage of residents used educational programs and/or word processing programs. A survey of the nursing home administrators identified three major benefits to residents: mental stimulation, increased family contact, and enjoyment from playing games. Barriers identified by the administrators included limited motor ability, lack of knowledge or interest, and insufficient cognitive skills to learn how to use the computer. Finally, 80% of the nursing home administrators in this study expressed interest in making computers and Internet access more available to residents.

Oliver, Wittenberg-Lyles, Demiris, and Oliver (2010) carried out a project to engage residents in long-term care in "virtual" sightseeing. Their study was built on the work of earlier researchers who have demonstrated the positive effects of activity programs in long-term care facilities. The authors tested the feasibility of using live video conferencing to establish communication between residents in a long-term care facility in Iowa and researchers in Athens, Greece. The overall goal of the study was to "open the world of travel for residents confined in long-term care settings and to engage residents in 'virtual' sightseeing of foreign settings" (p. 93). These authors documented that the residents who took part in this feasibility study became clearly engaged in the activity. They noted that through technology, nursing homes can offer residents a way to explore the world outside of their usual environment, and they challenged researchers to build an evidence base to demonstrate the long-term value of this initiative on clinical outcomes for residents.

Demiris et al. (2008) explored the potential of using video phone technology to improve quality of life for long-term care residents and distant family members. The authors hypothesized that video phone contact could reduce the feeling of social isolation and loneliness of residents in long-term care settings. They also identified a need to explore the relationship between social presence and social support. Ten long-term care residents and six family members were selected for the study. Participants were asked to conduct video calls once each week for 3 months. After completion of the study, participants reported a sense of closeness during the calls and reduced feelings of guilt. Video conferencing may be useful in reducing feelings of isolation in long-term care patients and distant family members. The authors propose that technology can redefine the role of distant caregiving for residents and family members in long-term care facilities. These two studies offer tantalizing glimpses into the possibilities of using technology to enrich the lives of people in long-term care.

Studies have been conducted to determine the use of technology in improving specific population outcomes. Brandon, Schuessler, Ellison, and Lazenby (2009) conducted a study to "determine the effect of an advanced practice nurse (APN)–led telephone intervention on hospital readmissions, quality of life, and self-care behaviors (SCBs) of patients with heart failure (HF)" (p. e1). The sample for the study was drawn from one cardiology group and most of the patients in the study were from vulnerable populations such as low-income groups. Participants were randomly assigned to either the control group or the experimental group. The controls received "usual" care. Usual care was provided through a cardiology clinic and consisted of education provided by a physician or RN on topics of exercise, sodium intake, medication counseling, and when to call a physician. The experimental group was educated by an APN according to SCB guidelines. During the intervention period, seven telephone calls were made to each patient. Calls were made weekly for 2 weeks then every 2 weeks for 10 weeks. At the conclusion of the study, heart failure–related hospital readmissions and SCBs were significantly lower in the intervention group and quality of life measures also improved in this group. This study demonstrates both the potential usefulness of using phone calls to increase personal contacts between patients and healthcare providers and the role of the APN in improving population outcomes.

Fry and Neff (2009) completed a systematic review in 2008 "to investigate the effectiveness of limited contact interventions targeting weight loss, physical activity, and/or diet that provided periodic prompts regarding behavior change for health promotion" (para. 2). They defined periodic prompts as those that use technology such as the Internet to send messages to participants. Nineteen studies met the criteria for inclusion and of those 13 were randomized trials. Twelve of the studies used weekly prompts and two used prompts every 2 weeks. Thirteen used e-mails as prompts, and seven used online tools in addition to prompts. Eleven of the studies reported generally positive results, suggesting that periodic prompts may be useful as a tool in programs designed to improve the nutritional status of patients. Fry and Neff emphasize that using technology for prompts is an emerging field and that additional studies are needed to fully demonstrate the effectiveness of using this type of approach.

Personal health records (PHR) are a set of Internet tools that can be used by consumers to coordinate their personal health information. They are used by individuals to keep track of their complete health histories including treatments and current medications. The information is maintained online and is accessible to the individual consumer and healthcare providers who have been granted access. PHR facilitate the sharing of up-to-date and accurate health records between consumers and their healthcare providers. Yamin et al. (2011) conducted a cross-sectional study of PHR use in a single health system. They compared consumers who activated a PHR with people who were offered the opportunity but did not activate a PHR. They found that "despite increasing Internet availability, racial/ethnic minority patients adopted a PHR less frequently than white patients, and patients with the lowest annual income adopted a PHR less often than those with higher incomes" (p. 568). They recommended designing interventions to increase the use of PHR by populations who need them. This is yet another example of the digital divide in healthcare and further illustrates the need to be aware of disparities among groups and the need to find ways to increase access to technologically underserved populations.

E-health is a growing field. The Internet can be a very helpful tool for APNs and their patients to track and monitor progress or to explore alternative practices for the common goal, to improve overall health. Populations are best served when their needs are met using a variety of approaches. Information can be provided between health provider and patient via teleconferencing, Web casts, podcasting (delivery of audio, text, pictures, and/or video to a computer or mobile device), and twitter (text-based messages sent through a social networking site). Communication devices range from tabletop home computers and lap tops to tablet computers and mobile phones. The examples cited in this chapter provide a window into the opportunities open to APNs to be creative in using technology to improve patient outcomes. Inherent in the fact that this is a relatively new way to provide care, there is a dearth of literature on long-term follow-up and replication of studies. There are also barriers to the use of new technologies such as inadequate competency, a poor match between clinical needs and the availability of devices, privacy issues, system downtimes, and disparities among groups related to availability and use patterns. Assessing populations for their patterns of Internet usage and other technologies is an important part of the APN's role. Equally important is designing interventions that make use of new technologies and measuring the impact on relevant population outcomes. Further research is needed to fully evaluate the advantages and disadvantages of using technology in populations to improve health.

E-RESOURCES THAT SUPPORT POPULATION-BASED NURSING

There are many resources on the Internet that support population-based nursing. The following list of Web sites is meant to provide an example of the information and resources that are available. Neither the list nor the descriptions of the sites are meant to be exhaustive. The intent is to provide APNs with an idea of what is available within different categories of Web sites and to pique the interest of APNs so as to encourage them to explore these sites, and more, on their own.

Government Resources

Government sites (which have *.gov* in the URL as mentioned earlier) are a rich source of information and resources for both consumers and health care professionals.

U.S. Department of Health and Human Services (HHS)
http://www.hhs.gov/

The HHS is the U.S. government's principal agency for protecting the health of all Americans. It provides essential services (such as Medicare) and administers more grant dollars than all other federal agencies combined. The site has a wealth of information on diseases and conditions. An excellent example is *Healthfinder.gov* which provides easy-to-understand information for consumers to stay healthy. *The Quick Guide to Healthy Living* explains in simple language recommendations for health screenings and tests. There is even a link for people to help find a physician, health center, or public library. A new addition to the HHS site is *StopBullying.gov,* which provides information on how children, young adults, parents, and educators can recognize, prevent, or stop bullying. A table provides specific information on how and where to get help for bullying (*http://stopbullyingnow.hrsa.gov/*). Another recent initiative of the HHS is the National Partnership for Action. This initiative includes a Health Information Disparities Workgroup. The goal of this workgroup is to create projects to combat the digital divide (HHS, 2011).

Centers for Disease Control and Prevention (CDC)
http://www.cdc.gov/

The CDC is a U.S. government agency. Organizationally, it is under the HHS. Its mission is to "collaborate to create the expertise, information, and tools that people and communities need to protect their health—through health promotion, prevention of disease, injury and disability, and preparedness for new health threats" (CDC, 2011). The site contains a wealth of information for consumers, health professionals, policy makers, researchers, and educators. The CDC offers a wide variety of helpful resources for these groups including publications on many health and safety topics, podcasts, and RSS feeds (RSS is the acronym for *Really Simple Syndication*, which is used to publish recent works such as blog entries, news headlines, audio, and video in a standard format and can be sent electronically to subscribers). The site includes many useful tools such as photos, a BMI calculator, and slide presentations that can be used for educational purposes. The CDC also publishes *Emerging Infectious Diseases* (EID), *Morbidity and Mortality Weekly Report* (MMWR), and *Preventing Chronic Disease* (PCD). These publications are free of charge and can be subscribed to on the CDC site. Also available on this site are data on a large range of topics including FASTSTATS A-Z and trends in U.S. health statistics.

The National Institutes of Health (NIH)
http://nih.gov/

The NIH is a U.S. government agency. Like the CDC, it is under the HSS. Its mission is to "seek fundamental knowledge about the nature and behavior of living systems and the application of that knowledge to enhance health, lengthen life, and reduce the burdens of illness and disability" (NIH, 2011). Its primary purpose is to support research for improving the health of the nation. It provides a wealth of material for teachers and students alike on science and health topics. It offers everything from brochures to fact sheets and prepared slide presentations on many health and science topics. *NIH News* provides updated information on U.S. health trends.

FedStats
http://www.fedstats.gov

FedStats provides access to the full range of official statistical information produced by the Federal Government. It links to more than 100 agencies that provide data and trend information on such topics as diseases, demographics education, healthcare, and crime (FedStats, 2011).

Agency for Healthcare Research and Quality (AHRQ)
http://www.ahrq.gov/

The mission of the AHRQ "is to improve the quality, safety, efficiency, and effectiveness of health care for all Americans" (AHRQ, 2010). The AHRQ provides information on health so that consumers and healthcare providers can make informed decisions and provide quality healthcare. The information is designed to be useful to consumers, policy makers, healthcare providers, and employers. The site includes extensive information and resources such as information on funding opportunities for research, databases, research findings, and a health information technology (IT) information tool.

The National Guideline Clearinghouse (NGC)
http://www.guideline.gov/

The mission of the NGC "is to provide physicians and other health profession-als, healthcare providers, health plans, integrated delivery systems, purchasers, and others, an accessible mechanism for obtaining objective, detailed information on clinical practice guidelines and to further their dissemination, implementation, and use" (NGC, 2011). Healthcare providers can search the NGC site to obtain up-to-date guidelines for the provision of evidence-based care. Also available on the site are guidelines syntheses that provide a comparative analysis of guidelines for similar topics.

Let's Move!
http://www.letsmove.gov/

Obesity is a national issue and there are related online sites springing up all over the Internet. One excellent resource for consumers and APNs alike is *Let's Move*, the online site for First Lady Michelle Obama's campaign against obesity. Read-ers can learn how to prevent childhood obesity, find nutritional facts, get ideas for being active, and learn how you can help schools and communities serve healthier foods to children. *Let's Move* is on Facebook where individuals can share stories and ideas. There are also connections to Twitter and Meetup (a social networking site that facilitates group meetings among people with common interests and goals).

Educational Sites

Nongovernmental Web sites are also a source of excellent information for healthcare providers and consumers. Sites with *.edu* in the address are owned by educational institutions. Many universities, particularly those that offer health-related degrees, have extensive resources available for people who are looking for information on health-related topics. A fascinating glimpse into the history of nursing is provided by the History of Nursing Archives, which is part of the Howard Gotlieb Archival Research Center at Boston University.

History of Nursing Archives, Boston University
http://www.bu.edu/dbin/archives/index.php?pid=401&holdings=nursingarchive

The History of Nursing Archives includes a collection of personal and professional papers of many nursing leaders including 250 letters of Florence Nightingale's. There are also records of schools of nursing, public health and professional nursing organizations, histories of various American and foreign schools of nursing, and early textbooks (History of Nursing Archives, 2011). These materials provide a fascinating look at the early years of nursing and public health.

Institute of Medicine (IOM)
http://www.iom.edu/

The IOM is an independent, nonprofit organization that works to provide unbiased and authoritative advice on health-related topics. It is an arm of the National Academy of Sciences. Its mission is to "advise the nation on matters of health and medicine" (IOM, 2011). It undertakes specific mandates from Congress, federal agencies, and independent organizations. The site makes available a complete list of its reports published after 1998. One such report is "The Future of Nursing: Leading Change, Advancing Health," commissioned by the Robert Wood Johnson Foundation and published in 2010.

Professional Organizations

Professional membership organizations are usually run as not-for-profits and work to further the interests of a profession and to protect the public. They are generally a rich source of information on the healthcare professions. They generally have *.org* in the address. APNs should search their specialty organizations for resources and information.

American Nurses Association (ANA)
http://nursingworld.org/

The ANA (2011) is the professional organization for registered nurses in the United States. It has 51 constituent (state) member nurses associations and is affiliated with 24 specialty nursing and workforce advocacy affiliate organizations. It publishes standards of nursing practice for general RN nursing and nursing subspecialty practices. The ANA also lobbies Congress and regulatory agencies on healthcare issues affecting nurses and consumers. The ANA publishes *American Nurse Today* and the *Online Journal of Issues in Nursing* (OJIN). The OJIN is a peer-reviewed, online publication. Only members have access to current issues but archived issues are available to anyone. The ANA also distributes the RSS, *ANA SmartBrief*.

The ANA teamed with seven other organizations and launched an online resource for consumers in 2011. The site, HealthCareandYou.org (*http://www.healthcareandyou.org/*) outlines the provisions in the Affordable Care Act and breaks down the Act's benefits by state. Healthcare providers can use the site to obtain information that will be useful for explaining the key points of the Affordable Care Act to patients, and the language and format are kept clear and simple for easy use by consumers (*The American Nurse*, 2011).

The American Nurses Credentialing Center (ANCC) is a subsidiary of the ANA. It sets the standards for professional certification, accredits continuing nursing education, and created and oversees the Magnet Recognition Program. Standards for certification and accreditation are published on the Web site (*http://www.nursecredentialing.org/default.aspx*).

American Public Health Association (APHA)
http://apha.org/

Founded in 1872, the APHA is a diverse membership organization of public health professionals. Its goal is to "protect all Americans, their families and their communities from preventable, serious health threats and strives to ensure community-based health promotion and disease prevention activities and preventive health services are universally accessible in the United States" (APHA, 2011). Among its goals are to increase access to healthcare, protect funding for core public health services, and eliminate health disparities. It publishes the *American Journal of Public Health* and *The Nation's Health*. These publications are available free to members and to nonmembers by subscription.

Not-for-Profit Organizations

A nonprofit organization uses its earnings to pursue its goals and have controlling members or boards instead of owners. Some examples are the American Heart Association (AHA), the American Cancer Society (ACS), and the Asthma and Allergy Foundation of America (AAFA). Many of these sites have an impressive amount of information and resources that they make available to the public. Most of these groups have *.org* in their URLs.

American Heart Association (AHA)
http://www.heart.org/HEARTORG/

The AHA has an extensive and eclectic library of information and resources for educators at all levels, consumers, and healthcare professionals. The site includes downloadable lesson plans, risk assessment tools, and free application software (apps) such as the Walking Path Mobile app. The AHA develops guidelines and course materials for first aid, basic life support, and advanced life support courses.

American Cancer Society (ACS)
http://www.cancer.org/

Like the AHA, the ACS provides extensive information and resources to both consumers and healthcare professionals. Its site includes information on the latest research in cancer prevention and treatment, information and resources for specific cancer topics, information on side effects of different treatments for cancer, and information on funding and paying for treatment.

Asthma and Allergy Foundation of America (AAFA)
http://www.aafa.org/

The mission of the AAFA is to improve the quality of life for people with asthma and allergic diseases through education, advocacy, and research (AAFA, 2011). Examples of its extensive online resources are an online "allergy forecast tool," information on its asthma and allergy certification program, an "ask the allergist" online tool, and extensive educational resources on allergies and asthma.

International Organizations

There are many international organizations described throughout this book. Perhaps one of the most powerful and influential is the World Health Organization (WHO).

World Health Organization (WHO)
http://www.who.int/

WHO (2011) is an arm of the United Nations. It provides leadership on global health matters, technical support to countries, and monitors and assesses health trends. Its Web site includes a multilingual page with publications and resources in many languages and on various health topics, and another page with evidence-based guidelines. There is also current information on disease outbreaks and world health trends. WHO publishes the *World Health Report*, *World Health Statistics Report*, and information for international travelers. The multimedia site includes podcasts and videos on various health topics. WHO news can be accessed on Twitter and via RSS.

Commercial Sites

Although only one is listed here, there are many commercial sites that provide balanced and transparent information. Do not dismiss Web sites because *.com* is in the address. Use the information provided in this chapter to evaluate all Web sites.

Medscape
www.medscape.com

Medscape (2011) is an online, peer-reviewed resource for health professionals. It features peer-reviewed original articles and provides both continuing medical education (CME) and continuing nursing education contact hours (CH). It also offers a customized version of the National Library of Medicine's MEDLINE database, a drug interaction checker, drug reference, and has free, downloadable apps for health professionals. All content in Medscape is available free of charge for professionals and consumers alike, but registration is required. Review the Web site for information on copyright restrictions and privacy protection.

Analytic Software on the Internet

Epi Info (Centers for Disease Control and Prevention—CDC)
http://wwwn.cdc.gov/epiinfo/

Epi Info is a collection of software tools that are available for free download through the CDC Web site. It can be used to create questionnaires and download data, and allows the user to perform advanced statistical analyses and geographic information system (GIS) mapping. GIS is a technological tool that allows users to map trends in disease or outcomes of interest using such markers as zip codes or city boundaries, and to integrate data into a geographic map that summarizes data to assist users in identifying trends based on geographic location. In health care, mapping can be used to show the geographical distribution of specific factors such as obesity or cancer types. By mapping these factors, patterns of occurrence can be identified and specific areas can be targeted for intervention.

The Visual Statistics System (ViSta)
http://www.uv.es/visualstats/Book/

The ViSta is a free, downloadable statistical system. ViSta can be used to calculate both descriptive and inferential analytic analyses. It performs both univariate and multivariate analyses. Go to the Web site to learn how to use the program, but be sure to review the copyright restrictions prior to usage.

SUMMARY

Technological innovation has led to a whole new lexicon for healthcare providers and also has provided new methods and opportunities for improving population outcomes. E-mail alerts, RSS, podcasts, video conferencing, and Twitter are efficient and cost-effective ways to "keep connected" and to deliver healthcare information to both consumers and healthcare professionals. E-health provides a means to bridge distances between patients and healthcare providers and is a creative option for providing patient care. In the fast moving world of healthcare technology provides a convenient way to keep up to date. Software applications (apps) that can be downloaded to mobile devices and updated on a regular basis make available immediate and important information (such as drug interactions/calculations) to APNs and other healthcare providers.

To provide excellent and up-to-date clinical care, APNs need to be technologically literate and willing to explore new ways to deliver health care. APNs should evaluate their Internet and other technological resources carefully and use them to advance their practices to provide the latest evidence-based care possible. They also need to stay current in their knowledge of the latest technology and guide their patients to resources that are valid and useful.

EXERCISES AND DISCUSSION QUESTIONS

Exercise 6.1 Find a Web site that would be helpful to the population that you serve. Using a search engine such as Google or Yahoo, type in the name of a disease or condition that is associated with a population to whom you provide care. Eliminate the Web sites that you find in your search that contain either *.gov* or *.edu* in the address. Evaluate the remaining sites and identify at least two that meet criteria for reliability and transparency using the guidelines in this chapter.

Exercise 6.2 Online databases are a rich source of information for healthcare professionals. Use the following CDC database to research the state that you live or work in.
Go to: *http://www.cdc.gov/nccdphp/burdenbook2004/toc.htm*

■ What is the burden of chronic diseases in your state?
■ How do the leading causes of death in your state compare to U.S. figures?
■ Identify five important risk factors that need to be targeted in your state.
■ Identify vulnerable groups for whom targeted services need to be provided.

Exercise 6.3 Select one vulnerable group identified in Exercise 6.2 and identify an outcome for improvement. Design an interventional study that incorporates the use of technology to improve that outcome.

REFERENCES

Agency for Healthcare Research and Quality (AHRQ) At A Glance. (2010). AHRQ Publication No. 09-P003, September 2010. Rockville, MD: Agency for Healthcare Research and Quality. http://www.ahrq.gov/about/ataglance.htm

American Association of Colleges of Nursing (AACN). (2006). *The essentials of doctoral education for advanced practice nursing.* Retrieved from http://www.aacn.nche.edu/DNP/pdf/Essentials.pdf

American Nurses Association. (2011). Retrieved from http://nursingworld.org/

American Public Health Association. (2011). Retrieved from http://apha.org/

Asthma and Allergy Foundation of America. (2011). Retrieved from http://www.aafa.org/index.cfm

Avdal, U., Kizilci, S., & Demirel, N. (2011). The effects of web-based diabetes education on diabetes care results: A randomized control study. *CIN: Computers, Informatics, Nursing,* 29(2), 101–106. 29TC29-34. doi:10.1097/NCN.0b013e3182155318

Brandon, A. F., Schuessler, J. B., Ellison, K. J., & Lazenby, R. B. (2009). The effects of an advanced practice nurse led telephone intervention on outcomes of patients with heart failure. *Applied Nursing Research, 22,* el–e7. Retrieved from EBSCOhost.

Centers of Disease Control and Prevention. (2011). *Vision, mission, core values, and pledge.* Retrieved from http://www.cdc.gov/about/organization/mission.htm

Demiris, G., Parker Oliver, D. R., Hensel, B., Dickey, G., Rantz, M., & Skubic, M. (2008). Use of videophones for distant caregiving: An enriching experience for families and residents in long-term care. *Journal of Gerontological Nursing, 34*(7), 50–55.

England, C. Y., & Nicholls, A. M. (2004). Advice available on the Internet for people with coeliac disease: An evaluation of the quality websites. *Journal of Human Nutrition and Dietetics, 17,* 547–559.

FedStats. (2011). Retrieved from http://www.fedstats.gov/

Fry, J., & Neff, R. (2009). Periodic prompts and reminders in health promotion and health behavior interventions: Systematic review. *Journal of Medical Internet Research, 11*(2), e16. Retrieved from EBSCO*host*.

Health on the Net Foundation. (2010). *The HON code of conduct for medical and health Web sites (HONcode).* Retrieved from http://www.hon.ch/HONcode/Webmasters/Conduct.html

History of Nursing Archives. (2011). Retrieved from http://www.bu.edu/dbin/archives/index.php?pid=401&holdings=nursingarchive

Holland, M. L., & Fagnano, M. (2008). Appropriate antibiotic use for acute otitis media: What consumers find using web searches. *Clinical Pediatrics, 47*(5), 452–456.

Institute of Medicine. (2011). Retrieved from http://www.iom.edu/Default.aspx?id=8089

Internet World Stats. (2010). *Usage and population statistics.* Retrieved from http://www.internetworldstats.com/stats.htm

McDaid, D., & Park, A. (2010). *Online health: Untangling the web.* Retrieved from http://www.bupa.com/healthpulse

Medical Library Association. (2011). *For health consumers.* Retrieved from http://www.mlanet.org/

MedlinePlus. (2011). *Evaluating internet health informatin: A tutorial from the national library of medicine.* Retrieved from http://www.nlm.nih.gov/medlineplus/webeval/webeval.html

Medscape. (2011). Retrieved from www.medscape.com

National Guideline Clearinghouse. (2011). Retrieved from: http://www.guideline.gov/

National Institutes of Health. (2011). Retrieved from http://nih.gov/

National Library of Medicine. (2011). *Health information.* Retrieved from http://www.nlm.nih.gov/hinfo.html

New website helps consumers understand health care law. (2011, March/April). *The American Nurse.*

Oliver, D. P., Wittenberg-Lyles, E., Demiris, G., & Oliver, D. (2010). Giving long-term care residents a passport to the world the Internet. *Journal of Nursing Care Quality, 25*(3), 193–197.

Pew Research Center. (2008). *Pew internet & American life project.* Retrieved from http://www.pewinternet.org/Reports/2009/8-The-Social-Life-of-Health-Information.aspx

Pew Research Center. (2011a). *Peer to peer healthcare.* Retrieved from http://www.pewinternet.org/~/media//Files/Reports/2011/Pew_P2PHealthcare_2011.pdf

Pew Research Center. (2011b). *Social media and young adults.* Retrieved from http://www.pewinternet.org/Reports/2010/Social-Media-and-Young-Adults/Part-4/1-Online-health-information.aspx?r=1

Schembri, G., & Schober, P. (2009). The Internet is a diagnostic aid: The patient's perspective. *International Journal of STD and AIDS, 20,* 231–233.

Schwartz, K. L., Roe, T., Northrup, J., Meza, J., Seifeldin, R., & Neale, A. V. (2006). Family medicine patients' use of the Internet for health information: A MetroNet study. *The Journal of the American Board of Family Medicine, 19*(1), 39–45.

Stone, T., & Jumper, J. (2001). Information about age-related macular degeneration on the Internet. *Southern Medical Journal, 94*(1), 22–25. Retrieved from EBSCO*host*.

Tak, S. H., Beck, C., & McMahon, E. (2007). Computer and Internet access for long-term care residents: Perceived benefits and barriers. *Gerontological Nursing, 33*(5), 32–40.

Underhill, C., & Mckeown, L. (2008). Getting a second opinion: Health information and the Internet. *Health Reports/Statistics Canada, Canadian Centre For Health Information = Rapports Sur La Santé/Statistique Canada, Centre Canadien D'information Sur La Santé, 19*(1), 65–69. Retrieved from EBSCOhost. http://www.californiahealthline.org/features/2011/wellness-cost-cutting-main-themes-at-health-2-0-spring-event.aspx#

U.S. Department of Health and Human Services (HHS). (2011). Retrieved from http://www.hhs.gov/

Weitzman, E. R., Cole, E., Kaci, L., & Mandl, K. (2011). Social but safe? Quality and safety of diabetes-related online networks [EPUB]. *Journal of American Medical Informatics Association*.

Wendel, M. L., Brossart, D. F., Elliot, T. R., McCord, C., & Diaz, M. A. (2011). Use of technology to increase access to mental health services in a rural Texas community. *Family and Community Health, 34*(2), 134–140.

World Health Organization. (2011). Retrieved from http://www.who.int/en/

Yamin, C. K., Emani, S., Williams, D. H., Lipsitz, S. R., Karson, A. S., Wald, J. S., & Bates, D. W. (2011). The digital divide in adoption and use of a personal health record. *Archives of Internal medicine, 17*(6), 568–574.

SEVEN

Concepts in Program Design and Development

Susan B. Fowler

Graduates of doctoral education for advanced nursing practice are expected to integrate nursing science with knowledge from other fields in order to provide the highest level of nursing care. They are also expected to develop and provide effective plans for "practice level and/or system-wide practice initiatives that will improve the quality of care delivery" (AACN, 2006, p. 11). In this chapter, the advanced practice nurse (APN) will learn how to design new programs by addressing factors related to planning and organizational decision making.

Nurse leaders are instrumental in using data to make decisions that lead to program development, implementation, and evaluation. Data used to drive decision making must be accurate, pertinent, and timely in order to be applied appropriately when designing a program. It is critical that a program be constructed in a way that takes into consideration all components that impact that program both internally and externally. Determining measures of success or desired outcomes when designing a program provides continuous check points for evaluation throughout program implementation. Program development, implementation, and evaluation will vary across geographic and practice settings because of the unique and varied characteristics of an APN's practice.

CONSUMER AND SOCIETAL TRENDS AND DEMANDS

Consumer and societal trends and demands provide information or data that drive the rationale for designing a specific program. It is not cost effective to support a program that does not meet an identified consumer need. A simple dictionary definition of a trend is the general direction in which something tends to move. In what direction is healthcare technology moving? In what direction are consumer attitudes and beliefs about disease prevention moving? Consumer and societal trends and demands are constantly changing, making it difficult to know to which trends or demands to pay attention and if they will continue and for how long. For example, in January of 2010, the following 10 trends were identified by Health Care Technology Online: (a) electronic medical record, (b) personal health record, (c) cost containment, (d) alternative care models, (e) Medicare fraud, (f) outbreak preparedness, (g) patient safety, (h) short supply of healthcare professionals, (i) storage and business continuity regarding data, and (j) physician groups joining healthcare systems for better access to technology. (Health Care Technology Online 2010). Did these trends continue in 2011? Will they continue through 2015? Is a program designed in 2010 based on these trends still needed and viable in 2011? Will it be needed in 2015? It is critical for APNs to examine on an ongoing basis the environment in which they practice to confirm the latest trends and demands or identify new ones.

Population demographics provide direction for population-based programs. Communities have their own unique identifying characteristics including age and racial and ethnic diversity. A program targeting the administration of influenza vaccines during influenza season may look different when implemented in an urban area such as New York City versus a rural community such as farmlands in Wisconsin. National information on changing population demographics and implications for healthcare providers can be obtained from national Web sites such the U.S. Department of Health and Human Services (DHHS) or the Centers for Disease Control and Prevention (CDC).

A starting point for developing a new program might originate in an organization where an APN is employed and can examine data that are already collected and easily accessible. For example, if designing a transitional care program from hospital to home it would be critical to gather information on the number of hospital discharges, number of discharges to home and/or other facilities (e.g., rehabilitation, nursing homes, etc.), demographics of clients discharged home, primary discharge diagnoses, rehospitalization rate, and time from discharge to rehospitalization. Review of the available data might reveal that there is a need for transitional programs for patients with certain diagnoses. Perhaps readmission rates for patients with heart failure are higher in the APN's facility compared to national benchmarks and that the rates are trending upward. Examination of the patient population (e.g., patient demographics, absence of insurance, access to a medical home, paucity of subspecialists, etc.) and processes involved in discharge and readmission can help guide the APN in developing a program to reduce the readmission rates while recognizing the characteristics of the patient population that may be contributing to the increase in these rates. A complete assessment of patient/consumer needs and characteristics and comparisons of population outcomes against standard benchmarks provide necessary information for the planning of new programs.

PROGRAM DEVELOPMENT

Justification

Justification for a program helps determine if it is reasonable or necessary. Information gained from investigating consumer and societal trends and demands contributes to this justification. If a program makes sense, nurse leaders have ammunition to argue their case. Justifying a program requires an understanding of and quantification of the planned scope of the program. Producing a well defined set of expectations and value propositions will make key stakeholders feel confident about approving and funding a program. The identification of a trend (such as increasing readmission rates for a particular population) is one justification for a program especially when the trend leads to increasing costs or morbidity/mortality. In addition, a literature search might reveal evidence that transitional programs for patients with heart failure are successful in preventing readmissions. Heart failure is the most costly diagnosis in the 65-year-old and older Medicare population (Sherwood et al., 2011). Several health indicators (including the readmission rates of patients with heart failure) are recognized as important indicators of poor quality of healthcare and are publicly reported through the Agency for Healthcare Research and Quality (AHRQ, 2004) in the Department of Health and Human Services.

Once a program is conceived and a literature review is completed, it is important to consider if the program is feasible. A feasibility study helps to frame the program structure and identify potential risks associated with the program. Basic questions need to be addressed and answered, such as:

- Are other programs in place that serve a similar purpose?
- Are there other alternatives to the proposed program?
- Is the program economically feasible?
- Does the program make financial sense? Constructing a cost-benefit table such as the one below can be used to list factors to consider when assessing economic feasibility.

	POTENTIAL COSTS	POTENTIAL BENEFITS
QUANTITATIVE		
QUALITATIVE		

- Is the program technically feasible?
- Is the program operationally feasible to implement?
- Is it possible to maintain and support the program once it is implemented?

Designing a program is different than implementing it; therefore, nurse leaders must determine whether or not the program can be effectively operated and supported. Critical issues need to be considered.

OPERATIONAL ISSUES	SUPPORT ISSUES
• What tools are needed to support the program? • What skills training does staff need? • What procedures or processes need to be created and/or updated?	• What support staff will be needed? • What program materials will staff use? • What training will staff be provided? • How will changes be managed?

▪ Is the program politically feasible considering strategic goals and administrative directives? Nurse leaders must be cognizant of the political landscape surrounding the program.
▪ Will the program be allowed to succeed?

The Centers for Medicare and Medicaid Services (CMS) have announced plans to tie reimbursement to certain key quality indicators. Readmission rates within 30 days for heart failure is one targeted indicator. Beginning in 2012, hospitals that are above the national average for 30-day readmission rates will see a decreased reimbursement rate of 1%, which will increase by 1% each year that the hospital is above the national average. Improving readmission rates makes good financial sense. The APN should assess the community to determine if other, similar programs exist that would compete with the proposed program, or if the proposed program could be built into an existing program. If a hospital has an existing community outreach department, the APN could use the existing structure to house a new program. In summary, justification of a program can be strengthened significantly by providing sound evidence such as a thorough review of the literature to establish the background of the problem and by examining current successful programs that may be applicable to the APN's population of interest. Additionally, following trends by using outcome measures that can be compared to national quality indicators as benchmarks that are followed over time with a goal to improve patient outcomes and cost savings is another successful approach to justifying a program. And finally, determining if the program is feasible will further strengthen the justification, as feasibility studies provide a systematic framework in which a program can be assessed and thoughtfully implemented or integrated into current practice.

Identification of Key Stakeholders and Players

Stakeholders

The term stakeholder is commonly used in the business arena and refers to a person, group, or organization that has a direct or indirect stake in an organization because they can affect or be affected by the organization's actions, objectives, and policies. The effect can either be positive or negative. Nurse leaders strive for stakeholders seeking positive effects who will support and facilitate successful program implementation and not thwart efforts. Furthermore, stakeholders can be internal and external, but in either case, there is a synergistic two-way relationship between the organization and its program and the stakeholders.

A list of questions can guide identification of key stakeholders:

■ Who will be affected by the program?
■ Who can influence the program but not be directly involved in its development, implementation, and evaluation?
■ What group is interested in the program's success and outcomes?
■ Who will be or could be impacted by the program?

There are many stakeholders in healthcare but there are five important and powerful stakeholders who should not be ignored: patients or clients, medical staff, agency management, professional staff, and the Board of Directors or Trustees. Think broadly when determining key stakeholders and also consider government agencies, professional groups or associations, present and prospective employees, local communities, the national community, the public-at-large, suppliers, competitors, the media, and future generations.

There may be considerable overlap of stakeholders' expectations including healthcare quality, support or adequacy of resources, and costs in terms of cost reduction and profitability. Publicly reported indicators impact consumers' image of a hospital's quality of care. The Board of Trustees may be concerned with the organization's image, which can directly impact a consumer's decision about where to seek care—or a physician's decision about where to admit patients.

The power or influence of stakeholders can vary as a result of the organizational makeup and the stakeholders' philosophy and values. Values drive needs and when a needs assessment is performed to justify a program, values should be addressed because expectations often arise from values. Understanding expectations of stakeholders and considering expectations when designing a program can result in stakeholder satisfaction and program success. The identification of program outcomes that stakeholders value can help win their support. Healthcare organizations have mission statements that reflect organizational values and, in many cases, these statements reflect the value placed on the development of community programs.

Key Players

Who are the key players in the program? The lead key player is the program administrator or manager. There are common responsibilities in this role, regardless of industry or setting, that include the following:

■ Identifies, researches, and solves program issues effectively.
■ Identifies the resources required for a program's success.
■ Oversees and directs team members.
■ Performs team assessment and evaluation.

- Recognizes areas for improvement and develops action plans.
- Documents and communicates operation of the program.
- Ensures that the program complies with standards, regulations, and procedures.
- Plans and sets timelines for program goals, milestones, and deliverables.

Makeup of the program team will depend upon the scope of the program. There are basically two types of staff involved in a program: (a) individuals providing direct program services and (b) staff that support direct providers and program implementation. The type of staff members needed to provide direct program services and how many depend upon the nature of services provided and number of program locations. The same is true for the type and number of support staff needed for program implementation and evaluation.

Regardless of the number and type of team members, the program manager or administrator plays a critical role in building a successful team. A team that is effective and focused contributes to the success of the program. A useful framework for building successful teams is described best by the acronym "together (T) everyone (E) achieves (A) more (M)." The origins of the model are difficult to trace, but its concepts are sound and used by many. Successful teambuilding requires attention to the following:

- Clear communication of expectations
- Team members' understanding of why they are participating on the team
- Commitment
- Competence
- Understanding of the program charter
- Control or sense of ownership
- Collaboration
- Communication
- Creative thinking
- Awareness of positive and negative consequences
- Coordination
- A cultural shift that is team-based, empowering, and enabling.

Stakeholders, team leaders, and team players all play a critical role in the success and/or failure of a program. Each member has a role and an expectation based on the anticipated outcome of a new program. Values sometimes play a role and it is important to share these values and address them early on to ensure success. Ultimately, commitment, communication, and collaboration are some of the most important characteristics a team requires for a successful program.

Structure

Program structure can be as simple or complex as desired as long as specific outcome measures and sustainability are considered in the planning phase. APNs must be careful when employing complex approaches to program structure as complex designs can lead to failure if discrete outcomes are not easily measured or if too many measures or variables are being studied. For example, a simple approach might structure the program around the following six areas:

1. WHAT
    *   What is the title of the program?
    *   What is the focus of the program?
    *   What are the goals of the program?
    *   What are the objectives of the program?
    *   What outcomes will be measured?
    *   What is the budget for the program?
    *   What is the timeline for program development, implementation, and evaluation?

2. WHERE
    *   Where will the program take place?
    *   Where is the program's base location?
    *   Where will staff be housed?
    *   Where will supplies or resources for the program be stored?

3. WHO
    *   Who are the stakeholders?
    *   Who is in charge of the program?
    *   Who are the staff members involved in program development, implementation, and/or evaluation?
    *   Who is the program attempting to reach?
    *   Who will fund this program?

4. WHEN
    *   When will the program be implemented?
    *   When will the program end?

5. WHY
    *   Why is the program needed (justification)?
    *   Why might the program succeed or fail?

6. HOW
    *   How will data be collected?
    *   How often will data be collected?
    *   How often will outcomes be examined?
    *   How will the program be developed? Implemented? Evaluated?
    *   How will the program sustain its funding or obtain future funding?
    *   How will the program's success be determined?

This structure is the "skeleton" on which a program can be designed and can serve as a reference when planning resources, budgets, staffing, and operational procedures. A program's structure consists of the program's goals and objectives, which follow directly from strategic planning. The plan should include a description of the resources needed to achieve the goals and objectives including necessary funding. A major component of these resources may include human resources described in terms of required skills and scope of practice. Technical resources for data, including its analysis and storage, will need to be considered when designing a program budget. Initial budget proposals for new programs usually estimate costs in broad categories. Final program budgets require careful attention to all aspects of program planning, implementation, and evaluation and should estimate yearly costs as closely as possible. Funding is determined after a program budget is created. The source may be a state or federal grant, or it may be self-financed through health insurance held by consumers or a combination of funding sources. Whatever the source (or sources) for financing costs, a method of funding must be identified before the program can move forward.

Outcomes

Outcomes are often defined by regulatory, governmental, or certifying agencies such as the Joint Commission, the AHRQ, and the American Nurses Credentialing Center (ANCC). The AHRQ, for example, has identified readmission rates (within 30 days) for patients with heart failure as an outcome measure of quality of care. The Joint Commission defines an outcome measure as the end result of a function or process in a patient population over a set period of time, often expressed as a rate or percentage.

The ANCC manages the Magnet designation program and describes outcomes as results, impacts, or consequences of actions. Agencies that have received the Magnet designation or are seeking it must compare data collected for a specific outcome against cohort groups at national levels and demonstrate that the majority of nursing units or practice arenas outperform the national benchmarks the majority of the time (ANCC, 2006).

Before establishing outcomes, one must revisit the mission and objectives of the program. What does the program do? Why does the program exist? Outcomes are the measurable results of the program objectives. They provide a method of evaluating the success of a program. State and national statistics can be used as benchmarks when examining outcomes. Comparisons to quality indicators (discussed in Chapter 2) can also serve as benchmarks to evaluate success or progress in a program. Outcomes should be established for short-term, intermediate, and long-term objectives. The mnemonic SMART provides a template for writing such objectives (CDC, 2011).

- *Specific*: The outcome is well defined and unambiguous.
- *Measurable*: Concrete methods and criteria for assessing progress are used.
- *Achievable:* The goal stretches you, but is reasonable given the program's resources and sphere of influence. Reasonable goals and objectives must be motivational; they should provide incentives for success of program staff and stakeholders.

■ *Relevant:* The outcome must be relevant to the program's vision, mission, and goals. Outcomes must also be relevant to all people affiliated with or impacted by the program.

■ *Time-framed:* The time period for accomplishing goals and evaluating outcomes is reasonable.

Outcomes can be incremental and subtle. Trying to turn personal or subjective experiences into concrete, specific, observable measures can be a daunting task. Hence, both quantitative and qualitative outcomes may be helpful and necessary.

Impact is another tool to measure program success in recent years. It uses qualitative and quantitative measures to establish its success by looking at broad-based outcomes. It is viewed in broader terms and is less specific than outcomes. *Impact* is defined as the difference in the changes in outcomes between those involved with the program and those not involved (Baker, 2000). It is the evaluation of the effects, both positive and negative, caused by a program. Impact evaluation is an effort to determine in broad terms, whether a program has the desired effects on individuals, households, and institutions, and whether those effects are attributed to the interventions associated with the program. The following are examples of how the *impact* of a transitional program for heart failure patients to reduce readmission rates might be articulated in quantitative and qualitative expressions:

■ Within 1 year of the inception of the program, the hospital's heart failure readmission rate was reduced and outperformed the national benchmark.

■ In a recent 10-month tracking period, more than 20 patients successfully completed the program.

■ A patient's wife describes its value this way: "Thank you so much for your excellent program! I sincerely believe you and your team deserve an award for excellence in patient care. I don't know what we would have done without your support and guidance."

■ The personal impact of the program and its professional staff is acknowledged by one participant "…the staff helped me realize I was not eating as well as I should and got me moving in the right direction. Also, I noticed that when I eat so many fruits and vegetables, I don't have room for so much junk food. Before this program I didn't realize how much salt was in the food I was eating."

Program outcomes illustrate what you want your program to do. Outcomes should provide information that can be used for quality improvement. After defining program outcomes, consider applying the following questions as a critique:

■ Is it clear what the program is assessing?
■ Is the outcome measurable?
■ Is the intended outcome measuring something useful and meaningful?
■ How will the outcome be measured?
■ Are the outcomes realistic for the time frame of the program?

Outcome data can be collected continuously throughout program implementation or at specific points in time, such as quarterly, or at the completion of a particular time-limited program.

When designing programs, outcome measures must be clear, concise, measurable, and easily compared to quality indicators when possible. They should be realistic and time delimited. Evaluation of the impact of a program can also be helpful when dealing with qualitative and quantitative measures. In summary, the outcomes selected should show the progress (or ineffectiveness) of a program and allow for objective evaluation.

Policies and Procedures

Well-designed policies and procedures (P&P) should document structure, processes, and outcomes and are essential for a successful program. They ensure compliance, manage risks, and drive improvement. P&P help describe the program—the way business is done, how situations are handled—provide legal protection, mandate compliance, and guide consistent performance. A program does not need a policy for every contingency, thus providing more latitude in operations. When developing P&P, the APN should consider the following:

- Writing of the P&P
- Providing administrative support and possible legal review.
- Reviewing and discussing of the P&P with the program staff.
- Ensuring P&P are supported by evidence.
- Interpreting and integrating the policies and procedures into program practices.
- Ensuring compliance with the P&P.

Using the earlier example, if a program was designed for transitioning patients with heart failure from hospital to home, it would require a review of the literature to determine evidence-based strategies that have been used by other organizations to prevent or delay readmissions. Program planners would also need to review state and federal regulations related to important factors such as reimbursement for services and zoning requirements for program facilities. The synthesis of evidence would provide a framework for development of P&P for clinical services and program implementation.

A carefully constructed P&P manual is critical for program success. It can be modeled after evidence-based protocols and can provide the framework for consistent training of staff and community outreach workers. P&P also serve as a guideline for staff to follow to ensure delivery of quality care and consistent practices in the program.

Marketing

The American Marketing Association (2011) defines marketing as "the activity, set of institutions, and processes for creating, communicating, delivering, and exchanging offerings that have value for customers, clients, partners, and society at large." Marketing involves activity and is not passive. It is a group effort involving a variety of individuals and groups, internal and external to the program or organization.

Marketing is process driven. Without processes, nurse leaders cannot plan effectively and can have difficulty determining what is working and what is not. A well-mapped out process is critical for success. Marketing is not advertising. Advertising is only one part of marketing. Market research is done through the identification of consumer and societal trends and demands.

Marketing is delivering on the promise made to key stakeholders. At the very least, the promise needs to be delivered. A nurse leader acting as a marketer can impress program customers and achieve desired outcomes.

The concept of "positioning" can be applied to a nurse-led program. Positioning is how you differentiate your program from the competition and present your brand in the marketplace. Positioning happens in one place—in the mind of the consumer—and occurs in a moment. You have to get the attention of the consumer who become interested in your program. The consumer will spend energy evaluating your program in relation to others and will make a choice to participate in your program or not. Ask yourself the following questions related to the concept of positioning (McNamara, 2010):

- Who is the target market?
- Who are the competitors for the program?
- What should be considered when setting the logistics of the program including costs?
- What should be considered when naming the program?

Marketing is an important component to consider in program design and development. It is not only important to be aware of your competitors but also to be aware of what will appeal to your audience (e.g., potential participants). A strong marketing campaign can lead to long-term successes not only for your program but future programs. Stakeholders will see the value in a well-constructed marketing plan, which ultimately is important for program sustainability.

Communication

If a tree falls in the forest, but no one is around to hear it fall, does it make a sound? This question highlights a realistic problem when communicating about a program. You may have the best program in the world, but if you do not communicate the benefits and features of the program to the right audience, how are consumers going to find out about it? How are stakeholders and program team members going to buy into the program?

Communication consists of a sender, a receiver, and a medium. Communication is important to marketing a program and can come in many forms. Consider the following basic questions when engaging in strategies to communicate about a program.

- Who will be responsible for communicating information about the program?
- What is the message being communicated?
- Who is the intended recipient of the communication?

The medium for the message can include verbal and nonverbal communication. Verbal communication may include word of mouth, telephone voice messages, and presentations at meetings. Communication through nonverbal means includes ads in newspapers, information on an organization's Web site, newsletters, posters, text messages, and e-mails.

Programs are successful only if they have participation of the target population. There must be buy-in by its members and without effective communication by a variety of modalities, this message may never reach the intended population. As noted earlier, there are verbal and nonverbal forms of communication; verbal communication is probably the most effective for some populations as the value of face-to-face interaction and relationship building cannot be replaced using nonverbal methods. With that said, many of these forms of communication require an investment of time and money, and these costs need to be included in the program budget.

Models for Program Design

The Logic Model

The *Logic Model*, developed by the W. K. Kellogg Foundation (2004), is commonly cited in the literature as a model for program planning. The model is used in program evaluation but is also useful and appropriate for program planning and management. It is a tool used to help shape a program. Additionally, logic models help leaders identify factors that may impact a program and enable them to forecast needed data and resources to achieve success. A logic model is a graphic display or "map" depicting the relationship among resources, activities, and intended results that identify underlying theory and assumptions.

The Logic Model is aligned with the scientific method. Just as an hypothesis is tested in research, program objectives are tested through program development, implementation, monitoring, and evaluation. The following steps outline the Logic Model program planning—clarifying program theory:

- Describe the problem(s) your program is attempting to solve or the issue(s) your program will address.
- Specify the needs and/or assets of your community that led your program to address the problem(s) or issue(s).
- Identify desired results by describing what you expect to achieve, short and long term.
- List factors you believe will influence change in the population or community.
- List successful strategies or "best practices" your research identified that helped address the targeted population and achieved results your program hopes to achieve.
- State assumptions underlying how and why the identified program will work.

The Logic Model provides a focus for leaders to articulate and clarify program progress. Goals are easily identified and assigned responsibilities for tasks and outcomes are clearly communicated. Key stakeholders and players visually see their roles and accountability. As a result, collaboration and communication are enhanced.

Lane and Martin (2005) have described the successful use of the Logic Model by three APNs in designing and evaluating a breast health program for rural, underserved women. According to the authors, "The Logic Model was most useful in outlining the program, guiding the first year, and identifying needed direction for the future of the program. It was at the heart of the program development and served as the visual schemata" (p. 110). A diagram of the completed Logic Model for this program can be found in Figure 7.1.

Developing a Framework or Model of Change

Another approach, built on the Logic Model and incorporating best processes from the literature that guides the development of programs to promote community change and improvement, is referred to as *Developing a Framework or Model of Change* (Community Toolbox, 2011). This model is an innovation of Community Toolbox, a public service of the University of Kansas. Community Toolbox is an online resource that provides information to people who are interested in promoting community health and development. Developing a Framework or Model of Change provides a road map for creating a new program by outlining the relationships among inputs such as resources, outputs or the proposed interventions, impact (i.e., immediate results), and outcomes including community or behavioral change. It is a 12-step process that organizes thinking and orients program development by intended outcomes. The steps include the following:

- Analyzing information about the problem or goal
- Establishing a vision or mission
- Defining organizational structure and operating mechanisms
- Developing a framework or model of change
- Developing and using action plans
- Arranging for community mobilizers
- Developing leadership
- Implementing effective interventions
- Ensuring technical assistance
- Documenting progress and using feedback
- Making outcomes matter
- Sustaining the work

Activities outlined in the Developing a Framework or Model of Change process can assist nurse leaders in bringing together diverse people to summarize collective thinking in an organized manner. As a result, a common understanding is created and commitment enhanced. Additionally, these steps, together, set the stage for strategic action with the likelihood of comprehensive interventions reflective of experience and research. Organized thinking through the Developing a

Define the problem.	Some rural women in the region lack knowledge about and access to malignancy screening techniques.

↓

Identify the intervention.	Create a model-based program to meet the malignancy screening needs of women in a rural community.

↓

State the goal.	Increase the knowledge and practice of malignancy screening techniques and increase linkages for rural women in this region by creating a cancer health network with initial focus on breast health.

↓

Outline key objectives.	1. Develop the infrastructure for the cancer heath network and establish linkages. 2. Provide annual screening opportunities, including education and referral information. 3. Identify and secure ongoing funding for the cancer health network to sustain annual screening.

↓

Determine desired outcomes.	1. Increase awarness of early detection screening techniques by rural women. 2. Increase the screening resource (i.e., access to and finances for) in the geographic area. 3. Increase community support for screening activities. 4. Stabilize a recognized program for providing the screening activities. 5. Track demographic data and screening results of the women participating in the program. 6. Disseminate the knowledge gained.

FIGURE 7.1   Logic Model.

Source: Lane, A., & Martin, M. (2005). Logic model use for breast health in rural communities. Oncology Nursing Forum, 32(1), 106. ONS disclaims any responsibilities for inaccuracies in words or meaning that may occur as a result of translation from English.

Framework or Model of Change approach results in a clear rationale for programs, which can facilitate funding opportunities, guide support staff, and direct the identification of outcomes and data collection. Using and developing best practices ensures that interventions will have the desired impact on outcomes and, more importantly, advance the science of healthcare. Several examples of how the model has been used to plan, develop, implement, and evaluate successful community programs are available on their online site (http://ctb.ku.edu/).

The Precede-Proceed Model

The *PRECEDE-PROCEED Model* of health program planning and evaluation is another design model evolved at Johns Hopkins University based on work by Green and Kreuter (1992). It is founded on epidemiological principles; social, behavioral, and educational sciences; and health administration. There are two fundamental propositions underlying this model: (a) health and health risks are caused by multiple factors, and (b) because of this, efforts to impact change must be multidimensional. The goals of the model are twofold: (a) to explain health-related behaviors and environments and (b) to design and evaluate interventions that influence both behaviors and the environment. The model is a continuous cycle. Information gathered in the PRECEDE steps drive actions in the PROCEED process, which in turn provide additional information for the PRECEDE process.

PRECEDE (*Predisposing, Reinforcing, and Enabling Constructs in Educational Diagnosis and Evaluation*) outlines the planning process that aids in the development of targeted and focused programs. PRECEDE consists of five steps:

1. Determine population needs.
2. Identify health determinants of these needs.
3. Analyze behaviors and environmental determinants of health needs.
4. Outline factors that predispose, reinforce, or enable behaviors.
5. Ascertain interventions best suited to change behaviors.

PROCEED (*Policy, Regulatory, and Organizational Constructs in Educational and Environmental Development*) guides program implementation and evaluation. PROCEED is a four-step process.

1. Implement interventions.
2. Evaluate interventions.
3. Evaluate the impact of the interventions on factors that supported the behavior as well as the behavior itself.
4. Evaluate outcomes.

Ahmed, Fort, Elzey, and Bailey (2004) used the PRECEDE-PROCEED Model to study the barriers that underserved women had to overcome in order to be screened for breast cancer. Once these barriers were identified, recommendations were made to improve healthcare system procedures. Table 7.1 summarizes how the model was used by these researchers.

Allegrante, Kovar, Mackenzie, Peterson, and Gutin (1993) used the PRECEDE-PROCEED Model to implement and evaluate a walking program for patients with osteoarthritis of the knee. They found success with their program and suggest that

---

TABLE 7.1   Application of the PRECEDE-PROCEED Model

CASE STUDY: USE OF THE PRECEDE MODEL TO EXPLORE HOW UNDERSERVED WOMEN OVERCAME BARRIERS TO MAMMOGRAPHY SCREENING. WHAT MUST PRECEDE THE OUTCOME?

PRECEDE

Step I: Determine population needs

The authors note that mammography can reduce breast cancer mortality and that rates of regular screening are very low in the general population. Efforts to improve rates have had varying results.

Step II: Identify health determinants of these needs

The authors conducted focus group discussions with women from underserved populations who themselves obtain regular screenings. The goal of the focus groups was to identify facilitators and barriers to mammography screenings.

Step III: Analyze behaviors and environmental determinants of health needs

Two themes emerged from the discussions. The first is related to the environment and the second to behavior: (a) The role of the healthcare system in preventive health behaviors and practices and (b) personal factors (the woman's responsibility).

Step IV: Outline factors that predispose, reinforce, or enable behaviors

The authors note that lack of insurance used to be viewed as one of the major barriers to obtaining mammography—but even with the removal of this barrier, rates remain low. The focus of this study was on the behavioral factors influencing mammography screening. The authors report that the women in the focus groups described characteristics that influence them to obtain regular screenings: (a) *awareness, knowledge, and trust*—they understood cancer risks; some had experiences related to family members with cancer; who had healthcare providers who were receptive and encouraging, (b) *personal responsibility*—they demonstrated attitudes that support proactive behaviors, and this behavior developed within their families or through interaction with others, and (c) *pride in self and satisfaction*—these women found satisfaction with being role models for others.

All of these factors preceded/influenced outcomes.

Step V: Ascertain interventions best suited to change behaviors

To increase screening rates in underserved populations, the authors recommend providing information on risks and the importance of mammography in early detection (education) and inviting adherent women to act as role models. They further emphasized the importance of involving the media in providing information, as many of the women in the focus groups reported getting their information about mammography from television.

Note: Adapted from Ahmed, N., Fort, J., Elzey, J., & Bailey, S. (2004). Empowering factors in repeat mammography: Insights from the storied of underserved women, *Journal of Ambulatory Care Management, 27*(4), 348–355.

the intervention strategies designed around this model are readily adaptable for a wide range of settings.

An Evaluation Framework for Community Health

Produced by The Center for Advancement of Community Based Public Health and based on work by the CDC, *Framework for Program Evaluation in Public Health* (2000) is another model that can be used for program development, implementation, and evaluation. This systematic approach involves procedures that are useful, feasible, ethical, applicable, and accurate. Evaluation is the driving force for planning effective programs, improving existing programs, and demonstrating results to justify investment in resources. The framework is comprised of six interdependent steps that build on one another and facilitate understanding of the program context, including its history, setting, and organization. The steps are as follows:

- Engage stakeholders
  - Those involved in the program, those served or affected by the program
- Describe the program
  - Program needs, expected effects, activities, resources, stages of program development, operational chart
- Focus the evaluation design
  - Program purpose, users, uses, questions, methods, agreements
- Gather credible evidence
  - Program indicators, sources, quality, quantity, logistics of data collection
- Justify conclusions
  - Program standards, analysis and synthesis, interpretation, judgments, recommendations
- Ensure use and share lessons learned
  - Program design, preparation, feedback, follow-up, dissemination, additional uses

Models serve as organizing frameworks for developing a program from beginning to end, including planning, implementation, and evaluation. Nurse leaders may tailor these models to guide them in the design and development of their own programs, can follow a specific approach outlined by each model, or can use various components from a number of models. All the approaches are strongly focused on outcomes or program results. Outcomes drive evidence-based practice and best practices and therefore are a critical part of program design and success.

Care Delivery Models

As societal and healthcare demographics change, the APN must consider new approaches to healthcare delivery. Implementing programs designed by nurse leaders requires innovation to promote health, decrease costs, and improve outcomes while maintaining quality, safety, and satisfaction.

Care delivery models or systems operationalize the philosophy, values, and mission of an organization and its programs. Values might focus on clinical practice, financial costs and viability, functional outcomes, and/or patient/client and provider satisfaction. Care delivery models and their programs must be value driven. Additionally, care delivery models identify who is accountable for expected outcomes and relationships among key stakeholders and players. Furthermore, care delivery models and frameworks provide rules and structures that define accountability and operational processes.

A white paper commissioned by the Robert Wood Johnson Foundation outlined innovative care delivery models (2008). Twenty-four models were identified and categorized into either acute care, bridging the continuum, or comprehensive care. Eight common elements or themes were noted throughout the models (Joynt, & Kimball, 2008):

1. Elevated roles for nurses: Nurse as care integrators
2. Migration to interdisciplinary care: Team approach
3. Bridging the continuum of care
4. Pushing the boundaries: Home as setting of care
5. Targeting high users of healthcare: Elderly plus
6. Sharpened focus on the patient
7. Leveraging technology in care delivery
8. Driven by results: Improving satisfaction, quality, and costs

How patient/client care, outlined in a specific program, is delivered will depend upon the type of care being provided. Regardless of the type of care or method of its delivery, nurse leaders need to incorporate the following concepts reflective of the common elements identified in the innovative care delivery model white paper:

- A specific population focus
- A team approach
- Consideration of the continuum of care including the home environment
- Strategies to engage the patient/client
- Teaching or education
- A focus on results or outcomes

The delivery of healthcare is an ever-changing process. Changes in the healthcare needs of a population should be addressed and reassessed on a regular basis to insure patients' needs are still being met. Programmatic changes may need to be made but the end result can lead to improved patient health, decreased costs, and overall improved patient satisfaction.

OVERCOMING BARRIERS AND CHALLENGES

The first step in overcoming barriers is assessing and identifying obstacles to program development, implementation, and evaluation. Insight into obstacles can pave the way toward developing action plans to overcome barriers and challenges. Is the challenge in the design of the program? Is the challenge the competition? Is the challenge related to resources including time? Is the challenge due to the data being collected or the process of data collection?

The plan–do–check–act (PDCA) model used in quality improvement can be used to identify obstacles and plan subsequent actions. In 1980, NBC-TV aired a program called, "If Japan Can... Why Can't WE?" It highlighted Japan's rise as an economic power from not just virtual but actual ashes. The program featured W. E. Deming, a statistician who taught quality control to Japanese manufacturers. That program and Deming are often credited with bringing quality improvement initiatives to the attention of corporate America (Walton, 1991). Deming believed that American thinking was too "linear" and that they should think in a more circular fashion. The PDCA model is a Deming creation based on work by Andrew Shewhart.

- *Plan*: Plan the change
- *Do*: Do it
- *Check*: Check the results—then tailor your action based on the results
- *Act*: Act to stabilize the change or begin to improve on the change with new information

An example of the successful use of the PDCA model to improve the quality of care in an acute care hospital is provided by Saxena, Ramer, and Shulman (2004). A collaborative team was formed in an acute care hospital and charged with improving blood-administering practices using the FOCUS-PDCA method. FOCUS is the acronym for Finding a process to improve, Organizing a team familiar with the process, Clarifying the current situation, Understanding causes of variation, and Starting the PDCA cycle. The hospital identified a need to improve blood-administering processes (F) and formed a collaborative team that included nursing representatives, quality improvement, and laboratory and pathology personnel (O). They reviewed all of the policies and procedures related to blood transfusions (C), had independent auditors assess current practices (U), then trained nurses to observe and assess the dispensing and administering of blood products to determine adherence to policy and procedure (S). They found that continuous, direct observational audits using the PDCA method improved compliance with policies and procedures, thus reducing risk related to transfusion error.

The PDCA model is a process. The point is to strive toward continuous improvement or quality through ongoing assessment and improvement. Quality improvement models such as this can provide a framework to assist APNs in addressing some of the barriers that may be encountered in program development.

SUMMARY

In this chapter, APNs and nurse leaders were given the tools to design and develop comprehensive programs that address multiple components of program development ranging from the identification of key stakeholders to marketing and communication strategies. Successful programs must incorporate knowledge from many fields in order to address issues related to the structure, process, and outcomes involved in program planning, development, implementation, and evaluation. Program models provide a standard and tested method for helping nurse leaders throughout the process of program implementation. Program designs that address consumer and societal trends are more likely to be successful and can lead to improved quality of care and ultimately improved patient outcomes.

EXERCISES AND DISCUSSION QUESTIONS

Exercise 7.1   Using data that can be found on the DHHS or the CDC Web sites, identify trends in population demographics and health in an area that you serve.

- What are the implications for healthcare providers?
- What type of healthcare services and programs are needed right now?
- What type of services do you believe will be needed in 10 years?
- From a demographic point of view, in 10 years, what will be the important characteristics of the population that you serve if you stay where you are right now?

Exercise 7.2   You work in a Family Center that is part of a large hospital system with a catchment area that covers three counties. In the course of your usual work, you note that there has been an increased rate of childhood communicable diseases in your community and a decrease in immunization rates. You want to convince your employer to start a program to increase vaccination rates in the community that you serve.

- How would you justify such a program?
- How would you determine the feasibility of the program?
- Who are the stakeholders?
- How would you create the structure of the program?
- Identify the program outcomes.
- Using the "SMART" method, write short-term, intermediate, and long-term objectives for the program.
- How might you use the PRECEDE-PROCEED Model to plan, implement, and evaluate the program?
- How will you market the program?

REFERENCES

Agency for Healthcare Research and Quality (AHRQ). (2004, July). *Prevention quality indicators overview*. AHRQ Quality Indicators. Retrieved from http://www .qualityindicators.ahrq.gov/pqi_overview.htm

Ahmed, N., Fort, J., Elzey, J., & Bailey, S. (2004). Empowering factors in repeat mammography: Insights from the storied of underserved women. *Journal of Ambulatory Care Management, 27*(4), 348–355.

Allegrante, J., Kovar, P., MacKenzie, C., Peterson, M., & Gutin, B. (1993). A walking education program for patients with osteoarthritis of the knee: Theory and intervention strategies. *Health Education Quarterly, 20*(1), 64–81.

American Association of Colleges of Nursing (AACN). (2006). *The essentials of doctoral education for advanced practice nursing*. Retrieved from http://www.aacn.nche.edu/ DNP/pdf/Essentials.pdf

American Marketing Association. (2011). Retrieved from http://www.marketingpower .com/AboutAMA/Pages/DefinitionofMarketing.aspx

American Nurses Credentialing Center (ANCC). (2006). *Magnet recognition program®️ FAQ: Data and expected outcomes*. Retrieved from http://www.nursecredentialing.org/ FunctionalCategory/FAQ/DEO-FAQ.aspx

Baker, J. L. (2000). *Handbook for practitioners: Evaluating the impact of development projects on poverty*. Washington, DC: The World Bank.

CDC Division for Heart Disease and Stroke Prevention. (2011). *Evaluation guide: Writing smart objectives*. Retrieved from http://www.cdc.gov/dhdsp/programs/nhdsp_ program/evaluation_guides/docs/smart_objectives.pdf

Center for Advancement of Community Based Public Health. (2000). *An evaluation framework for community health*. The Center for Advancement of Community Based Public Health, University of North Carolina. Retrieved from http://www.cdc.gov/eval/eval-cbph.pdf

Community Toolbox. (2011). *Overview and evidence base-developing a framework or model of change*. Retrieved from http://ctb.ku.edu/en/promisingapproach/tools_bp_sub_ section_37.aspx

Green, L. W., & Kreuter, M. W. (1992). CDC's Planned approach to community health as an application of PRECEED and an inspiration for PROCEED. *Journal of Health Education, 23*(3), 140–144.

Health Care Technology Online. (2010, January 14). *10 Health care IT trends to watch in 2010*. Retrieved from http://www.healthcaretechnologyonline.com/article.mvc/10-Health care-IT-Trends-To-Watch-In-2010-0001

Joynt, J., & Kimball, B. (2008). *Innovative care delivery models: Identifying new models that effectively leverage nurses*. Robert Wood Johnson White Paper submitted to: Human Capital Team. Retrieved from http://innovativecaremodels.com/docs/HWS-RWJF-CDM-White-Paper.pdf

Lane, A., & Martin, M. (2005). Logic model use for breast health in rural communities. *Oncology Nursing Forum, 32*(1), 105–110.

McNamara, C. (2010). *Designing and marketing your programs*. Retrieved from http:// managementhelp.org/np_progs/mkt_mod/market.htm

Saxena, S., Ramer, L., & Shulman, I. (2004). A comprehensive assessment program to improve blood-administering practices using the FOCUS-PDCA model. *Transfusion Practice, 44*, 1350–1356.

Sherwood, A., Blumenthal, J., Hinderliter, A., Koch, G., Adams, K., Dupree, S., Bensimhon, D., ... O'Connor, C. (2011). Worsening depressive symptoms are associated with adverse clinical outcomes in patients with heart failure. *Journal of the American College of Cardiology, 57*(4), 418–423.

Walton, M. (1991). *Deming management at work.* New York, NY: Perigee Books.

W. K. Kellogg Foundation. (2004). *Using logic models to bring together planning, evaluation, and action: Logic model development guide.* Retrieved from http://www.uwsa.edu/edi/grants/Kellogg_Logic_Model.pdf

Eight

Evaluating Practice at the Population Level

Barbara A. Niedz

*E*arly in their careers, nurses often have an enthusiasm and energy that focuses on helping one patient at a time. Over the years, that focus broadens as the more experienced nurse embraces a role that is more expansive and addresses issues at a population level. As advanced practice nurses (APNs) serve as administrators, leaders, educators, and managers, the scope of practice widens even further. Quality nurse professionals expand their view to the entire organization and across departments. Nurses have, over the years, moved in many diverse directions. We not only care for patients at the bedside but in their homes, businesses, schools, prisons, rehabilitation settings, as well as in outpatient and mental health facilities. As nurses, we care for patients with attention to increasing complexity because of advances in medical science and in nursing practice. Oversight responsibilities for clinical outcomes at the population level are a critical part of advanced practice nursing.

The advancement of many educational opportunities for nurses has moved our profession into new and exciting places. The advent of the advanced practice licensure designation has opened doors for nurses that did not exist 20 years ago. Nursing has become proactive and more responsive to the needs of the healthcare environment and to the needs of our patients. Our potential to influence the health of patient populations has expanded accordingly.

The purpose of this chapter is to determine ways and means to evaluate population outcomes and to evaluate systems' changes as well as effectiveness, efficiency, and trends in care delivery across the continuum. Strategies to monitor healthcare quality are addressed as well as factors that lead to success. Most importantly, these concepts are explored within the role and competencies of the APN.

MONITORING HEALTH CARE QUALITY

Nurses have been concerned about the quality of patient care for many years. Although our definitions of quality have varied through the years, the heart of this discussion is our collective desire to continuously improve patients' health and the management of various disease states, regardless of where a given patient fits on the continuum.

Definitions of Quality and Theoretical Models

Just as nurses care for one patient at a time, initial models for quality dealt with individual patient reviews. Donabedian (1980) defines quality in broad terms: "Quality is a property that medical care can have in varying degrees" (p. 3). His definition holds that "attributes of good care ... are so many and so varied that it is impossible to derive from them either a unifying concept or a single empirical measure of quality" (p. 74). This notwithstanding, Donabedian's (1980) model of structure, process, and outcome addressed how quality can be maximized in organizations and continues to be used today to structure research on quality methods throughout the globe (Chen, Hong, & Hsu, 2007; Handler, Issel, & Turnock, 2001; Schiller, Weech-Maldonado, & Hall, 2010; Wubker, 2007).

Nash, Reifsnyder, Fabius, and Pracilio (2011) explain that the concept of population health includes an integrated system of care across the continuum. The population health model "seeks to eliminate healthcare disparities, increase safety, and promote effective, equitable, ethical and accessible care" (p. 4). Accordingly, they explain that quality is defined in terms of clinical data and economic and patient-centered outcomes. In their view, "quality is founded on evidence based medicine" (p. 5). Finally, their model describes the relationship between quality of care and the cost of care; if the quality of care improves, the cost of care is reduced (Nash et al., 2011).

Juran (DeFeo & Juran, 2010) offers a definition of quality that is both parsimonious and applicable across disciplines. Juran defines quality in terms of the customer and explains that a product or service has quality if it is "fit for use" in the eyes of the customer. Goonan (1995) and Dienemann (1992) have applied Juran's definition to healthcare scenarios. Patients, as consumers of healthcare products and services, fit the definition of customers, regardless of the payment source. Juran (DeFeo & Juran, 2010) explains that for a product or service to meet the needs of the customer, it must have the right features, and it must be free from deficiencies. In Juran's view (2010), new features (like new cardiac surgical equipment or the capacity to provide outpatient dialysis) may require capital and operating expense. Deficiencies or defects in our healthcare products or services always contribute to the cost of poor quality. The cost of one hospital-acquired infection has been estimated as $15,000 by McCaughey (2006) and may range from as low as $500 to as much as $50,000 (Hassan, Tuckman, Patrick, Kountz, & Kohn, 2010). Hospitals are no longer reimbursed for the cost associated with the development of a third or fourth degree pressure ulcer in a patient, if that ulcer was hospital acquired and not present on admission. The Centers for Medicare and Medicaid (CMS), which functions under the aegis of the United States Department of Health and Human Services (DHHS), promulgated rules to this effect in 2008 (see http://www.cms.gov/HospitalAcqCond/). The development of a hospital-acquired third or fourth degree pressure ulcer is also included in the National Quality Forum's list of "never events" ("The Power of Safety," 2010). In recent years, CMS has dictated by law and regulation that hospitals will not be reimbursed for care related to 14 of these "never event" conditions that occur during an inpatient admission (http://www.cms.gov/HospitalAcqCond/). Other preventable outcomes that contribute to the cost of poor quality have consequences that go beyond dollars and cents. Deficiencies that result in complications and even death arise from poor systems and human failures. These have gotten significant and appropriate attention through the patient safety movement (Institute of Medicine [IOM], 1999, 2001).

Through the Joint Commission and the National Patient Safety Goals (The Joint Commission and CMS, 2010), attention to hospital and other healthcare organizational venues for patients has resulted in significant strides toward reducing deficiencies. The importance of improving quality by avoiding the "never events" and reducing deficiencies has reinforced the necessity of accurate and thorough documentation and medical decision making by all healthcare providers.

While Juran's definition of quality does have merit and application in healthcare (Kaplan, Disgaard, Truesdell, & Zetterholm, 2009; Meurer, McGartland-Rubio, Counte, & Burroughs, 2002), capturing ways and means to measure both outcome and process indicators of quality has emerged from an evidence-based approach. For example, research has shown that in order to decrease the incidence of hospital readmission rates in patients with congestive heart failure (CHF), patient discharge instructions from the hospital should minimally capture key components including the following: (a) knowledge of medications, (b) the importance of weight tracking, (c) diet control, (d) what to do if symptoms worsen, (e) activity level, and (f) follow-up care (http://www.qualitymeasures.ahrq.gov/content.aspx?id=16253&search=chf). Lack of any of these components is clearly seen as a "deficiency" and should be captured in data across patient sets in hospitals (see http://www.jointcommission.org/specifications_manual_for_national_hospital_inpatient_quality_measures/). Thus, measurement mechanisms emerge from Juran's definition of quality (2010), which also fit with Donabedian's (1980) framework of structure, process, and outcome, and Nash's (Nash et al., 2011) view of population health.

Organizational Models for Excellence

Nurses provide the backbone of healthcare organizations, whether inpatient, outpatient, rehabilitation, home care, community health, or telephonic services. As such, understanding the organizational framework that can maximize positive outcomes and minimize deficiencies through the role of the nurse has value.

Both Defeo and Juran (2010) and Donabedian (1980) put the concept of quality into the framework of an organization. Care of a patient across the wellness-illness continuum requires consistent and cogent processes and systems. Accordingly, Donabedian's view is that healthcare organizations require appropriate structure and key processes. Taken together, the structure and processes assist the organization in producing desired outcomes for their patients (Donabedian, 1980). Juran characterizes organizations as high functioning and marked by positive outcomes if features are maximized and deficiencies are minimized. In order to accomplish this, organizations plan for control and continuously improve quality. Both clinical and service quality characteristics are defined in terms of customers' needs and expectations. Others have made similar observations in applying Juran's organizational model in healthcare organizations (Best & Neuhauser, 2006; Goonan & Scarrow, 2010; Maddox, 1992). In 1987, the federal government instituted the Malcolm Baldridge Award, which recognizes those organizations that demonstrate principles characteristic of high performance and achieve significant business results through quality improvement techniques (2010–2011 Malcolm Baldridge Award Criteria, 2010). This award is based on seven key guiding principles and embodies the theoretical model of quality that Juran honed throughout his career (DeFeo & Juran, 2010; http://www.nist.gov/baldrige/publications/hc_criteria.cfm). In the late 1990s, this award was opened to healthcare organizations. Since 2002, there have been 11 winners of the Baldridge Award in the healthcare division (http://patapsco.nist.gov/Award_Recipients/AwardRecipients.cfm?sector=Health%20Care).

In order for organizations to maximize positive outcomes and minimize deficiencies, planning must take on a strategic focus. Leadership and governance have responsibility and oversight for quality and are essentially responsible for organizational planning. Quality planning, according to Juran (DeFeo & Juran, 2010), provides depth, breadth, and scope of how the product or service is designed, developed, and implemented. Key quality characteristics in the form of measurable goals and objectives for the organization and for patient outcomes are designed in the system or process before that product or service begins.

Once that product or service is in operation, customers' needs and expectations (whether in the form of clinical quality, customer satisfaction, core business processes, or utilization of healthcare resources) can be understood, defined, and measured. External benchmark comparison data can be helpful in goal setting and in evaluating the extent to which a product or service meets customers' expectations. Juran (DeFeo & Juran, 2010) explains that all products and services are delivered to the customer employing various processes and systems. High-performing organizations design processes and systems to meet customer needs consistently, reducing variation in outcomes and minimizing defects. Juran calls this piece of the puzzle "quality control."

W. Edwards Deming (Moen & Norman, 2010) developed similar theories of quality and consistently modeled the theme of reducing variation and building quality into a product or system so that there is less requirement to depend upon inspection (after the fact). Deming's model was also influenced by the work of other quality giants, like Shewhart and Feigenbaum (Guru Guide, 2010). Ishikawa

(Guru Guide, 2010) paved the way for Japan's economic turnaround after World War II, largely based on the work of both Juran and Deming, who were sent by the U.S. government to support Japan after the war. These models rely heavily on the theory that all of quality is measurable and that reducing variation in processes holds a vital role in reducing the incidence of defects and ultimately, ensuring better outcomes.

Berwick, Godfrey, and Roessner (1990) were preeminent in applying these theoretical models to healthcare. Six leading healthcare organizations were armed with a national demonstration grant from the Robert Wood Johnson Foundation; within this seminal work, the authors cataloged the experiences of these organizations in applying this theoretical approach to quality. Their experiences clearly indicate that the models and tools had merit and value in reducing defects, improving processes, and maximizing outcomes (Berwick, Godfrey, & Rossener, 1990). This landmark work demonstrated that what had been shown repeatedly in manufacturing and in service industries throughout the country (and, in fact, worldwide) could be repeated in healthcare and laid the groundwork for potential application throughout the healthcare industry.

Deming (Moen & Norman, 2010), Juran (2010), Crosby (Guru Guide, 2010), and others explain that reducing variation is a continuous task, even when a given product or service is exceeding the needs of customers and especially when a given product or service is not competitive in the marketplace. The *Six Sigma* movement (DeFeo & Barnard, 2004; Pyzdek, 2003) emerged from a quality improvement initiative at General Electric in the 1980s, which set out to reduce defects or deficiencies to less than 3.4 defects per 1,000,000 opportunities. In essence, this model for quality improvement and planning is built on the work of Juran, Deming, Crosby, Ishikawa, Feigenbaum, and others (Guru Guide, 2010). While it is clear that Donabedian's work is theoretically sound, it also resonates with this thinking. Kaplan, Bisgaard, Truesdaell, and Zetterholm (2009) applied the model to a population health issue. Many others have applied the Six Sigma theoretical model to healthcare processes. The application of this model for process improvement has significant application across the spectrum of healthcare processes (Corn, 2009; Drenckpohl, Bowers, & Cooper, 2007; Fairbanks, 2007; Stankovic & DeLauro, 2010; Yun & Chun, 2008). To illustrate the application of process improvement theory and the use of Six Sigma models, consider the studies presented in Exhibit 8.1.

The patient safety movement in healthcare has given rise to a wider application of the Six Sigma model. In addition, the language of defects and deficiencies, although developed out of manufacturing and other types of product development, has resulted in consistent thought that complications heretofore considered risks of procedure or hospitalization are now considered preventable (Courtney, Ruppman, & Cooper, 2006). The patient safety movement in the United States emerged largely because of the Joint Commission (TJC, 2010) for their focus on sentinel events (Joint Commission Resources, 2003). In addition, the consensus report of the IOM "To Err is Human," published by the IOM in December, 1999, shines a light on the potential for preventable errors. One of the most telling comments early in the book explains that there are between 44,000 and 98,000

EXHIBIT 8.1
Examples of Process Improvement Theory and the Use of the
Six Sigma Models

1. Corn (2009) described the history of the model, and its application in healthcare, (Drenckpohl, Bowers, and Cooper, 2007).

2. Bowers and Cooper (2007) used the method to reduce errors related to breast milk identification processes in the neonatal intensive care unit (NICU).

3. Fairbanks (2007) applied Six Sigma and Lean methodologies, which is a variation of Six Sigma model, focusing on eliminating waste and "nonvalued added" steps in a given process to improve operating room delays in throughput (Womack & Jones, 2003).

4. Stankovic and DiLauro (2010) used the model to improve timeliness and reduce errors in the laboratory, in processing specimens.

5. Yun and Chun (2008) applied the design aspect of Six Sigma to telemedicine services processes.

preventable medical errors annually in the United States, which lead to patient death (IOM, 1999). The variability in the range is significant. Measurement mechanisms did not exist at that time to provide accurate descriptions of these sentinel events. In the language of the process improvement gurus, these are defects and deficiencies. Applying these theoretical models to healthcare has tremendous potential in accurately describing the quality of care, but improving outcomes through attention to process.

Kaplan and Norton (1996; 2001) take measurement in organizations a step further and link progress against the strategic planning cycle to organizational goals and objectives. Their "balanced scorecard" model lends itself well to healthcare and has been applied internationally (Chu, Wang, & Dai, 2009; Moulin et al., 2007; Potthoff & Ryan, 2004; Yap, Siu, Baker, Brown, & Lowi-Young, 2005). In fact, the Malcolm Baldridge Award has several specific criteria (http://www.nist.gov/baldrige/baldrige_120310.cfm). One of the most important criteria is the recognition of "results" that fashion the measurement and improvement of quality across organizations and systems. A well-defined scorecard at the enterprise level, which is balanced across several categories relating to the customer's experience, is a useful and important tool for senior leadership and governance. As we move into a discussion about planning, controlling for, and improving quality across the entire patient population, understanding theoretical models for process improvement and application of these models becomes not only useful and accepted but necessary and, most importantly, leads to improved outcomes of care.

Process Improvement Models and Tools

The literature is replete with evidence of various process improvement models. They have many commonalities. Deliberate and thoughtful applied use can result in reduction of defects and deficiencies to levels that meet and exceed customers' expectations, whether those expectations surround clinical quality, customer satisfaction, core business process, or utilization of healthcare resource expectations. The "Plan, Do, Check, Act" (PDCA) Process Improvement Model (Moen & Norman, 2010), the Juran Six Step Quality Improvement Process Model (DeFeo & Juran, 2010), or Six Sigma's Define, Measure, Analyze, Improve, and Control (DMAIC) Model all have common features, and they are all problem-solving models that drive toward measurable improvement when used properly. They can facilitate a thought process and require a team initiative. They will work whether the problem is related to clinical quality, customer satisfaction, core business processes, or utilization of healthcare resource. They work inside and outside of healthcare, whether the problem is simple or complex, and whether one is concerned about the care of patients or making widgets. Exhibit 8.2 describes characteristics that are commonly found in process improvement models.

EXHIBIT 8.2
Characteristics and Commonalities of Process Improvement Models

1. The problem is defined in measurable terms.

2. The problem is stated in terms of the customer's needs and expectations.

3. External comparative benchmark data are sometimes drawn on to help set the goal for the project.

4. Members of the team have well-defined responsibilities.

5. Most teams should have 6–10 members. Larger teams may not be able to control the problem process and might need to break into smaller groups to be effective. Smaller teams may have inadequate representation to fully address all facets of the problem.

6. The team includes an executive sponsor to usher the project as a priority in the organization.

7. Other team roles include business process owner as team leader, internal or external consultant as facilitator, and clearly described roles for remaining team members.

8. There is an analysis phase. This phase employs both qualitative and quantitative methods to arrive at barriers, obstacles, and root causes of the problem.

(continued)

Exhibit 8.2 *(continued)*

9. The analysis phase should be well supported with qualitative data (like a cause-effect diagram) and quantitative "theory testing" data (like a diagnostic study of the root causes of the process problem).

10. Remedies are designed that address both the qualitative and quantitative barriers.

11. A plan for piloting or testing the remedies is well defined, engages the full team, considers the cost of implementation and decision making therein, and defines whether or not all are sufficient to achieve the desired improvement.

12. A measurement mechanism is designed to evaluate the effectiveness of the change strategy and the degree to which an additional remedial plan is needed.

13. A mechanism for evaluating ongoing data collection, day to day and month to month, is put in place, to ensure that the gains are held constant.

14. In order to provide an effective use of a process improvement model, the focus must be clear and well defined. Teams must sometimes winnow down a larger project to its smaller component parts. At the end of a successful process improvement project, it may be necessary to go back and revisit other improvement opportunities, which may have been set aside from the focal interest.

All process improvement models have these common characteristics. In addition, a variety of tools support the quality professional along the process improvement path. Tools like process flow charting, barriers and aids charts, cost-benefit analyses, data collection tools and statistical methods, SIPOC (Suppliers-Inputs-Process-Outputs-Customers) analysis, project planning tools, lean thinking, and many others provide useful insight and drill closer to improvement goals (DeFeo & Barnard, 2004; Pyzdek, 2003; Womack & Jones, 2003).

Population-Based Models

On a continuum from health and wellness products to complex care management, a variety of population-based models have emerged over recent years (Exhibit 8.3). Patients move across a continuum from good health to end of life and enter a variety of settings in doing so. Programs are designed to offer both telephone care and field-based approaches to prevention, disease management, care coordination, case management, and care integration. Patients are identified through predictive models and other stratification methods. Outreach is defined within various levels of acuity and may include frequency of patient contact depending upon clinical assessment, decision making, and care planning. Motivational interviewing and health education are primary strategies, but a hallmark of all of these programs is a change in health behaviors, which leads to desired outcomes. Preventive strategies, such as smoking cessation, as well as care coordination strategies, such as identifying a medical home and ensuring medical transportation to an outpatient facility, combined with condition-specific strategies in the presence of various chronic disease states to reduce the incidence of emergency department (ED) usage for primary care and reduce inpatient admissions are all examples of ways to improve access to care in the hopes of ensuring overall quality of care (Fetterolf, Holt, Tucker, & Khan, 2010; O'Toole et al., 2010; Rice et al., 2010). Research has shown that disease and case management programs are effective in reducing the trajectory of chronic disease, by providing less utilization of healthcare resources and providing enhanced satisfaction with ability to perform activities of daily living, improved functional status, and day–to-day management of chronic disease (Baicker, Cutler, & Song, 2010; Bedell & Kaszkin-Bettag, 2010; Govil, Weidner, Merritt-Worden, & Ornish, 2009; Lamb, Toye, & Barker, 2008).

EXHIBIT 8.3
Population Health Models

1. *Health and Wellness (H&W):* These programs are primarily telephonic and may have a biometric screening component; program awareness and patient education materials are often part of a direct mail campaign. These programs aim at identifying patients with significant health risk and encourage patient participation in screening. Smoking cessation, weight reduction, and preventive care visits are examples of desired outcomes for this patient population. Although significant health risks may emerge here, this patient population is largely well without the presence of diagnosed disease states.

2. *Disease Management (DM):* These programs are likely to be telephonic, field based, or a combination of both. Patients qualify for a DM program on the basis of identified disease states, singly or in combination. Most DM programs target at least five or six disease conditions: persistent asthma, chronic obstructive pulmonary disease (COPD), coronary artery disease (CAD), diabetes mellitus, congestive heart failure (CHF), and depression. Other programs are broader and capture high-cost, high-risk patients with varied chronic disease states. DM programs often have a care coordination component, which provides such practical considerations as a medical home, transportation to the outpatient clinic or doctor's office, a funding source for medication management, etc. Examples of outcomes for this

(continued)

Exhibit 8.3 *(continued)*

patient population include but are not limited to the following: (a) ensuring that a diabetic patient gets a HbA1c test done at least annually, (b) ensuring that a patient with persistent asthma has a prescription for controller medications, and (c) confirming that a CHF patient knows the importance of daily weights and what to do if symptoms worsen. DM programs may include a care coordination component, which targets patient needs surrounding their physical ailment. For example, providing the patient with transportation to the doctor or clinic for routine or outpatient care can significantly reduce the overuse of emergency medical services (EMS) and emergency departments (ED). Similarly, when discharging a patient from the inpatient setting who has CHF and an ejection fraction of less than 40%, we ensure that the patient is appropriately prescribed an angiotensin-converting enzyme (ACE) inhibitor and knows the importance of weighing themselves daily. Care coordination ensures that the patient has the means and wherewithal to have that prescription filled, a scale at home or the means to purchase one, and transportation to the doctor's office to fulfill their discharge plan.

3. *Case Management (CM):* These programs capture patients who have complex needs and multiple health conditions. These patients are often high risk and high cost and come to the surface in stratification and predictive models because of overutilization of EDs and multiple admissions because of poor outpatient management or lack of a medical home. When the total population is viewed, these patients account for a small percentage of the total in volume, but account for in excess of 60% of the total healthcare dollar. Models that integrate care across various specialties for a given patient set (e.g., patients with severe mental illness who also have multiple medical disease conditions) are emerging.

One of the most interesting recent trends in population-based care management is *care integration. Care integration* is a concept that is well known to nurses, but may not be as familiar to other health professionals. Here is an example: A patient is admitted to an inpatient acute care hospital with a significant drug overdose, subsequent to an attempted suicide. This long-standing behavioral health (BH) patient has been managed "on and off" by a variety of BH professionals and has been receiving various psychotropic medications. In addition, the patient has a medical history that includes long-standing diabetes and coronary artery disease; other healthcare professionals have managed this aspect of the patient's healthcare. In fact, the medical professionals have not been in touch with the BH professionals, at the patient's request. In the ED, the BH professionals' role is preempted as the patient's overwhelming medical needs are the priority. When the patient is admitted to the intensive care unit, a host of consultants are brought to the case, and after being "cleared medically," the patient is transferred to the inpatient BH unit. Care is sometimes fragmented, and the BH needs are addressed separately and apart from the medical needs of the patient. The primary care physician may not be involved until after discharge and may not have a clear sense of the many issues that play a role in the complete care of this patient. Although there is no question about the prioritization of care, there is also no integration of care. The patient's experience is divided into two distinctly different phases, in some ways compromising effective use of healthcare resources. This is where the importance of the medical home comes into play. Length of stay is clearly segmented into two sequential phases rather than managed in parallel. While this inpatient example is a familiar one, lack of *care integration* also is a common problem on the out-patient side of the care continuum. Processes of care that appropriately integrate care have been somewhat problematic in the U.S. healthcare system in the past. In recent years, there has been some recognition that care integration needs to improve quality of care, resolve access issues, and reduce overutilization of health-care resources (Gill, Swarbrick, Murphy, Spagnolo, & Zechner, 2009; Godchaux, 1999; Santos, Henggeler, Burns, Arana, & Meisler, 1995).

Two recent initiatives bring these ideas into sharp perspective. The first is the concept of the patient-centered medical home (PCMH). Within this model, care integration services are well defined, and the process of bringing care to the patient where, when, and how they need it becomes not only possible but also practical. The National Committee for Quality Assurance (NCQA) promulgates standards that well describe this initiative (http://ncqa.org/tabid/1302/Default. aspx). Accountable care organizations (ACOs) are another model that incorporates these ideas into organized systems of care with providers, PCMHs, and hospitals partnering together. This is a program furthered by the CMS (http://www.cms. gov/PhysicianFeeSched/downloads/10-5-10ACO-WorkshopAMSessionTran-script.pdf).

Nurse-Sensitive Process and Outcome Indicators at the Population Level

Many authors have promulgated ways to organize measures, as taken together they represent a picture of quality. Kaplan and Norton (1996; 2001) suggest four generic categories that could work for any organization, including organizations that focus on healthcare. These perspectives include the following: (a) internal business processes, (b) customer focus, (c) learning and growth, and (d) financial (Kaplan & Norton, 1996; 2001). The NCQA places the Healthcare Effectiveness Data and Information Set (HEDIS) measures into categories as well. The HEDIS categories include the following: (a) effectiveness of care, (b) access/availability of care, (c) satisfaction with the experience of care, (d) use of services, and (e) cost of care (HEDIS, 2010).

While the list of possible indicators to measure population health and popu-lation health nursing may seem endless, four categories of measures, metrics, and indicators emerge. These broad categories include clinical quality, customer satisfaction, core business processes, and utilization of healthcare resources. Loosely based on Kaplan and Norton (1996, 2001) and the NCQA HEDIS frameworks, an organizing framework for evaluating population health nursing emerges. As these categories are of use in organizing our thinking regarding quality in the inpatient setting, they also have merit in outpatient settings, and as we consider care of the entire population with a given disease condition, these categories continue to add value to this discussion as an organizing framework. For the purpose of this discussion, the words "measures," "metrics," and "indicators" are used interchangeably. As we have put forward a definition of quality that is "measurable," our measures are quantifiable, a set of metrics that indicate the presence or absence of quality and degrees on that continuum.

Whenever possible, standardized data definitions are essential. This sets up a level playing field for comparisons. Since the late 1990s, data sets, external comparisons, and guidance for standardized numerator and denominator have emerged across the patient continuum of care. As our industry has become more accountable to the public for outcomes, this kind of standardization has been essential, facilitating external comparisons on the basis of datasets. In addition, these numerators and denominators are described in detail, right down to the technical specifications. These technical specifications describe what types of codes are included in the numerator, and which are included in the denominator. These codes have become widely accepted, the application of which results in fair and appropriate comparisons and rankings. Various groups (both governmental and private) have defined measures, specified the technical mechanics of counting and determining rates, and applied these measures across the industry. These include, but are not limited to, the following: (a) CMS http://www.cms.gov/center/quality.asp, (b) TJC http://www.jointcommission.org/, (c) the Agency for Healthcare Research and Quality (AHRQ, 2010) http://www.ahrq.gov/qual/, (d) NCQA http://ncqa.org/, and (e) the National Quality Forum (NQF, 2010), http://www.qualityforum.org/

Measures have also emerged over time. As our foray into this area of accountability for outcomes has been heightened by legislators, policy makers, and the public-at-large, the connection between the cost of poor quality in healthcare and healthcare reform has become more explicit. While it might require capital and operational outlay of funding to develop a specific product or service with the right features within the healthcare industry, the cost of poor quality adds a substantial burden to the cost of healthcare. For example, when a patient in a hospital setting experiences a delay in obtaining a diagnostic procedure that is essential to the appropriate management of that patient's disease state, this core business process can delay decision making and lead to a longer hospitalization for the patient. This delay may also lead to disease progression and result in complications that otherwise might have been prevented. Another question that should be addressed is whether the delay is because of the type of insurance, underinsurance, or lack of insurance. As discussed in Chapter 2, an important component of APN practice is the need to recognize and address issues related to healthcare disparities.

When patient safety is compromised in hospitals, the result can be substantial. The example of delayed diagnostic testing may not only hinder the determination of a patient's diagnosis but may also lead to patients receiving inaccurate medications or treatments, or a patient identification mix-up can result in loss of life. Over time, we should be able to identify the impact of the cost of poor quality by capturing and quantifying these indicators of quality in the aggregate. Sorting out "what counts and what does not" helps to provide clarity and a clearer view of quality across the board.

Clinical Quality

Nurse-sensitive indicators of population health that relate to clinical quality can be seen in a number of the metrics recognized by external organizations with available external benchmarks. In the HEDIS (NCQA, 2010 http://ncqa.org/tabid/59/Default.aspx) dataset created and maintained by the NCQA, there are several benchmarks that relate to chronic disease conditions. Nurses who are in the field or on the phone in telephone call centers reach out to patients with the intention of helping them wade through the various resources made available to them through private and public means to manage their overall health, given the presence of various disease states. The most common disease states managed by disease management (DM) programs include the following: (a) diabetes mellitus, (b) persistent asthma, (c) COPD, (d) CAD, and (e) CHF. Other chronic disease conditions also may be of interest. In CM programs, the complexity of care is heightened by the number and acuity of the chronic conditions coexisting in a patient's profile. Social problems, housing, transportation, and pharmacy costs often emerge in case management programs. Similarly, the emphasis from a clinical quality perspective in health and wellness (H&W) programs is on preventive care, early recognition of emerging disease, and the use of appropriately placed screening tools.

Exhibit 8.4 lists several examples of clinical quality measures that are sensitive to the APN role at the population health level in disease management, case management, and lifestyle management or H&W programs, whether their intervention is on the telephone, in person, or in a field-based model.

Utilization of Health Care Resources

In a global sense, collectively nurses who work in DM, CM, and H&W programs direct patients to the use of healthcare resources in the most cost-effective way. In the context of population health, the most expensive healthcare resources include the use of the ED and acute care inpatient stays. By making sure that the patient's discharge plan coming out of the inpatient setting is fully executed, we can predict that patients will lessen the need for repeat hospitalization. By ensuring that patients have their transportation and other care coordination needs met, we can have more confidence that there will be less utilization of the EMS system for a ride to the local ED to have their primary care needs met. The two metrics that

EXHIBIT 8.4
Sample Nurse-Sensitive Clinical Quality Measures in DM, CM, and H&W Programs (HEDIS, 2010)

1. HEDIS comprehensive diabetes care (CDC): Does the patient have at least one HbA1c level drawn in a 12-month period?

2. HEDIS ASM asthma care: Does the patient diagnosed with persistent asthma have prescriptions for the right constellation of medications?

3. AHRQ prevention quality indicator CHF: What is the inpatient admission rate per 100,000 (at the population level) for CHF?

4. AHRQ prevention quality indicator COPD: What is the inpatient admission rate per 100,000 (at the population level) for COPD?

5. HEDIS CMC coronary artery disease: Does the patient diagnosed with CAD and LDL level of >100 have a prescription for a statin (or HMG-CoA (3-hydroxy-3-methylglutaryl-coenzyme A) reductase inhibitors)?

6. HEDIS CAP: Does the child between the ages of 0 and 15 months have at least six well-child visits?

7. HEDIS AAP: Does the woman aged 35 or older have an annual Pap smear to screen for cervical cancer?

are the most useful and sensitive to the nursing role in DM and CM programs are admissions per 1,000 members and ED visits per 1,000 members. Measuring the impact of lifestyle management programs in terms of their impact on preventing ED usage and inpatient admissions is a little longer term. In some ways, this work is an extension of the work that nurses have participated in for years, in Utilization Management (UM) programs in hospitals, for health plans, and for other providers of healthcare benefits. However, DM, CM, and H&W nurses take UM to the next step and ensure that patients have the means, insight, and knowledge to carry out their healthcare needs with some degree of independence and autonomy. By reviewing care needs and targeting the right level of care and service and matching it to the appropriate venue, we reduce the inappropriate use of these very costly services.

An evaluation of the utilization of healthcare resources is often included in a given DM or CM contract as a "return on investment" (ROI) analysis as evidence of financial performance. The bulk of the healthcare dollar resides in the use of primarily two resources: ED visits and inpatient stays. Both may be misused in the absence of an effective medical home or access to primary care. At the population level, measuring the impact of population health models on utilization of these two key healthcare resources is a very important component of any population health evaluation method. Three possibilities present themselves in an ROI evaluation; rigorous methodology is a component of well-designed DM and CM models. First, an estimation of cost avoidance involves using historical data to predict the number and percentage of ED usage and inpatient admissions in a given patient population that are likely to occur after a year of DM intervention. For example, after one year of investment in a telephonic nursing DM program, it is fair to predict that patients will be better linked into a medical home and be better positioned to avoid admissions for preventable primary care conditions (like uncontrolled diabetes, asthma, or even CHF). These strategies also have the potential to prevent the use of EDs for primary care. Another method to evaluate ROI is to predict a trend and trajectory based on the baseline history of a given set or population of patients. A typical dataset for comparison is a 12-month period of time, used as the starting point or baseline for comparisons moving forward. A third option is to calculate the ROI of a DM, population health nursing program and posit that with this intervention, certain specific events will not occur (e.g., a reduction in the following: readmission rates, the number of patients with multiple admissions in a given year, or patients with admissions for ambulatory sensitive conditions [ASC]). These are also described by AHRQ as Preventive Quality Indicators or PQI (see www.ahrq.gov for more information on these important indicators).

Customer Satisfaction

Patients have for many years been identified as important consumers of healthcare products and services and accordingly have been defined as "customers" and important stakeholders in DM and CM organizations (NCQA, 2009; URAC, 2009). Accordingly, key metrics that are sensitive to the nursing role can tell us something about the degree to which our patients, as customers, have had a positive experience with our nurses, whether those nurses practice in hospitals or in DM organizations. How frustrating is it when a customer makes a telephone call to any company and ends up in a hold queue for a long period of time? Two call center metrics are often cited as important: (a) average speed of answer (ASA) and (b) call abandonment rate (ABN) (Cross, 2000; Del Franco, 2003; Formichelli, 2007; Gustafson, 1999). This literature is replete with guidance on how long it should take to answer inbound telephone calls in order to meet or exceed customers' expectations. The industry standard for ASA is less than 30 seconds and the industry standard for ABN is less than 5%. That is, less than 5% of calls should be lost when a customer abandons the call because of a prolonged waiting time (Cross, 2000; Del Franco, 2003; Formichelli, 2007; Gustafson, 1999). Akin to waiting for a response to a call light in an inpatient setting, in a call center setting, this is a primary source of customer dissatisfaction. Ensuring that staffing levels (for both licensed and nonlicensed staff members) are appropriate, and that technology provides adequate tools for observing the call queue, and using data down to the level of the staff member are all important oversight supervisory functions, which deliver telephonic DM or CM care in a way that meets and exceeds customer satisfaction.

Monitoring, managing, and measuring complaints are another way to tap into the customer's experience. Customer complaints, whether from patient as customer or provider as customer, can be an insightful means to understanding patterns and trends of care delivery and can be the key to improvement. Customer complaints can be very serious and can lead to a written complaint or a formal grievance when a patient is unhappy with the resolution offered in the moment. Customer complaints that are resolved by the nurse on the call are important to document and are worth tracking. Sometimes, complaints come into a DM call center that might be serious, but the target of the complaint is not the DM organization. In this case, these complaints are also valuable indicators of quality and should be referred to an appropriate authority or organization. Again, tracking and trending the nature of the complaint and the agency or organization to which the complaint was referred (rather than resolution) may be all that is required.

Various techniques are available for tracking patient, provider, and client satisfaction for DM programs. Annual surveys are the most frequent vehicle, and the Care Continuum Alliance (CCA), formerly known as the Disease Management Association of America (DMAA), provides patient and provider surveys to organizational members of the CCA (http://carecontinuum.org/). These surveys have established reliability and validity. They include items that measure the overall satisfaction of the patient with the services provided by the DM organization, but also tap into the "likelihood to recommend." Satisfaction with the skills and techniques employed in the service of DM by the individual nurse can also be assessed. Accordingly, these items are "nurse sensitive." Examples include items that evaluate the nurse's willingness to "listen" as well as provide information that can influence the patient's behavior in the interest of better management of specific chronic disease states.

Measuring customer satisfaction through a survey process has long been established as an important function, whether that measurement occurs in a hospital, or in a total population health setting such as a DM program. Hospitals are familiar with prominent vendors for patient satisfaction monitoring like Press Ganey™ Associates (http://www.pressganey.com/index.aspx), Healthstream® Research, (http://www.healthstreamresearch.com/Pages/Default.aspx), and many other research groups that specialize in healthcare survey processes. In recent years, the CMS has mandated the use of an agreed upon set of questions administered in a consistent way regardless of vendor. In the inpatient venue, the CMS survey entitled the "Hospital Consumer Assessment of Healthcare Providers and Systems" (HCAHPS) is widely applied (http://www.cms.gov/HospitalQualityInits/30_HospitalHCAHPS.asp). Although individual vendors like Press Ganey™ offer comparisons based on various methods, the HCAHPS survey offers broad comparisons across the country on an agreed set of questions, worded the same and applied using the same, mandated research methods.

The CCA also provides a survey targeted at physicians and other providers of healthcare services that evaluates the extent to which the DM organization provides services to them, in the interests of their patients. Annual surveys of providers as customers can also be insightful to a DM organization.

Phone automated surveys and interactive voice response (IVR) surveys are also available, and a variety of telephone services provide this capability. This type of data collection and these methods have been used extensively because they provide timely feedback that is relevant on an ongoing basis. Phone automated surveys provide a data stream on 6 to 8 items more frequently than once a year, so that monitoring the impact of intervention on customer satisfaction is more timely.

In recent years, the CMS have launched a customer satisfaction survey that taps into a given patient's level of satisfaction with the benefits and administration of their health plan (HP). This tool entitled the Consumer Assessment of Health care Providers and Systems (CAHPS) has been developed in conjunction with the NCQA (2010). Technical specifications on the use of this survey tool can be found in Volume 3 of HEDIS (2010). Some of these measures do evaluate patients' health behaviors (for example, if the patient has obtained a flu shot), and their overall experience with the healthcare industry in general. Although the CAHPS tool does not specifically measure DM or CM, some of the items on the instrument may be nurse sensitive and may be of value because of available comparative data, and because some HPs bundle DM into their services. For example, some of the questions on the adult CAHPS tool refer to specific aspects of care rendered by the doctor or other healthcare provider (nurses are not included as a separate type of healthcare provider). Other questions refer to the extent to which advice has been offered by healthcare providers on smoking cessation and on hypertension and cholesterol management, all of which may relate to the nursing role in disease prevention/management or health and wellness programs which encourage self-care management.

Core Business Processes

Nurses are supported in many ways by the systems and processes through which they provide care. While this is true in any direct care setting, it also has merit in telephone care and field-based DM and CM programs. In hospitals, patient acuity is often considered in defining a staffing model; the same is true in DM programs, even though many more patients are included in the model. At the same time, nurses are supported by job descriptions that are accurate and competency based; they are evaluated on their performance on a regular and ongoing basis. This is sound human resource practice, regardless of the setting or care type. Similarly, productivity levels are very important in all settings in which nurses practice. Can a given nurse manage a patient care assignment that is appropriate to the setting and meet all of the patient care requirements in a given time frame? This important question in the DM and CM industry might be answered by examining not only how many patients can be cared for per nurse per day, but how many active minutes of the day the nurse is on call. While in hospitals, outpatient settings, and rehabilitation facilities, there is a "hands on" nature to the care; in telephonic DM programs, both "calls per nurse per day" and "talk time in minutes" are direct measures of nursing productivity. Clinical quality and utilization of healthcare resource outcomes may be the best overall indicators of the quality of care, but these indirect measures also have merit. In other words, for a nurse to be effective in managing the care of an entire population of patients, across the continuum of care, volume and focus matter. In order to measure overall effectiveness of a group of nurses in DM programs, these measures of core business processes, when taken with clinical quality, customer satisfaction, and utilization of healthcare resources, can add to the panel of metrics that add depth and understanding to managing the care of hundreds of thousands of patients across an entire population.

Other measures that are reflective of core business processes have value in evaluating the role of the nurse. In population health, DM, and CM processes, APNs are interested in finding those patients for whom they can have an impact on their healthcare behaviors and make a difference in the way in which they manage their day-to-day care. A diabetic patient with advanced comorbidities, who has not been in an ED or admitted (even for short- or long-term complications) to an inpatient facility, may not have obvious gaps in treatment (i.e., this patient is well managed without any help from the DM nurse). Suppose that a given diabetic patient is well managed (on his or her own), has an annual checkup with their physician, and their last HbA1c was less than 7%. This patient may have very little actionable need for a conversation with a nurse in a DM program other than an introduction, consent, a condition-specific assessment, written materials, and encouragement to stay the course. Contrast this to a newly diagnosed 55-year-old patient with a HbA1c of over 11%, with poor nutritional habits, who has just started on insulin and was just discharged from the hospital for "uncontrolled diabetes." This patient has more actionable needs and is at risk for readmission, if no DM assessment and intervention is put into place. Finding these patients, teeing them up for the nurse, and ensuring that we have accurate call information are all strategies that are collectively called "patient identification" and "acuity stratification" processes. Oftentimes, DM and CM companies use sophisticated information technology processes to identify patients for the nurse to call. A resulting "engagement rate" (CCA, 2011) that measures the percent of patients who are identified with one or more of the disease conditions under study and the percent of patients who complete an enrollment and condition-specific assessment process with a nurse are useful indicators of the degree to which the DM and/or CM programs are reaching the intended population. This is a type of volume indicator, which, when taken together with productivity metrics, can provide some evaluation of the impact of the role of the nurse on population health in DM and CM programs.

In summary, about 20 to 25 metrics in the four categories of (a) clinical quality, (b) customer satisfaction, (c) utilization of healthcare resources, and (d) core business processes taken together would provide an organization with a keen and parsimonious panel of metrics. This panel of metrics described earlier in this chapter provides the reader with possibilities for evaluating the totality of any given population health nursing program, whether DM, CM, or all three program types. Kaplan and Norton (1996; 2001) describe this idea of panel of metrics to guide the strategy of the organization as "the balanced scorecard." The examples provided earlier and from these four categories fit the evaluation need in DM, CM, and

H&W programs, but neither the categories nor the example metrics are the only possibilities. In general, metrics and measures should be easily found using existing measurement mechanisms and standardized data definitions, which can be compared against national standards and are representative of the nurse's role in improving the health of the population. A parsimonious set is useful; it is often the case that in healthcare we measure too many things. In tracking countless indicators without intention or purpose, we lose the ability to make the measures meaningful and may miss the overall strategic goals of the organization.

Data Sources

Administrative datasets have been criticized in the past for not providing useful information and for not serving as accurate measures of quality (Case-mix Measurement and Assessing Quality of Care; 1987). However, a broader understanding of the usefulness of claims data has emerged in more recent times, particularly when evaluating quality at the level of the population (Jha, Wright, & Perlin, 2007; Schatz et al., 2005). In DM, the ICD9 codes, demographics, and patient experiences as captured through a claims process provide an outline of care that is rich in both identifying patients with the most actionable need and finding patients with those gaps in treatment. Years ago, evaluation of quality required detailed and sometimes tedious chart review with random samples of charts pulled from various patient types; today, the effective use of claims data is providing a rich source of information on the effectiveness of a DM program in shaping patients' health behaviors and habits over time (HEDIS, 2010).

In most DM programs, some type of documentation is required to track the patient's progress with an educational approach and to measure the degree to which behavior is shaped. So, while it is most important for the nurse to document an educational session on, for example, the importance of asthma controller medications, it may be just as important to hold a three-way call with the patient's primary physician to identify the need to move from frequent use of a short-acting beta agonist to an inhaled corticosteroid and to document this action. The measure of the true outcomes (such as the claim for the prescription or no documented ED visits for the remaining year) may come through that administrative dataset later on, but the role of the nurse is and should be accurately captured in written or electronic documentation. The review of the nurse's documentation from a clinical perspective is no less important in call center and field-based DM programs than it is in the hospital, in an outpatient or a direct care, home setting. This documentation needs to be audited on a regular and ongoing basis; this supervisory function can also provide rich evidence of the productivity and role of the nurse. It is an important precursor to those outcomes, which may be measured through claims or other sources.

Patient self-reported data may also be useful, but this source of information may be risky as it introduces bias (e.g., recall bias, information bias, etc., [see Chapter 4]). Patients' recollection of a given result may be colored by their own resistance to a change in health behavior, by their lack of knowledge or by very strong denial defense mechanisms that develop along what may be a very difficult path. Consequently, there are times when self-report data may not be useful at all. In the NCQA DM Accreditation with Performance Measurement award, there are certain measures that must include actual laboratory results, and patient self-report is not permitted. Data collection methods using the HEDIS "hybrid" method require actual provider-held chart reviews (for a random sample) or data on laboratory results that come directly through a link to the laboratory that performed the test. Two examples that exemplify the use of laboratory data include the collection of HbA1c annual results in the patient with diabetes and the annual LDL levels in the CAD patient. The HEDIS technical specifications provide a depth of rigor on these data collection methods that is intense and appropriate. On the other hand, HEDIS recognizes that claims data on flu shots are very unreliable. Appropriately, patients are offered flu shots on a seasonal basis at health fairs, county-run clinics, during an inpatient stay, or at a local pharmacy (Pollert, Dobberstein, & Wiisanen, 2008). It may be the case that in these venues, there may be no claim submitted for the flu shot, considerably reducing the accuracy of the claims data on the incidence of obtaining flu shots in various patient populations. In most cases, the accuracy of the data on whether or not a patient has received or has not received a seasonal flu shot may be maximized by asking them. Self-report may be the best source of data available but is still not ideal. Data sources abound for key metrics in a panel of indicators that are both nurse sensitive and descriptive of population health nursing.

Quantitative Strategies for the Evaluation of Outcomes

One significant advantage to the study of health at the population level is the rich source of sample size and electronic data availability. Certainly, nursing's role in population health is enhanced by nursing's ability to measure and track key characteristics of the patient population that are indicative of clinical quality and utilization of healthcare resources. Administrative datasets and access to an electronic medical record (EMR) in a given venue or an electronic health record (EHR) that has the potential to "follow" the patient across various inpatient and outpatient settings have enhanced our collective ability as a profession to evaluate nursing's role in providing care and service.

Data Availability

The advent of the universal electronic billing process became a reality many years ago in the United States with the advancement of Medicare legislation. CMS, known at the time as the Health Care Financing Authority (HCFA), launched an electronic billing process for hospitals in the early 1990s. The electronic format emerged from a device called the "universal bill." This universal bill issued in 1992 (UB92) was the first vehicle to provide a rich source of demographic, diagnostic, and procedural data. In more recent years, ways and means to measure quality through this dataset and other claims from individual providers, from outpatient venues of all types, as well as rehabilitation settings and other post-hospital venues, have been continually refined. Known as claims data, this information does provide some practical application. Although the usefulness of these data has been qualified and challenged over time, there is a fair amount of consensus that the information included in claims can indeed be rich and useful in determining the overall health of a given population of patients with certain chronic conditions (e.g., CHF, CAD, asthma, COPD, and diabetes) and with nursing's role, regardless of venue, in influencing outcomes for these patients (Case-mix Measurement, 1987; Jha, Wright, & Perlin, 2007; Schatz et al., 2005).

Because of the very nature of lifestyle management (health and wellness), and DM and CM programs, the potential for data collection on large datasets becomes possible. While there may be appropriate methodological considerations for appropriate hypothesis testing, developing processes for determining the impact of the nursing role on outcomes becomes possible without extensive and tedious chart review and manual data collection.

Electronic systems for facilitating both EMR and EHR also raise the bar for potential outcomes research related to nursing's role in population health. In H&W, DM, and CM programs, the documentation that captures the nursing role in providing guidance for patients' self-management of their disease conditions is captured in a way such that this "self-reported" data on milestones for patient care management can be used for electronic reporting, theory testing, and hypothesis evaluation. For example, nurses who participate in smoking cessation programs as a result of their involvement in lifestyle management and H&W programs interact with patients telephonically to ascertain their progress with smoking cessation. Though our ability to evaluate whether or not the patient is using an aid may be facilitated if pharmacy claims are forthcoming (Does the patient have a prescription for a smoking cessation aid?), we have no idea whether the patient filled the prescription and is taking it without a self-report. Additionally, the patient's report on 7-day prevalence (Have you smoked a tobacco product in the past 7 days?) is the type of data only available through self-report or direct observation.

Hybrid data collection is a method proffered in the HEDIS data collection model. For some of the metrics, securing the data may require samples of outpatient charts with designated data collectors to provide specific data that is not available through electronic means. Here is an example. Some programs may have the ability to secure electronic results of laboratory data. The HEDIS measure called "comprehensive diabetes care" (CDC) includes 10 components. One measure includes the extent to which patients who have the diabetes diagnosis were able to secure a HbgA1c test within a 12-month period. This HEDIS metric can easily be compiled through quantitative methods if claims data are available. However, unless laboratory data are also available, the actual value of the HbgA1c is not forthcoming. An alternative to this is found in the hybrid method of data collection. HEDIS provides for a method of random sample selection and sample size.

Data collectors are deployed and collect the needed information by hand. For this measure and for several others in the HEDIS dataset, patient self-reported data are not acceptable. In order to be able to sort out the impact of a nursing DM strategy on patients' ongoing diabetes management, it is essential to be able to determine not only whether the patients have an annual HbgA1c test performed but what results were forthcoming, and to be able to sort out patients with good control (less than 7%) from patients with poor control (greater than 9%). Without actual laboratory results in an electronic feed or hybrid data collection, claims data are limited in providing this insight.

The CMS has, over time, refined billing practices and requirements for appropriate documentation in the electronic invoicing processes for inpatient facilities and independent providers of care. Accordingly, changes have refined our ability to capture useful information in claims but also in provider practices and to make connections for patients across the continuum of care. Incentives have been developed in recent years to reward positive practices and to better align payment with outcomes. For example, years ago UM practices for Medicare required payment for the appropriate patient placement and level of care in an acute care venue, whereas individual provider reimbursement for an inpatient stay occurs regardless of denied payment to the facility. When TJC and CMS aligned their processes around the core measures project, holding hospitals accountable for process of care measures (like getting the acute myocardial infarction [AMI] patient with ST elevation to the catheter laboratory within 90 minutes of arrival to the hospital), no incentive was permitted to the cardiologist or emergency physician who facilitated the 90-minute outcome. Similarly, keeping a patient in the hospital longer for a hospital-acquired complication (like removal of a retained instrument) had no consequences in the past. In 2009, CMS began a drive to hold reimbursement to hospitals that demonstrate these "never events" (CMS, 2010 and 2010a; http://www.cms .gov/center/quality.asp). As a result, 14 conditions were identified in this category. Similarly, in 2006, a drive by CMS to "pay for performance" was launched, encouraging individual providers to capture data in their billing practices that demonstrate patient outcomes and preventive measures in their outpatient practices with a resultant financial reward (http://www.cms.gov/pqri/). For example, for providers who can demonstrate (through their CMS billing) that a certain percentage of their diabetic patients have had a HbA1c test done annually, and that a significant proportion of that patient population has results below 7%, additional reimbursement would be provided.

The ease of access to administrative datasets and claims data has appropriately led to legislation that is intended to protect the integrity of these electronic data. The Health Care Information Portability and Accountability Act (HIPAA) was passed in 1996 and has resulted in a number of requirements across the country and in any venue or service related to the patient's right to confidentiality and privacy protections. Highlights of these regulatory requirements include the following concepts: (a) annual training for all staff members (whether involved in patient care or not) regarding protected health information, (b) signed business associate agreements ensuring that these protections transverse various vendors and clients, and (c) adequate auditing, policies, and procedures are in place to ensure that the extent and spirit of the regulations are met (Brown, 2009).

National Trends and Health Care Reform

Data availability whether from electronic, self-report, or hybrid data have changed the nature of the healthcare landscape, and the accessibility and reliability of these data have been influenced by powerful market pressures. Certainly, CMS has had a significant impact on the availability of care in the United States since its Medicare legislation in the 1960s first guaranteed healthcare as a right to all Social Security recipients over the age of 65 (http://www.ssa.gov/history/tally65.html). In recent years, evolving legislation links the issue of availability of healthcare to the quality of healthcare, and recognizes the inherent relationship between cost and quality. As quality improves, the cost of care is reduced. As measurement mechanisms and the availability of data have developed over the past 20 years, so has the collective wisdom. At the end of 2009, it was almost impossible to pick up a newspaper or read about the latest political debate without time and attention brought to "healthcare reform." Though pundits deconstruct the key elements of the current need for healthcare reform, all agree that the cost of providing healthcare in the United States has escalated. One can only hope that accessibility has improved for increasing segments of our society, but there are still significant disparities throughout regions of the country with a shortage of both primary care and subspecialty providers. There continues to be broad disagreement over the way in which healthcare reform was enacted, despite legislation passed in 2010. Regardless of the raging debate, data availability as a result of claims, patient self-report, hybrid data collection, and as a result of pay for provider (P4P) initiatives make the measurement of quality considerably more elegant, more reliable, and clearer than it has ever been in the United States in estimating the impact of nursing's role in improving population health.

Standardized Data Definitions and Comparative Databases

A theme that is consistent in this chapter is that measurement methods have evolved for the better over the course of the past 20 to 30 years. Clearly, the information technology age and the availability of administrative datasets have made this possible. In addition, clinicians have provided adequate guidance through professional organizations on both process and outcome indicators of quality and have developed data definitions that have methodological rigor and standardization (http://www.qualitymeasures.ahrq.gov/; http://www.ahrq.gov/clinic/cpgsix .htm). This agreement and standardization gives rise to the potential for comparisons on a "level playing field."

Standardized data definitions are made available by the NCQA (HEDIS volumes 1, 2, and 3 which are available for purchase at www.NCQA.org) and include detailed technical specifications. NCQA is a leader in the field and provides not only technical specifications and guidance on hybrid data collection and sample size, but also certifications for HEDIS auditing capabilities. In addition to this functionality, the NCQA provides annual data comparisons with actual percentile rankings on the HEDIS measures for Medicare, Medicaid, and commercial lines of business. These are published on their Web site annually. Purchase of the *Quality Compass* makes regionalized comparisons possible and provides the percentile ranking comparisons a little sooner than they become public.

The AHRQ (www.AHRQ.gov) provides technical specifications as a free service for many of their measures and provides the technical specifications and free software for either SPSS (2011) or SAS (2011)[1], which facilitates access to actual comparative database information. Another interesting Web site provided by AHRQ is called the "National Clearinghouse for Indicators." This Web site provides search capabilities on various topics including specific disease states and conditions and provides a collection of hundreds of metrics submitted by various specialty groups, some of which are international. The indicators are provided in a standardized format, but the technical specifications are not nearly as detailed as those provided by NCQA through its HEDIS initiative and through AHRQ. The format includes information about the name of the indicator, the owner or author, the broad inclusions in the numerator and the denominator, with typically extensive bibliographic support from the evidence-based literature on why this indicator accurately describes some aspect of clinical quality for a given condition or disease state (http://www.qualitymeasures.ahrq.gov/). This national clearinghouse includes metrics from private and public groups including but not limited to the National Quality Forum (http://www.cms.gov/center/quality.asp), CMS (http://www.cms.gov/), TJC (http://www.jointcommission.org/), and specialty groups such as the American College of Cardiology, the Society of Thoracic Surgeons and many others.

Evaluation Using Qualitative Strategies

Significant strides in nursing have been made that did not exist 40 years ago to improve measurement methods and use quantitative means to evaluate population health. This notwithstanding, qualitative methods are a source of rich and useful information in this evaluation process.

---

[1]SPSS and SAS are both powerful statistical software programs that permit data mining, and statistical analysis with a full range of descriptive, inferential (both parametric and nonparametric), and trending capabilities. They are available for purchase and used extensively in large organizations, government programs, and academic institutions. Individuals can also purchase various modules and needed statistical analytic capabilities. See http://www.spss.com/ and http://www.sas.com/

Accreditation and Certification

Accreditation and certification programs offer a systematic review of a given organization's ability to provide evidence of compliance with standards. Standards define the required elements to accreditation success, and these organizations provide both rigor and agreed-upon methodologies in pursuit of organizational distinction. Though many would argue that the process itself is more quantitative than qualitative, most would agree that the result is a credential that is desirable, often sought after, and sometimes a mandate. Most accreditation and certification programs provide various levels of review and accept both depth and breadth in terms of evidence permitted. Regardless of the type of program reviewed, these accrediting bodies have a number of common elements.

The use of standards to measure quality and effectiveness is the hallmark of an accrediting program. Whether evaluation of a given program is housed in a facility (like an acute care hospital that is accredited through TJC) or a DM program that is made up of telephonic call centers, accreditation or certification is considered to be a measure of quality. For example, TJC's certification program for CHF is offered in conjunction with the American Heart Association and offers this certification based on standards and outcomes (http://www .jointcommission.org/certification/heart_failure.aspx). As nurses practice and provide nursing care within and throughout these facilities and programs, accreditation is an indirect measure of the quality of nursing practice. The processes used within an accrediting program are also variable, but are often characterized by common features: (a) written documentation is submitted for review, (b) site visits are comprised of overview of the program, its capabilities and outcomes, and staff interviews, and (c) chart reviews of some kind are included in the accreditation process validating that as nurses we provide evidence-based care.

As part of the accreditation process, there is hardly a time when an organization must not produce metrics that are sensitive to the nursing role, demonstrate patient characteristics, and quantify patient outcomes. The accrediting process becomes qualitative as the evaluation of the quality program may or may not show actual improvement in defined patient care indicators. Many accrediting bodies are not prescriptive in the application of their standards; this is in no way a detracting characteristic. In fact, the latitude in the application of the standards (the "how") is often desirable as there are many ways to achieve the same outcome. Examples of accrediting bodies and the type of programs that they accredit or certify are provided in Exhibit 8.5. This list is not intended to be exhaustive, but simply illustrative. Each includes standards that posit to evaluate the outcome of nursing care in some way.

Community Advisory Boards

As DM, CM, and UM programs have within their essential construct the total health of the population at large as a key benefit, oftentimes representative members of that patient population are sought after to provide insight into the effectiveness of

EXHIBIT 8.5
Examples of Accrediting Bodies and the Types of Program They Accredit

1. The Joint Commission (TJC) accredits acute care hospitals and provides certification to a number of specialty hospitals and programs, many of which have a patient focus that goes well beyond the patient's inpatient experience. Accordingly, these accreditation programs have an influence on the health of the total patient population and nursing's role within. TJC is often designated by state licensure for hospital review. TJC holds deemed status for CMS; hospitals seeking to achieve or maintain provider status must be both accredited and licensed. Find more information about TJC at http://www.jointcommission.org/

2. The National Committee for Quality Assurance (NCQA) offers numerous recognition, accreditation, and certification programs, including but not limited to health plans, utilization management programs, DM programs, HEDIS auditing, and many other types. Information regarding the fine programs offered by this organization can be found at http://www.ncqa.org/

3. The Utilization Review Accreditation Committee (URAC) formally adopted the acronym URAC in 1996. It is an organization with a long track record in offering accreditation for total population health. UM, DM, and CM programs and other types of accreditation that are related to the nursing role in total population health are among the many types offered. More information on this organization can be found at http://www.urac.org/

4. The Commission on Accreditation of Rehabilitation Facilities (CARF) is yet another organization with a focus on evaluating quality of various programs including behavioral health services across the rehabilitation continuum, durable medical equipment providers, aging programs, and other program types. The CARF Web site provides a wealth of useful information on this important body: http://www.carf.org/Accreditation/

5. DNV NIAHO: This organization provides an accreditation based on the International Organization for Standardization (ISO) 9000 and achieved deemed status from CMS in September, 2008 (http://www.dnv.com/industry/healthcare/). Though this organization specializes in managing risk for many types of industries, a recent focus on healthcare and CMS-deemed status has opened a new option for accreditation. This organization has focused on accrediting hospitals, primary stroke centers, and critical access hospitals. More information can be sought at http://www.dnvaccreditation.com/pr/dnv/default.aspx

these programs and the usefulness of these programs as benefits. These committees or boards meet on a regular basis (as frequently as quarterly to as seldom as annually or "ad hoc," depending upon the need) and provide qualitative insight as to the impact of the program on patients' lives, as well as providing insight into enhancements. Telephonic services, written materials, field-based options, communication devices, and program changes are often reviewed with these boards to anticipate patient response. Similarly, insight into program results that requires community viewpoint might be the type of feedback sought from a community advisory board. Certainly members of the benefit program (patients and families) and local community groups representing the various segments of the community affected by the benefit might be included in the membership roster.

Provider Advisory Committees

Providers across specialties and venues, from nurses to physicians or from community health clinics to hospitals, are key components to the overall success in improving the health of the patient population in its entirety. Telephonic nursing provides options for care that did not exist in the past. In addition, quantitative methods have the potential to supply providers with data on their care practices that may or may not demonstrate improvement in patient outcomes. Providing feedback to physicians in a systematic and patient-centered way is a strategy that can be of tremendous benefit. Consequently, devising a vehicle to enhance communications with healthcare providers in a formal setting such as through committees can be of significant value.

Provider advisory committees come in all shapes and sizes and meet with varying frequency. Shalala (2010) advises that APNs who are in private practice represent an important enhancement to our ability to extend primary care capacity across the country (http://www.rwjf.org/pr/digest.jsp?id=10662&topicid=1318). Representative providers, including APNs, can "weigh in" on data presentation; they can provide advice on ways and means to make sound use of these data in a global way, as well as helping to anticipate reaction. These forums serve as educational opportunities on the role of the DM program and the ways in which it can enhance practice management, as well as the ways that an EHR across the continuum of care can enhance communication processes among all members of the healthcare team as well as maximize patient outcomes. Provider advisory committees provide depth to a DM program that is not easily found through quantitative methods.

SUMMARY

APNs play an increasingly important role in evaluating the quality and effectiveness of healthcare delivery systems. As APN roles have expanded into this area, it is paramount that APNs understand the ways and means to evaluate population health outcomes, as well as the systems of care that provide population health services. Various definitions of quality have been presented, and several theoretical frameworks are available for evaluating quality. Nurse-sensitive indicators of quality can be described using the following categories: (a) clinical quality, (b) utilization of healthcare resources, (c) core business processes, and (d) customer satisfaction.

Population-based models including disease management, case management, and care coordination are relevant to advanced nursing practice. Application and use of process improvements models are becoming an integral part of population-based nursing at all levels. Both quantitative and qualitative methods can be used to measure the quality and the effectiveness of programs. There are also a number of strategies available to help ensure the successful collaboration of community members and providers to ensure a strong medical home model. More information emerges day to day on these new and exciting ideas, which add depth to our healthcare system, reduces fragmentation, improves outcomes, and reduces the cost of care.

EXERCISES AND DISCUSSION QUESTIONS

Exercise 8.1 **Case Study**: Measuring quality often depends on one's definitions, and it is quite appropriate to provide a glossary of terms to ensure a common understanding. Imagine that you are a clinical director at an organization with a contract for Medicaid Disease Management in a rural Midwestern state. You have oversight responsibility for eight registered nurses who serve in the capacity of health coaches in a telephone call center located in an office setting in the state's capital. Your patients live in very rural areas of the state, there are no urban settings, and there are few primary care providers who accept Medicaid. However, there are five primary hospitals spread throughout your state, a number of 25 bed "critical access" hospitals, and a few federally qualified health centers (FQHCs). Your disease management (DM) program consists of a focus on five disease conditions: congestive heart failure (CHF), chronic obstructive pulmonary disease (COPD), asthma, diabetes, and coronary artery disease (CAD). Your program is guided by a very competent medical director, who is a physician, and you report to an executive director, who is also an APN. You have sound information technology (IT) support, and the state sends claims data weekly with eligible patients who have already been identified with one or more of the various disease states for entry into your DM program. Consider your customer (the state in the Midwest) and the role of the telephone nurse and answer the following questions for discussion.

■ What are some examples of customer's expectations that might emerge from this contract?

■ How might the state define quality in measurable terms? At the end of the 3-year term? On an ongoing basis?

■ What would represent the features of your program?

■ What patient outcomes might be considered of value to your customer?

■ What would constitute a deficiency?

Exercise 8.2 **Case Study**: As an APN, you are serving in the capacity as the executive director of an office that proudly holds commercial contracts with health plans all over the country to provide DM and CM services to their members. In approximately 40 different contracts, some large and some small, your site houses a telephone call center with over 40 registered nurses "on call" with patients in health plans across the country. Your leadership team is made up of a full-time medical director, six supervisors in both clinical and nonclinical roles, and another 40 people who serve various administrative and nonclinical functions. You have access to claims data for every contract, and a fully functioning electronic medical record (EMR) for your DM and CM documentation. Most of your contracts are 3-year contracts.

■ Brainstorm at least three metrics for each of the four categories that we have discussed in this chapter.

■ Consider goal setting. What will you set for annual goals for clinical quality outcome measures selected in the above?

■ How will you track your nurses' progress on the core business process measures?

■ What resources will you consider to capture data on customer satisfaction?

■ Your contracts are, for the most part, 3 years in length. At the end of the first year, describe where you would like to go with HEDIS measures when compared to the rest of the commercial PPO and HMO patients? The second year? The third year?

Exercise 8.3 **Case Study**: Imagine that you are the vice president for quality improvement in a national disease management company with contracts and interests in 26 states across the country. Your health coaches are registered nurses who work in telephone call centers across the country, and focus on patients with gaps in their treatment program. These nurses work under the supervision of clinical managers, who are also RNs with advanced degrees. Quality managers in these local sites are seeking your input and guidance on a matter of measurement. In addition, your company is preparing a balanced scorecard and is interested in monitoring quality in four categories: clinical quality, utilization of healthcare resources, core business processes, and customer satisfaction. Your contracts consistently include patients with diabetes mellitus, chronic obstructive pulmonary disease, congestive heart failure, asthma, and coronary artery disease. You serve primarily commercial clients with health maintenance organizations (HMO) and a preferred provider organization (PPO). You will need access to the Internet for this exercise.

- Name at least two clinical qualities or utilization of healthcare resource (condition-specific) metrics for each of the five above mentioned conditions. Choose at least two HEDIS metrics.
- Consult the NCQA Web site and the available data that provide percentile rankings. If you were to set a quality goal for the coming year at the 75th percentile using HEDIS guidance for commercial PPO plans, what average score for your two selected HEDIS clinical metrics would your contracts each need to achieve?
- Think about how these measures "connect" to the RN/health coach role. What functions does the nurse perform in the day to day on the call with a patient that drives toward the outcomes you have chosen to measure in the first item in this exercise?

Exercise 8.4   **Case Study**: As an APN, you have an expanding role as an actively practicing primary care clinician. You are in private practice with two other similar APNs and a primary care physician. Your practice has a large number of Medicaid recipients who have, as a benefit, eligibility and enrollment in a disease management program. Your practice has achieved recognition by the NCQA for diabetes care in your practice (http://www.ncqa.org/tabid/139/Default.aspx). You do not know much about the DM program (at all), but you know that (a) you have been contacted by a nurse on the phone representing the needs of your patients, (b) you have seen some data on your patient outcomes (and they are not as high as you would expect them to be), and (c) your practice has been invited to serve on a provider advisory committee. You are really pressed for time in your busy practice but you are intrigued. You have decided to participate. Consider the following questions in making a contribution.

- What questions would you bring to the table?
- How would you like to see the agenda take shape?
- Would you be expecting contract hours for your participation? Why or why not?
- Your practice is already recognized by the diabetes association with "provider status." How can these data possibly be correct?

REFERENCES

2010–2011 Malcolm Baldridge Award criteria. (2010). Retrieved from http://www.nist .gov/baldrige/baldrige_120310.cfm

Agency for Healthcare Research and Quality. (2010). http://www.ahrq.gov/qual/

Baicker, K., Cutler, D., & Song, Z. (2010). Workplace wellness programs can generate savings. *Health Affairs, 29,* 304–311.

Bedell, W., & Kaszkin-Bettag, M. (2010). Coherence and healthcare cost—RCA actuarial study: A cost-effectiveness cohort study. *Alternative Therapies, 16*(4), 26–31.

Berwick, D. M., Godfrey, A. B., & Roessner, J. (1990). *Curing healthcare: New strategies for quality improvement.* San Francsisco, CA: Jossey-Bass.

Best, M., & Neuhauser, D. (2006). Joseph Juran: Overcoming resistance to organizational change. *Quality and Safety in Health Care, 15,* 380–382.

Brown, J. (2009). *The healthcare quality handbook, 24th edition.* Pasadena, CA: JB Quality Solutions, Inc.

Care Continuum Alliance. (2011). http://carecontinuum.org/

Case-mix measurement and assessing quality of hospital care. (1987). *Health Care Financing Review Annual Supplement,* pp.39–48.

Chen, C. M., Hong, M. C., & Hsu, Y. H. (2007). Administrator self-ratings of organizational capacity and performance of healthy community development projects in Taiwan. *Public Health Nursing, 24,* 343–354.

Chu, H. L., Wang, C. C., & Dai, Y. T. (2009). A study of a nursing department performance measurement system: Using the balanced scorecard and the analytic hierarchy process. *Nursing Economic$, 27,* 401–407.

CMS. (2010a). Retrieved at http://www.cms.gov/HospitalAcqCond/

CMS. (2010b). *Quality of care center.* Retrieved from: http://www.cms.gov/center/quality.asp

Corn, J. B. (2009). Six sigma in healthcare. *Radiologic Technology, 81*(1), 92–95.

Courtney, B. A., Ruppman, J. B., & Cooper, H. M. (2006). Save our skin: Initiative cuts pressure ulcer incidence in half. *Nursing Management, 37*(4), 36, 38, 40.

Cross, K. F. (2000). Call resolution: The wrong focus for service quality? *Quality Progress, 33*(2), 64–67.

DeFeo, J.A., & Barnard, W.W. (2004) Juran Institute's Six Sigma; Breakthrough and Beyond. New York: McGraw Hill.

DeFeo, J. A., & Juran, J. M. (2010). *Juran's quality handbook: The complete guide to performance excellence* (6th ed.). New York, NY: McGraw-Hill.

Del Franco, M. (2003). Cutting back on call abandonment. *Catalog Age, 20*(7), 59–60.

Dienemann, J. (Ed.). (1992). *Continuous quality improvement in nursing.* Washington, DC: American Nurses Publishing.

Donabedian, A. (1980). *The definition of quality and approaches to assessment.* Ann Arbor, MI: Health Administration Press.

Drenckpohl, D., Bowers, L., & Cooper, H. (2007). Use of the six sigma methodology to reduce incidence of breast milk administration errors in the NICU. *Neonatal Network, 26,* 161–166.

Fairbanks, C. B. (2007). Using six sigma and lean methodologies to improve OR throughput. *AORN, 86*(1), 73–82.

Fetterolf, D., Holt, A. E., Tucker, T., & Khan, N. (2010). Estimating clinical and economic impact in case management programs. *Population Health Management, 13,* 73–82.

Formichelli, L. (2007). By the numbers. *Multichannel Merchant, 24*(4), 44–45.

Gill, K. J., Swarbick, M., Murphy, A. A., Spagnolo, A. B., & Zechner, M. R. (2009). Co-morbid psychiatric and medical disorders: Challenges and strategies. *Journal of Rehabilitation, 75*(3), 32–40.

Godchaux, C. W. (1999). Case managers drive care integration. *Nursing Management, 30*(11), 32B–32C, 32F–32G.

Goonan, K. J. (1995). *The Juran prescription*. San Francisco, CA: Jossey-Bass.

Goonan, K. J., & Scarrow, P. (2010). Interview with a quality leader: Kate Goonan and performance excellence. *Journal for Health care Quality, 32*(3), 32–35.

Govil, S. R., Weidner, G., Mrritt-Worden, T., & Ornish, D. (2009). Socioeconomic status and improvements in lifestyle, coronary risk factors and quality of life: The multisite cardiac lifestyle intervention program. *American Journal of Public Health, 99,* 1263–1270.

Guru guide. (2010). Six thought leaders who changed the quality world forever. *Quality Progress, 43*(11), 14–21.

Gustafson, B. M. (1999). A well staffed PFS call center can improve patient satisfaction. *Health care Financial Management, 53*(7), 64–66.

Handler, A., Issel, M., & Turnock, B. (2001). A conceptual framework to measure performance of the public health system. *Amercian Journal of Public Health, 91,* 1235–1239.

Hassan, M., Tuckman, H. P., Patrick, R. H., Kountz, D. S., & Kohn, J. L. (2010). Cost of hospital-acquired infection. *Hospital Topics, 88*(3), 82–89.

HEDIS. (2010). *Narrative, technical specifications, and survey measurement* (Vols. 1–3). Washington, DC: NCQA. http://ncqa.org/tabid/59/Default.aspx

Institute of Medicine (IOM). (1999). *To Err is human; building a safer health system. A consensus report*. Retrieved from http://iom.edu/Reports/1999/To-Err-is-Human-Building-A-Safer-Health-System.aspx

Institute of Medicine (IOM). (2001). *Crossing the quality chasm: A new health system for the 21st century.* http://iom.edu/~/media/Files/Report%20Files/2001/Crossing-the-Quality-Chasm/Quality%20Chasm%202001%20%20report%20brief.pdf

Jha, A. K., Wright, S. M., & Perlin, J. B. (2007). Performance measures, vaccinations, and pneumonia rates among high-risk patients in Veterans Administration healthcare. *American Journal of Public Health, 97,* 2167–2172.

Joint Commission Resources (JCR). (2003). *Root cause analysis in healthcare; Tools and techniques* (2nd ed.). Oakbrook, IL: JCR.

Kaplan, R. S., & Norton, D. P. (1996). *The balanced scorecard*. Boston, MA: Harvard Business School Press.

Kaplan, R. S., & Norton, D. P. (2001). *The strategy-focused organization*. Boston, MA: Harvard Business School Press.

Kaplan, S., Bisgaard, S., Truesdell, D., & Zetterholm, S. (2009). Design for six sigma in healthcare: Developing an employee influenza vaccination process. *Journal for Health care Quality, 31*(3), 36–43.

Lamb, S. E., Toye, F., & Barker, K. L. (2007). Chronic disease management programme in people with severe knee osteoarthritis: Efficacy and moderators of response. *Clinical Rehabilitation, 22,* 169–178.

Maddox, P. J. (1992). Successful implementation of a CQI process. In J. Dienneman (Ed.), *Continuous quality improvement in nursing* (pp. 115–124). Washington, DC: American Nurses Publishing.

McCaughey, B. (2006). Saving lives and the bottom line. *Modern Health care, 36*(5), 23.

Meurer, S. J., McGartland-Rubio, D., Counte, M. A., & Burroughs, T. (2002). Development of a healthcare quality improvement measurement tool: Results of a content validity study. *Hospital Topics: Research and Perspectives on Health care, 80*(2), 7–13.

Moen, R. D., & Norman, C. L. (2010). Circling back: Clearing up myths about the Deming cycle and seeing how it keeps evolving. *Quality Progress, 43*(11), 22–28.

Moulin, M., Soady, J., Skinner, J., Price, C., Cullen, J., & Gilligan, C. (2007). Using the public sector scorecard in public health. *International Journal of Health Care Quality Assurance, 20,* 281–289.

Nash, D. B., Reifsnyder, J., Fabius R. J., & Pracilio, V. P. (2011). *Population health; creating a culture of wellness.* Sudbury, MA: Jones and Bartlett Learning.

National Committee for Quality Assurance (NCQA). (2009). Standards and guidelines for the accreditation and certification of disease management. Washington, DC: NCQA.

National Committee for Quality Assurance (NCQA). (2010). http://ncqa.org/

National Quality Forum (NQF). (2010). http://ncqa.org/

National Quality Forum (NQF). (2010. June). The power of safety: State reporting provides lessons in reducing harm, improving care. *Quality connections.* Retrieved from http://www.qualityforum.org/Publications/2010/06/Quality_Connections_The_Power_of_Safety_State_Reporting_Provides_Lessons_in_Reducing_Harm,_Improving_Care.asx

O'Toole, T. P., Buckel, L., Bourgault, C., Blumen, J., Redihan, S. G., Jiang, L. M., & Friedmann, P. (2010). Applying the chronic care model to homeless veterans: Effect of a population approach to primary care on utilization and clinical outcomes. *American Journal of Public Health, 100,* 2493–2499.

Pollert, P., Dobberstein, D., & Wiisanen, R. (2008). Jumping into the healthcare retail market: Our experience. *Frontiers of Health Services Management, 24*(3), 13–21.

Potthoff, S., & Ryan, M. J. (2004). Leadership, management, and change in improving quality in healthcare. *Frontiers of Health Services Management, 20*(3), 37–40.

Pyzdek, T. (2003). The Six Sigma Handbook. New York: McGraw Hill.

Rice, K. L., Dewan, N., Bloomfield, H. E., Grill, J., Schult, T. M., Nelson, D. B., ... Niewoehner, E. (2010). Disease management program for chronic obstructive pulmonary disease: A randomized controlled trial. *American Journal of Respiratory Critical Care Medicine, 182,* 890–896.

SAS. (2011). http://www.sas.com/

Santos, A. B., Henggeler, S. W., Burns, B. J., Arana, G. W., Meisler, N. (1995). Research on field-based services: Models for reform in the delivery of mental healthcare to populations with complex clinical problems. *American Journal of Psychiatry, 152,* 1111–1123.

Schatz, M., Nakahiro, R., Crawford, W., Mendoza, G., Mosen, D., & Stibolt, T. B. (2005). Asthma quality-of-care markers using administrative data. *Chest, 128,* 1968–1674.

Schiller, K. C., Weech-Maldonado, R., & Hall, A. G., (2010). Patient assessments of care and utilization in Medicaid managed care: PCCMs vs. PSOs. *Journal of Health care Finance, 36*(3), 13–23.

Shalala, D. (2010). *Group recommends expanding nurses' role in primary care.* Retrieved at http://www.rwjf.org/pr/digest.jsp?id=10662&topicid=1318

SPSS. (2011). http://www.spss.com/

Stankovic, A. K., & DeLauro, E. (2010). Quality improvements in the preanalytical phase: Focus on the urine specimen flow. *MLO: Medical Laboratory Observer, 42*(3), 20, 22, 24–27.

The Joint Commission (TJC). (2010). http://www.jointcommission.org/

The Joint Commission and CMS. (2010). *Specifications manual for national hospital inpatient quality measures.* Retrieved at http://www.jointcommission.org/specifications_manual_for_national_hospital_inpatient_quality_measures/

URAC. (2009). Case Management Standards, Version 4.0. Washington, DC: URAC.

URAC (1996). Retrieved from http://www.urac.org/accreditation/

Womack, J. P., & Jones, D. T. (2003). *Lean thinking.* New York, NY: Free Press.

Wubker, A. (2007). Measuring the quality of healthcare: The connection between structure, process and outcomes of care, using the example of myocardial infarction treatment in Germany. *Disease Management & Health Outcomes, 15*, 225–238.

Yap, C., Siu, E., Baker, G. R., Brown, A. D., & Lowi-Young, M. P. (2005). A comparison of systemwide and hospital-specific performance measurement tools. *Journal of Health care Management, 50*, 251–263.

Yun, E. K., & Chun, K. M. (2008). Critical to quality in telemedicine service management: Application of DFSS (design for six sigma) and SERVQUAL. *Nursing Economic$, 26*, 384–388.

NINE

Building Relationships and Engaging Communities Through Collaboration

Barbara A. Benjamin

There is an old African saying, "One silver bracelet does not make much jingle." Let us consider this adage when we think community health assessment (CHA). The primary purpose of building relationships and engaging communities through collaboration is to facilitate a dialog to aid in the assessment, planning, action, and evaluation of challenging care-based issues through program design and development. By working with the community, healthcare professionals have the opportunity to collaborate on issues relevant to the community to ensure sustainability and long-term success of community-based programs. This type of collaboration fosters bidirectional communication, understanding, and knowledge in the quest to ensure compassionate, quality, and culturally sensitive interventions.

Elizabeth Lenz (2005) in an article "The Practice Doctorate in Nursing: An Idea Whose Time Has Come" chose to define advanced practice nursing at the doctoral level to include management of care for individuals and populations, administration of nursing and healthcare organizations, and health policy formulation and evaluation. The practice-focused doctorate is an important alternative to research-focused doctorates in nursing. The choice to use a second approach was based, in part, on a long-standing conceptualization of nursing practice as having two related domains: the direct and the indirect, with the latter defined as activities that are carried out in support of the provision of direct care. Furthermore, Lenz felt that the decision to define nursing practice more inclusively than hands-on care is based on recognition of the authority and responsibility to make decisions that influence nursing and healthcare. In addition, ultimately patient outcomes often reside at the system level (i.e., with nursing administrators and policy makers). According to Lenz, there is an increasing need for insightful and visionary nursing leadership in practice; there must be a place at the decision-making table for the nurse. To paraphrase Lenz, the ability to make decisions at the community level requires that the APNs who work in the community (prepared at the doctoral level) be part of the higher level of care management and policy decision making in concert with the community-based consortium of healthcare policy makers. Lenz (2005) states, "It [Doctor of Nursing Practice degree] is increasingly the credential that is needed for credibility in leadership positions" (para. 24).

Darlyne Bailey (1992) defines a community-based consortium as "a partnership of organizations and individuals representing consumers, service providers, and local agencies or groups who identify themselves with a particular community, neighborhood, or locale and who unite in an effort to collectively apply their resources to the implementation of a common strategy for the achievement of a common goal within that community" (72). It is necessary for community-based APNs to know the community and to interact with its leaders toward a common healthcare goal when making healthcare decisions at the community level.

In order for the APN to practice at the level inclusive of all of the particulates described by Lenz, that nurse must know the community. The CHA is the most effective and efficient method used to know that community. Shuster and Goeppinger (2008) state that "Community assessment is one of the three core functions of public health nursing" (p. 351).

IDENTIFYING COMMUNITY NEEDS

Why Assess the Community?

Community assessment and analysis is a cornerstone of effective care and is the first step in community practice. There is an essential incentive for conducting a community assessment. A thorough assessment should identify the community needs by recognizing the diversity of the community and understanding the community's goals and listening to their priorities. Assessment can help to identify what works and what does not work and can help to address perceived advantages and disadvantages by both parties, thus meeting the needs of that community through collaboration.

Any plan to meet the needs of the community that is derived from a CHA may truly be considered an evidence-based practice plan. According to the Department of Health and Human Services (DHHS), addressing health improvement is a shared responsibility of federal, state, and local governments, policy makers, business, healthcare providers, professionals, educators, community leaders, and the American public (U.S. DHHS, 2000a,b). Therefore, if health improvement is the goal, all segments of the community must be involved in a community health assessment, a collaborative effort.

A community health assessment may focus on a community as defined by its geopolitical boundaries (e.g., towns, cities, counties) or on a defined population or an aggregate of a community. Aggregates are subpopulations within the larger population, a collection of individuals having one or more characteristics in common (Stanhope & Landcaster, 2008). Community health assessments are most often conducted for geographical communities. These assessments can be used to identify populations that need more intensive study of specific problems that require an aggregate assessment. A comprehensive community assessment addresses the characteristics of the community's physical environment, infrastructure, and population characteristics. It is through this type of assessment that the APN can begin to identify the strengths and weaknesses of a community. This information will be required when the time comes to work with community members to achieve mutually agreed upon goals for improvement in targeted outcomes.

Conducting the Assessment

The APN who works in the community in collaboration with the principal players in the healthcare environment of the community has many options when deciding what method is best for the community that is being assessed. Assessment can be done by any number of methodologies and can include assessment tools, surveys, focus groups, and windshield surveys. Information found in online databases and Web sites is an invaluable resource for every community-based APN. Online databases can provide a plethora of knowledge including but not limited to:

- geographical composition of the community;
- vital statistics such as births, deaths;
- morbidity, mortality, communicable diseases;
- housing, migration, population density;
- education, employment;
- marriages, divorces, adoptions;
- health services provided; and
- insurance companies, accidents, police, and fire reports.

The experienced APN will use a combination of methods to obtain an evidence-based CHA. By using research from online resources, as well as a combination of quantitative methods (e.g., searching databases), or qualitative methods, (e.g., focus groups and surveys), the APN can accomplish a fuller, richer, more powerful CHA (Hanchet, 1988) (Figure 9.1).

Anderson and McFarland (2008) suggest that CHA is not a "solo job." No one should attempt to assess a community alone. The APN should involve many people in the assessment because all stakeholders within a community have something to offer. The APN who can mobilize an interdisciplinary team of administrators, policy makers, and members in public service such as police and fire departments, educational facilities, and health departments, will have a diverse resource of knowledge to access for a CHA. And by working together on the assessment, the initial steps taken toward an early collaboration will improve the chances of achieving targeted outcomes (American Association of Colleges of Nursing [AACN], 2004a).

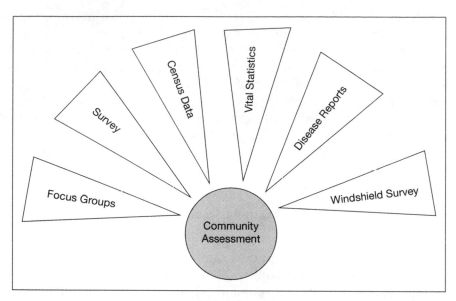

FIGURE 9.1 Symphony to Achieve a Comprehensive Community Assessment. Graphic by Ariel Haney, 2011.

The APN might decide to customize an assessment tool to suit the needs of a specific community. Anderson and McFarlane, in their text *Community as Partner Theory and Practice in Nursing* (2008), suggest in their plan for the assessment of a community that many essentials need to be included in the assessment. Among these essential factors are the history of the community, demographics, ethnicity, vital statistics, values, beliefs, and religion. It is also essential to include physical environment of the community, the health and social services provided within that community, and the safety and political environments. Anderson and McFarlane (2008) considered all of these factors in an assessment plan for a town called Rosemont. By using these factors Anderson and McFarlane developed a community assessment wheel that includes communication, human and social services, politics and government, safety and transportation, education, physical environment, recreation, and economics. From that wheel they devised an assessment tool. They note that even when using all parts of their model, a community assessment is never complete and they recommend that assessments should be done in increments in order to better manage the enormity of the task. The APN should stop at predetermined intervals, synthesize the data that have been collected, and use the accumulated information to identify potential areas for intervention. These authors feel that while no CHA is ever complete, their model provides a framework for success and the basis for creating a plan for successful intervention.

During the analysis and evaluation phase of the assessment data, the APN may discover that further information is needed. The scope of the data collected may be large but certain parts may be missing. For example, if the APN is interested in childhood obesity and needs more information on the scope of the problem in the community, it may be essential to assemble a group of parents within the community to better assess the problem. This subgroup of the population can meet using an open discussion methodology, in which the parents discuss their concerns about childhood obesity in their own community. Qualitative information derived from community members can be as valuable as, or in some cases, more valuable than quantitative information. An additional benefit is that allowing parents to derive their own conclusions about the root of the problem may yield a significant amount of insight into this community's values and needs. This may also lead parents to consider solutions that work best for their own family and communities, which is more likely to ensure long-term buy in and success.

Assessment Tools

Most community health textbooks contain examples of CHA tools. Angeline Busby, in her textbook *Orientation to Nursing in the Rural Community* (2000), details a comprehensive plan for a CHA, inclusive of phases of assessment with objectives and activities for completion of the assessment. Busby's phases include:

> Organize and establish community-provider partnerships
> Review, analyze and understand existing data
> Collect additional community data
> Analyze and interpret community data
> Develop a community health plan
> Implement community health plan
> Evaluate the implementation and outcome of the plan.
>
> (pp. 50–51)

For the process phase, she lists the types of assessment as well as primary and secondary sources. She stresses the importance of engaging partners in the CHA process and having the community take responsibility for planning, implementing, and evaluating the action plans that are developed to deal with the community's health-related concerns. For Busby, the CHA goes well beyond collecting data. Importance is placed on bringing communities together to solve local problems. (Busby, 2000).

Anderson and McFarlane, in their text *Community as Partner: Theory and Practice in Nursing* (2008), state that a CHA is "a process: it is the act of becoming acquainted with the community" (p. 217). They quote Hancock and Minkler (1997) "For Health Professionals concerned with ... community building for health, there are two reasons for (conducting) community health assessments: information is needed for change, and it is needed for empowerment" (p. 1400).

A community-based consortium is defined as a partnership of organizations.

For three decades, *Healthy People* has provided a comprehensive set of national 10-year health promotion and disease prevention objectives aimed at improving the health of all Americans (see Chapter 2 for more background). It is grounded on the notion that establishing objectives and providing benchmarks to track and monitor progress over time can motivate, guide, and focus action. *Healthy People 2020* will continue in the tradition of its predecessors to define the vision and strategy for building a healthier nation with a focus on reducing disparities.

According to *Healthy People 2020*, the determinants of health are individual biology and behavior, physical and social environments, policies and interventions, and access to quality healthcare. These determinants have a profound effect on the health of individuals, communities, and the nation. An evaluation of these determinants is an important part of developing any strategy to improve health (U.S. DHSS, 2008).

Truglio-Londrigan and Lewenson, in their text *Public Health Nursing: Practicing Population-Based Care* (2011), used a systematic approach to design a Public Health Nurse Assessment Tool (PHNAT). The PHNAT is thorough and inclusive. The authors feel that their tool provides a systematic method for community assessment and "offers a kaleidoscope way to view the individual, family, community system and population." The authors further suggest that use of the online versions of their tool "further facilitates the use of this tool because it can be more easily manipulated and implemented in that format" (Truglio-Londrigan & Lewenson, 2011, p. 56).

Healthy People 2020 updates that model to include "a feedback loop of intervention, assessment, and dissemination of evidence and best practices that would enable achievement of *Healthy People 2020* goals." This updated model adds monitoring and evaluation to the graphic. *Assessment* is considered by both the nursing profession and *Healthy People 2020* to be the cornerstone of effective care. Collaboration was also considered invaluable in the development of this Action Model (Figure 9.2) "The *Healthy People* process is inclusive; and its strength is directly tied to collaboration" (DHHS, healthypeople2020@hhs.gov). This assessment tool like the others mentioned earlier stresses community collaboration as necessary for a successful community assessment.

ASSESSMENT METHODOLOGIES

Focus Groups

CHA can be enhanced through the use of focus groups. Through the focus group format, community members can provide input about what they feel their community needs. Sometimes specific stakeholders in a community such as

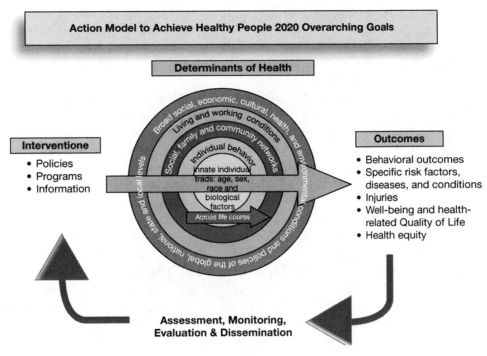

Figure 9.2 Action Model to Achieve *Healthy People 2020.*
Overarching Goals. *Source:* U.S. DHHS (2008, p. 7).

members of government, designees from police or fire departments, clergy, and representatives from senior or youth groups form the focus group. More often the focus groups are open meetings to which all members of a community are invited. Several community destinations such as churches or public libraries provide appropriate settings, and a variety of meeting times optimize the opportunities for community members to participate.

A focus group should have a well-prepared moderator to lead the group. The moderator should guide the group so that it does not stray from the issues or topics being addressed, and the moderator should ask explicit questions that are specifically worded to elicit public input. Without a moderator, focus can be lost and the discussion may become tangential and too diffuse to extract useful information. An experienced moderator can actually prompt or cue the members in a way that elicits innovative and constructive ideas with creative solutions. The use of an experienced moderator is essential to keep the focus group members on task. Many times, these meetings are recorded to avoid missing any thoughts and ideas or nuances from the community. Butler, DePhelps, and DePhelps (1994) suggest selective community members who have relevant knowledge can provide the needed information through a focus group approach. During focus group discussions, it can sometimes become apparent that the project that has been targeted by the APN may not be important to or a high priority for the community and that often leads to a change in project focus. This should not be considered a negative outcome of a focus group but a success as it is important for the community to buy into the project in order to have long-term sustainability. It is appropriate for community members to prioritize their needs.

A school nurse intervention program for inner-city Mexican American children was planned by Cowell, McNaughton, and Ailey (2000) using data obtained from focus groups. The focus groups, conducted in Spanish, focused on mothers of Mexican American children attending a local elementary school. The mothers were asked to discuss what nursing services they would like and where these services should be located. The problems these mother identified included discipline, domestic violence, substance abuse, and unemployment. The mothers also discussed their problems with American culture. As a result of the focus groups, home visits by nurses were planned with interventions designed to address the identified problems. It is important to note that the needs of the community were assessed and addressed by the focus group. This led to a mutually agreed upon solution with a good chance for success because participants felt that they were heard. Programs designed with input from focus groups that include community members have a better chance of addressing a community's needs and wants, and a higher likelihood of success than programs developed without community input.

Surveys

Surveys form an excellent matrix for the collection of information about a population. Usually in a CHA survey, questions are asked to a sample of the community's population, and the responses generate information either numerically (quantitative) or written (qualitative) about the topics under examination. Surveys can be distributed to community members via face-to-face interaction, e-mail, telephone and/or mail. They can also be distributed through schools and churches, and in some cases through the local newspaper. An excellent site for survey development can be found at http://cru.cahe.wsu.edu/CEPublications/wrep0132/wrep0132.html. The authors of this Web site, Andranovich and Howell (2008), provide step-by-step instructions on survey development and administration as well as collation of results. Several commercial electronic methodologies such as Survey Monkey (www.surveymonkey.com) are also available and some require a fee for their usage. Many of these online resources can help guide the APN in survey development and distribution.

Lundy and Janes (2009), in their text *Community Health Nursing: Caring for the Public's Health*, discuss the use of a survey to discover the rates of drug use among long-haul truck drivers and the influence of the drugs on truck accidents and fatigue. Thirty-five truck drivers were surveyed at truck stops and loading facilities across cities and towns in Queensland, Australia. Truck drivers reported high rates of usage of prescription medications, over-the-counter drugs, and amphetamines. They also reported that they were motivated to use drugs because of peer pressure, socialization, and the need for relaxation, in addition to wanting to fit the image of a truck driver. The data collected through the survey identified those social factors that must be considered when developing drug prevention and treatment programs for truck drivers. This is an example of how surveys can be useful for describing the characteristics of a population. Surveys, however, are not useful when trying to establish a cause-and-effect relationship. In this case, there are three potential variables—peer pressure, socialization, and the need for relaxation that cannot be easily controlled. After a literature review is performed, if no relationship is evident in the literature, additional studies may need to be performed to evaluate the impact of these variables on drug usage in truck drivers. Regardless, the use of surveys can establish a pattern of behaviors and attitudes that may need to be addressed in the assessment phase. By carefully reviewing the literature and history of similar population-based interventions, the experienced APN can approach this problem with evidence-based solutions or establish new solutions using the information obtained in the assessment.

Windshield Survey

A windshield survey refers to the means that information can be obtained about a community by driving through it. It is an excellent tool for getting an overall feel or impression of a community. The APN can use a windshield survey to view the amount of open space, the number and types of retail stores and commercial developments, and the type and condition of housing. Walking through the community can yield similar results (Stanhope & Lancaster, 2008). The PHNAT tool of Truglio-Londrigan and Lewenson (2011) is useful when doing a windshield survey as it provides a comprehensive matrix for describing the physical environment of the community.

One CHA windshield survey that undergraduate students conducted in a small industrial town revealed a large number of taverns. Upon visiting the taverns, the students discovered that many of the men who patronized them smoked cigarettes. They learned that it was the usual custom for the men in this community to stop at these places on their way home after work in the local industries to enjoy some socialization. A review of local health department data also revealed a high incidence of oral cancer in this town. This is an example of how a windshield survey, combined with other health-related data, can be used to identify potential areas for intervention in a community.

Databases

Essential #3 of the AACN *Position Statement on the Practice Doctorate in Nursing* (2004) states that graduates of DNP programs should be able to use information technology and research methods appropriately to: collect appropriate and accurate data to generate evidence for nursing (p. 12). Some useful databases for the APN who works in the community include the following: the census, state and local health department vital statistics, and databases maintained by local police departments and school systems. Valuable information on health indicators is also available in the *Morbidity and Mortality Weekly Report*. A comprehensive discussion for locating population data is presented in Chapter 2 of this text. The CHA is further enhanced when data are collected from a variety of sources.

Census Data

As required by the United States Constitution, the United States Census Bureau conducts a census of the entire population every 10 years. While basic data are collected on everyone, a selected sample of the population is surveyed in greater detail using the "long form." That data provide a plethora of community characteristics (e.g., age, sex, race, education, employment, income) and better describe the makeup of communities. The information gathered is compiled and analyzed and reported to the nation. It should be noted that low-income and migratory populations are often under-represented in the data. Ervin (2002) writes that the importance of census data as a source of information is invaluable. She states that the census is a rich source of information and can provide details that will help identify important community characteristics (e.g., culture, socioeconomic characteristics). Census information is available at www.census.gov.

Disease Reports

The Centers for Disease Control and Prevention publishes the *Morbidity and Mortality Weekly Report* (http://www.cdc.gov). The APN may want to subscribe to this free publication. The data within these reports are often not available elsewhere and can be invaluable sources of information (Ervin, 2002). Morbidity and mortality data are also available from the DHHS and CDC Web sites. Information on notifiable diseases, specific topics such as registries, adverse drug reactions, injury surveillance, occupational health, and birth defects is available from these two government agencies. Most of this information is available on the Internet and is provided at little or no cost. This information can be valuable and useful in enhancing the APN's understanding of a community. It can also help the APN generate new and innovative ideas in survey design or development of a focus group questionnaire (refer to Chapter 2 of this text for suggestions on retrieval of data).

Health Department Vital Statistics

Vital statistics are an excellent source of data and are easily obtainable. While considered "dry" by many community assessors, data on births, deaths, marriages, and divorces are vital statistics within the community and are collected on an ongoing basis. As explained in the example of the college students who combined data obtained through a windshield survey with discussions with residents and morbidity statistics, combining quantitative data from databases with more personal and qualitative CHA methods can help to clarify community needs. There is a wide spectrum of quantitative information on populations available on the Internet. Information from health departments in combination with information gleaned from other sources such as surveys or focus groups provides solid data for the development of specific interventions (i.e., high mortality rates because of breast cancer in a community might suggest the need for an increase in breast screening and mammography) (Ervin, 2002). This information is also useful for comparing data before and after interventions to determine if a community intervention is successful (Ervin, 2002).

BUILDING RELATIONSHIPS

Collaboration: Community Partnership

Although one musical note may have no meaning, add a few notes and then a few more and it becomes a melody that can be sung and enjoyed. A community is made of many people, and the APN must have a comprehensive understanding of those people in order to build a trusting relationship. Understanding a community's culture is essential to program success.

Traditionally, a "community" has been defined as a group of interacting people living in a common location. The word is often used to refer to a group that is organized around common values and is attributed with social cohesion within a shared geographical location, generally in social units larger than a household. The word "community" is derived from the Old French *communité* which is derived from the Latin *communitas* (*cum*, "with/together" + *munus*, "gift"), a broad term for fellowship or organized society (Community, 2010) (for more information on defining populations and subgroups refer to Chapter 1).

Community involvement is the foundation of a successful CHA. The members of the community including the people, the government, the health department, the churches, the local businesses, to name but a few, all need to be involved. Who are the leaders in the community? Who are the people who are respected and trusted and can engage community members? This is not always a political leader but can be a church member, a parent, a community advocate, etc. Many communities do not have an inherent trust in "outsiders" who come into their community. There may be a history of people who have started programs only to leave without providing community members with the tools (financial or otherwise) to sustain programs after they are gone. The APN will have more chance of success in building programs by working with and being guided by a trusted member of the community than starting programs without first seeking the input and trust of the community.

It is also imperative that communities are not viewed as having a "problem." Communities want to feel they are productive and cohesive and do not want someone to tell them how to fix their problems. They want partnership and understanding of who they are and what they stand for. When approaching a community, it is essential that you identify the community's strengths and weaknesses. By knowing the strengths, you can establish more trust from community members because they do not want to only be defined by their problems. This mutual understanding can build trust and cooperation. It requires listening by both parties involved; education should be bidirectional. Program leaders such as the APN should provide the community and its members with the tools to sustain programs on their own. A sense of independence and self-sufficiency is important for long-term success. This is the ultimate form of partnership—one that is build upon trust, cooperation, and communication.

Building Relationships and Engaging Communities Through Collaboration: An Example

The concept of community collaboration can be understood by looking at Lee County, North Carolina. As has been discussed earlier, there are many methods for creating a profile of a community. A community health (CHA) assessment using a survey was used in this North Carolina County. First, a general overview of the community was provided by a combination of geographical information and vital statistics. Lee County is located in the geographical center of the state, covering 259 square miles, and it is one of the smallest counties in North Carolina. The county is comprised of eight townships and has had a population increase of 13.2% since April of 2000. It continues to grow at a steady rate. According to the U.S. Census, the 2005 population for Lee County was 55,704. The per capita income, while slightly lower than the North Carolina average, has been increasing since 2000. Lee County has maintained an unemployment rate slightly higher than the rest of the state since 2000. Employment opportunities are a concern among all groups, especially Hispanics. This collection of vital statistics from the U.S. Census provides a snapshot of the strengths of the community, as well as some areas that could be targeted for intervention. But for a truly comprehensive view of the area, a variety of community assessment tools are needed to fully assesses and address the community's needs.

The CHA Task Force

The lead in this CHA was a task force composed of the members of the Health Department, the supervisor of school nurses for Lee County, and the members of the Healthy Carolinians Partnership in Lee County known as the Community Action Network (LeeCAN). The LeeCAN is a partnership with representation from government agencies, civic groups, citizen groups, and members from the faith-based communities. The mission of the LeeCAN is "to increase awareness and resources to effectively address health and safety issues in Lee County through a collaborative community effort" (Mary B. Oates, Supervisor of School Nurses, Lee County, personal communication, September 2010).

Lee County Survey

To ensure adequate community participation, primary data for the CHA were collected through the use of a community survey that was distributed as both an online questionnaire, a paper/pencil questionnaire, and through "open house" and "community forum" type events. Local churches, volunteer fire departments, and local businesses also distributed information about the survey. The survey was available in the local newspaper.

Members of the CHA team first looked for an appropriate instrument for collecting information. A CHA should measure the variables of interest consistently, dependably, and accurately (Burns & Grove, 2004). The questionnaire selected was originally used in three other North Carolina counties—Montgomery, Moore, and Richmond—as the tool for their CHA. As a result, the questionnaire has been validated for use as a health assessment data collection tool. Montgomery, Moore, and Richmond Counties are all in Lee County's incubator group (http://www.sph.unc.edu/nciph/aboutus/maps.htm). This allows Lee County data to be compared with data from other counties that are in the same incubator group.

The survey had a total of 28 questions. Demographic questions included gender, race/ethnicity, zip code of residence, age, marital status, number of people living in household, number of children in the home aged 18 years or younger, education levels, and employment status. In addition to demographic questions, the survey also included questions that asked respondents their perceptions about community problems or issues, specific health-related issues, access to healthcare and insurance, and prevalence of diseases and disability.

Lee County Community Health Opinion Survey

This survey is part of the CHA currently in progress in Lee County. "This survey is in the public domain. Community health assessment is the process of learning about the health status of our community. We will use this information to identify needs/concerns about our community and then develop ways to address those needs" (Mary B. Oates, Supervisor of School Nurses, Lee County, personal communication, September 2010) (Exhibit 9.1).

EXHIBIT 9.1
Lee County, North Carolina, Community Survey

1. Thinking about your community, what kind of place is it to live? (check only one)

   ___ Excellent ___ Good ___ Fair ___ Poor

2. In your opinion, does your community have a problem with any of the issues listed below? (Please check whether you think it is no problem, a minor problem, a major problem or I do not know.)

LIVING IN OUR COMMUNITY	NO PROBLEM	MINOR PROBLEM	MAJOR PROBLEM	I DO NOT KNOW	PRIORITY
Traffic safety					
Affordable, safe housing					
Employment opportunities					
Recreational programs and facilities					
Education and training for adults					
Water supply and quality					
Racial/ethnic discrimination					
Legal services					
Crime					
Air quality					
Animal control					
Public transportation					
Food safety					
Solid waste disposal					
Terrorism (biological, chemical)					
Quality education (K-12)					

(continued)

Exhibit 9.1 *(continued)*

3. Now, out of the above list, please rank your top five concerns with "1" having the highest priority, and "2" being next and so on.

4. How long have you lived in Lee County?
_____ less than 1 year _____ 1–5 years _____ 6–10 years
_____ more than 10 years _____ my whole life

5. In your opinion, are the issues below a problem in your community?

LIVING IN OUR COMMUNITY	NO PROBLEM	MINOR PROBLEM	MAJOR PROBLEM	I DO NOT KNOW
Alcohol abuse				
Illegal drug use/substance abuse				
Tobacco use				
Driving/riding without seatbelts				
Homelessness				
Sexually transmitted diseases				
Poor eating habits				
No physical activity/exercise				
Family violence				
Child abuse				
Juvenile delinquency				
Suicide				
Work safety				
Youth access and use of weapons				
Teen pregnancy				
Men's health				

6. In your opinion, do people in your community have a problem finding/using these services?

HEALTH AND HUMAN SERVICES:	NO PROBLEM	MINOR PROBLEM	MAJOR PROBLEM	I DO NOT KNOW
Routine health care				
Hospital services				
Dental care				

(continued)

Exhibit 9.1 *(continued)*

HEALTH AND HUMAN SERVICES:	NO PROBLEM	MINOR PROBLEM	MAJOR PROBLEM	I DO NOT KNOW
Mental health care/counseling				
Emergency medical care				
Pharmacy/drug stores				
Drug and alcohol treatment				
Health education programs				
Transportation to health care				
Health insurance coverage				
Enrolling in Medicaid/ Medicare				
Food assistance ($ or food)				
Housing assistance				
Electricity, fuel, or water bills				
911 emergency services				
Long-term care facilities				
Care for pregnant women				
Childhood immunizations				
After school care				
Child care for infants/ preschoolers				
Car seats for infants and children				
Home health care				
Parenting skills education				
Adult day care/respite care				
Nutrition help				
Medical equipment				

7. Why do you think people may not use the services in Question 6? Please give us your opinion by checking the appropriate answer.

HEALTH AND HUMAN SERVICES:	NO PROBLEM	MINOR PROBLEM	MAJOR PROBLEM	I DO NOT KNOW
Person's dislike of the provider				
Cost of services				

(continued)

Exhibit 9.1 *(continued)*

HEALTH AND HUMAN SERVICES:	NO PROBLEM	MINOR PROBLEM	MAJOR PROBLEM	I DO NOT KNOW
No information about services				
Lack of transportation				
Inconvenient times				
Lack of childcare				
Inconvenient locations				
Language barriers				
Wait too long for service				
Concerns about confidentiality				
Quality of service				
Prior bad experience				
People were not friendly				
Lack of handicap access				
Reluctance to go for help				
Racial/ethnic discrimination				

8. In the past year, have there been any health-related services you or a member of your household have needed but have not been able to find in your community?

Yes   No

If you answered "yes" to the above question, list those services on the line below.

_____

9. Are you covered by a health insurance plan? Yes   No

If "yes," what type of coverage do you have?

____ Medicare (includes supplemental policy) ____ Medicaid ____ Private insurance ____ Other

Does everyone living in your household have health insurance? Yes   No

If you have private insurance, who pays the premium cost?

____ My employer pays the majority of the cost

____ I (or my family) pay the majority of the cost

____ Employer and I (or my family) each pay about half

(continued)

Exhibit 9.1 *(continued)*

10. Where do you go for routine health care when you are sick?

    ____ Doctor's office ____ Hospital emergency room ____ Free clinic

    ____ Health department ____ Chiropractor ___ Other_____

    ____ Urgent care ____ I do not seek health care

11. Where do you get most of your health-related information about your health?

    ____ Friends and family __ Doctor/nurse/pharmacist

    ____ Newspaper/magazine/TV __ Help lines (telephone)
    __Health Department __ Church__

    School __ Internet __ Hospital __Free clinic
    __ Other _____

12. In your opinion, does your community have a problem with any of these diseases or disabilities?

DISEASES AND DISABILITIES	NO PROBLEM	MINOR PROBLEM	MAJOR PROBLEM	I DO NOT KNOW
Lead poisoning				
Breast cancer				
Lung cancer				
Prostate cancer				
Other cancers				
Diabetes				
Heart disease				
High blood pressure				
HIV/AIDS				
Pneumonia/flu				
Stroke				
Mental health problems				
Dental problems (adult)				
Dental problems (child)				
Learning and developmental disabilities				
Bulimia/anorexia				
Adult asthma				
Childhood asthma				

(continued)

Exhibit 9.1 *(continued)*

DISEASES AND DISABILITIES	NO PROBLEM	MINOR PROBLEM	MAJOR PROBLEM	I DO NOT KNOW
Adult obesity				
Childhood obesity				
Depression				
Diseases people get from animals (rabies, West Nile):				
Arthritis				

In order to understand the results of this survey, we need to know more about you.

The answers to these questions will be kept strictly confidential. We do not ask for your name on this survey.

13. What is your zip code? _____

14. What is your age? (please check one)

    ____ 0–17 ____ 18–34 ____ 35–54 ____ 55–64 ____ 65–74 ____ 75 or older

15. Are you male or female? (please circle)

16. What is your current marital status? (please check one)

    ____ Single, never married ____ Married ____ Separated
    ____ Divorced ____ Widowed

17. What is your race/ethnicity? (please check)

    ____ White ____ Black ____ Native American ____ Asian/Pacific Islander

    ____ Hispanic/Latino ____ Other_____

18. How many people live in your household? _____

    How many children living in your home are 18 years old or younger?_____

    How many adults are 65 and older? _____

19. What was your household income last year? (please check one)

    ____ Less than $10,000 ___$10,000–19,999
    ___ $20,000–29,999 ____ $30,000–49,999

    ____ $50,000–74,999 ___$75,000 or more

20. What is the highest level of schooling you have completed?

    ____ Less than12th grade ___ High school graduate or equivalent (GED)

(continued)

Exhibit 9.1 *(continued)*

_____ Vocational training

_____ Associate degree in college ___ 4-year college degree (bachelors')

_____ Advanced degree in college (master's, doctorate)

21. Are you a member of a faith organization? Yes   No

22. What is your employment status?

_____ Employed full-time _____ Employed part-time _____ Retired

_____ Unemployed _____ Disabled _____ Student _____ Homemaker

23. What is your job field?

_____ Agricultural (farming, ranching)

_____ Business and Industry (banking, retailer, plumber, attorney, factory)

_____ Government (city manager, county officer, police)

_____ Education (teacher, principal, professor)

_____ Health (physician, nurse, administrator)

_____ Student

_____ Homemaker

_____ Other _____

Survey Results

The data were analyzed and reviewed by an advisory team from Lee County Public Health and members of the LeeCAN. Health-related concerns in Lee County have been noted as a result of this process. According to Mary Oakes (Mary B. Oates, Supervisor of School Nurses, Lee County, personal communication, September 2010), respondents of the survey report that the most prevalent health-related problems for the county are the following:

- Access to mental health services
- Access to dental care
- Teen pregnancy
- Crime in the county
- Poverty levels
- Migrant children whose parents are no longer in seasonal migrant jobs

The top five disease entities identified through this CHA as a "major problem" in Lee County (Lee County Community Health Assessment, 2006) were

1. High blood pressure
2. Adult obesity
3. Diabetes
4. Childhood obesity
5. Heart disease

In this case, the CHA was being used as a tool for improving and promoting the health status of Lee County residents. It engaged community members by having them identify their needs and in doing so raised their awareness of areas that needed improvement. The information garnered from the CHA also assisted community agencies in planning their program goals and objectives and in determining priority health issues. A further benefit has been its usefulness in identifying community resources (Lee County Community Health Assessment, 2006).

The information that has been collected through the CHA has been of great value. It identified the priorities of community participants and in doing so helped members of the collaborative identify those areas in the community that must be addressed. The process of collecting the information was invaluable as it built relationships and engaged the community in the process. The data obtained were useful for writing grant proposals. Additionally, data were used to leverage an increase in funding available to address specific county priority issues (Mary B. Oates, Supervisor of School Nurses, Lee County, personal communication, September 2010).

Lee County Reassessment

After reviewing the results of the survey, it was noted that certain areas of Lee County had a poor rate of return of their surveys. Lee County only has two incorporated areas, the City of Sanford and the Town of Broadway. Lemon Springs is an area of aggregated population outside of these two areas. The town of Broadway in Lee County has just over 1000 residents. The Lemon Springs area in Lee County is a small community; however, it is not incorporated into a town. Very few surveys (less than 10) were received from these areas. Several factors were cited as possible barriers to returning surveys (Mary B. Oates, Supervisor of School Nurses, Lee County, personal communication, February 2011):

■ Language barriers: Some community members are not able to read English or are illiterate.
■ A sense of trust: Anything that comes from the Health Department or even the government is viewed with suspicion by some members of these communities.
■ Complacency of community members: This is an identified problem.

Focus Groups

Because of the small number of surveys from Lemon Springs and Broadway, the assessment team felt another method was needed to gain input from these communities; a qualitative approach, using focus groups, was employed. Focus groups were held in each of these areas. Community leaders were identified and invited to attend. Topics were preselected from the surveys, and a moderator familiar with the CHA process and not actively involved in the data collection was chosen. The meetings were held on a weekday in a central location during midday; food was provided. No record of attendees was kept in order to maintain anonymity. Some of the population came for intrinsic reasons. The population that responded to the focus group meetings needed some incentive to do so as this might be the only way to get the responses; door prizes and refreshments were provided (Mary B. Oates, Supervisor of School Nurses, Lee County, personal communication, February 2011).

Focus Group Results

The focus groups unearthed valuable information. Common themes were as follows: affordability of health insurance, lack of specialty care in Lee County, and the need to educate residents about public health services. Specific concerns of the focus groups were drugs and the subsequent negative impact in their communities. In addition, more activities or community facilities were requested to cater to older adults and children. The groups generally felt their community was a good place to live. However, there were concerns in the community about drugs, fear of criminal activity, and funding for community services, such as law enforcement, mental health service, fire, and assistance for the disabled. Participants stated that the local hospital had a very long emergency room wait time, and they could go to another hospital in a nearby county and get better and faster service. Participants offered concerns regarding a lack of mental health services, especially after normal business hours for problems such as drug detoxification.

Focus group participants felt services were needed to "help the ones who need help," because most drug addicts are "good people who have gotten in a bad place." They stated more training was needed for local clergy on how to counsel addicts and how to refer them to available services. Participants stated that they wanted to know how to teach children about avoiding drug usage and to provide parents who have problems with help. They also commented about the need for the unemployed to have access to training that matches available employment in the area. Additionally, transportation was noted as "always an issue," and more public transportation was needed to access healthcare in the community.

The qualitative data collected from the focus groups provided rich information that coincided with results from the completed surveys. This combination of information obtained from surveys and focus groups was used to develop action plans to target the issues identified by community members as priorities.

Other Resources

The CHA survey and the focus groups, while helpful in revealing residents' perspectives about health and quality of life issues in Lee County, did not provide a comprehensive picture of health-related issues. To validate the survey findings and to fill gaps in information, secondary data sources were also used. Data were pulled from reports and queries from the North Carolina State Center for Health Statistics and the North Carolina Department of Health and Human Services.

In addition to the survey and the focus groups, resources used by Lee County included the following (Lee County Community Health Assessment, 2006):

- Statistical data from the North Carolina State Center for Health Statistics
- North Carolina Department of Health and Human Services
- North Carolina Division of Public Health: Office of Minority Health and Health Disparities
- North Carolina Department of Public Instructions
- 2000 Census Data
- Sanford/Lee County Strategic Services
- Center for Health Services Research, University of North Carolina
- Community Level Information of Kids: Annie E. Casey Foundation
- Employment Security Commission of North Carolina
- North Carolina Office of the Governor (LINC)
- North Carolina Child Advocacy Institute
- North Carolina Crime Statistics: North Carolina State Bureau of Investigation

SUMMARY

To paraphrase Busby, the CHA process extends beyond collecting community data; it includes establishing rapport among partners and is an ongoing process. Community programs are most successful when community members participate in the planning, implementation, and evaluation of programs that address local health concerns (Busby, 2000). The case study found at the end of this chapter provides the APN with another example of a successful collaboration. Building relationships and engaging communities through collaboration is a rewarding experience for the APN. The CHA must be totally inclusive and reflect the collaboration necessary to create an accurate and comprehensive depiction of the community. It is also a dynamic process and should incorporate multiple methods to assess and address a community's needs.

The CHA should be readdressed at regular intervals to identify changing needs. With the information obtained through a well-designed CHA, the APN has the data needed to develop evidence-based projects that meet the needs of the community. Working with community leaders is critical for success, especially in engaging community members in the process. Only then can community programs be developed and integrated into a successful healthcare plan for the community.

EXAMPLE CASE STUDY

A university had a contractual relationship to provide healthcare services with an underserved urban community, physically located near its catchment area. The School of Nursing (SON) intended to engage in the community with the goals of providing health promotion services, health education, and primary care to improve the health of the community, as well as provide a site for student clinical education. Beyond the high-level agreements that were in place, a relationship had to be forged between SON faculty, administrators, students, and community members in order to realize the goals of the SON. Mutual goal setting was needed in order to fully develop a partnership that would be "real" and "realistic," not just an agreement on paper. SON held meetings with various community groups, interested in engagement, as part of the assessment process. Elements of the assessment process can be related to the Action Model to Achieve Health People 2020 goals. In the assessment phase, conversations between the SON and multiple community partners centered on fit of organizational culture, timing of services, need for health services, and feasibility. Some of the organizations that the SON had conversations with had needs for health services that were far beyond what undergraduate and graduate nursing students could provide; others proved to have a different culture. A collaborative learning model was sought, one in which community members and students could learn from each other. Multiple projects were anticipated, with different characteristics, and service provisions.

One relationship that developed was between the SON and a church nurse group. During the assessment and initial collaboration stage, several common elements were found. First, the fit of the culture, a major purpose of the church nurse group was health promotion and education, mirroring the community health and primary care focus of the nursing curriculum. Members of the church nurse group were not professional nurses; by and large, they were caring individuals who were called to care for the sick and address health concerns in their church community. Second, timing was important. Classes for the SON were held at night, and church nurse meetings were held at night, as well. The timing fit so well into student's schedules that no class rotation had to be rearranged. The services of health promotion and education were handled by the undergraduate students; concomitantly, graduate nurse practitioner students rotated through a clinic setting to provide direct primary care–related services under the auspices of the university's nursing care center. A small foundation grant was secured to offset some of the anticipated costs associated with the program—church suppers, educational material, supplies, and advertising. Thus, the feasibility of the partnership was assured.

A premise of the collaboration was that addressing individual behaviors would impact the health of the community at large. This premise was held by both the church members and SON faculty and students. The relationship between the two groups deepened as discussions were held on what health behaviors the two groups would address. The format of the program was to include education sessions in a church supper format and health fairs, and referrals to clinics for acute care problems. The SON faculty and students proposed a curriculum based on health disparities addressed in Healthy People 2010, the standard at that time. The church nurse group counters proposed topics that they felt were the most pressing concerns in the community. Discussion shifted away from the federal guidelines to the real issues of health in community.

An example of tailoring the health program to the needs of the community was the diabetes screening program. The church nurses identified uncontrolled diabetes as a problem and wanted to do a health fair that included mass finger sticks to identify persons with high blood sugars. This strategy is not in the health promotion guidelines, but was adapted to a successful health fair. Community members came to the health fair; church nurses provided information on where to get low cost or free diabetic supplies in the community, had some supplies on hand, and exhorted people to "keep their sugar under control." Student nurses provided one-on-one counseling for known diabetics, answering questions about medication, diet, and exercise. The mass screening of 100 community members yielded four people with blood sugars well over 500 mg, and they were referred to the nursing center for immediate follow-up. Student nurses worked to ensure individual privacy, while the community members saw the screening as a "family affair," with each person responsible for their neighbor's health. This unorthodox approach to health promotion education and screening caused a buzz in the community and paved the way for a multi-year health promotion project and ongoing relationships.

Evaluation of the program occurred at individual, group, and community levels. The success of the relationship was evident in the personal relationships that developed between students, faculty, and community members.

Based on Kotecki, C. N., (2002). A health promotion curriculum for faith-based communities. *Holistic Nursing Practice, 16*, 61–69.

Kotecki, C. N., (2002). Incorporating Faith based partnerships into the Curriculum. *Nurse Educator, 27*(1), 13–15.

EXERCISES AND DISCUSSION QUESTIONS

Exercise 9.1 Using a professional journal, the newspaper, or the web, locate an article that describes the development of a community partnership. Select a partnership that focuses on health and has a least three partners, if possible.

■ Based on your reading of the chapter, identify what strategies may have been implemented during the community assessment phase by the partners.

■ Identify any assessment tools described in the chapter that were used or should have been used.

■ What databases would be appropriate to access and to demonstrate the need for the partnership?

■ If the partnership focuses on health disparities, what epidemiologic studies should have been conducted? What would suggest that the partnership was based on evidence, relationship, or politics?

■ Apply the Action Model to Achieve *Healthy People 2020* goals to the described partnership. What elements of the model can you identify?

REFERENCES

American Association of Colleges of Nursing. (2004a). *AACN Position Statement on the Practice Doctorate in Nursing*. Washington, DC: AACN. Retrieved fromwww.aacn.nche.edu/DNP/DNPPositionStatement.htm

Anderson, E. T., & McFarland, J. (2008). *Community as partner theory and practice in nursing*. Philadelphia, PA: Lippincot Williams & Wilkins.

Andranovich, G., & Howel, R. E. (2008). *The community survey: A tool for participation and fact finding*. Retrieved from http://cru.cahe.wsu.edu/CEPublications/wrep0132/wrep0132.html

Bailey, D. (1992). Using participatory research in community consortia development and evaluation: Lessons from the beginning of a story. *American Sociologist, 23* (4), 71–82.

Busby, A. (2000). *Orientation to nursing in the rural community*. Thousand Oaks, CA: Sage Publications.

Burns, N., & Grove, S. K. (2004). *The practice of nursing research conduct, critique and utilization*. Philadelphia, PA: W. B. Saunders.

Butler, M., DePhelps, L., & DePhelps, C. (1994). *Focus groups: A tool for understanding community perceptions and experiences. Community Ventures: Partnerships in Education and Research Series, WREP 0128*. Pullman, WA: Washington State University.

Community. (2010). *Oxford English Dictionary (OED) Online*. Retrieved from http://oed.com/

Cowell, J. M., McNaughton, D. B. & Ailey, S. (2000). Development and evaluation of a Mexican immigrant family support program. *Journal of School Nursing, 16*, 4–7.

Ervine, N. E. (2002). *Advanced community health nursing practice*. Upper Saddle River, NJ: Prentis Hall.

Hanchett, E. S. (1988). *Nursing frameworks and the community as client: Bridging the Gap*. Norwalk CT: Appleton & Lange.

Hancock, T., & Minkler, M. (1997). Community health assessment or healthy community assessment: Whose community? Whose health? Whose assessment? In M. Minkler (Ed.), *Community organizing and community building for health* (pp. 139–156). New Brunawick, NJ: Rutgers University Press.

Lee County community health assessment. (2006). Sanford, NC: Lee County Public Health Assessment Team and LeeCAN.

Lenz, E.R. (2005). The practice doctorate in nursing: An idea whose time has come. *Online Journal of Issues in Nursing, 10* (3), Manuscript 1. Retrieved from www.nursingworld.org/MainMenuCategories/ANAMarketplace/ANAPeriodicals/OJIN/TableofContents/Volume102005/No3sept05/tpc28_116025.aspx

Lundy, K. S., & Janes, S., (2009). *Community health nursing: Caring for the Public's Health.* Boston: Jones and Bartlett.

Shuster, G., F., & Goeppinger, J. (2008). Community as client: Assessment and analysis. In M. Stanhope & J. Lancaster (Eds.), *Public health nursing: Population-centered healthcare in the community* (7th ed., pp. 339–372). St Louis, MO: Mosby Elsevier.

Stanhope, M., & Lancaster, J. (Eds.). (2008). *Public health nursing: Population-centered healthcare in the community* (7th ed.). St Louis, MO: Mosby Elsevier.

Truglio-Londrigan, M., & Lewenson, S. B. (Eds.). (2011). *Public health nursing: Practicing population-based care.* Boston: Jones & Bartlett Publishers.

U.S. Department of Health and Human Services. (2000a). *Healthy People 2010 (Vol.1).* Washington, DC: U.S. Government Printing Office.

U.S. Department of Health and Human Services. (2000b). *Developing healthy people 2020: Public comment on draft objectives for healthy people 2020.* Washington, DC: U.S. Government Printing Office. Retrieved from http://www.healthypeople.gov/HP2020/

U.S. Department of Health and Human Services. (2008). *Phase I report recommendations for the framework and format of healthy people 2020.* Retrieved from http://www.westbridge.org/assets/HP2020_PhaseI_Report.pdf

TEN

Challenges in Program Implementation

Janna L. Dieckmann

*T*he role of the nurse in healing includes compassionate and quality care not only for the individual, but also the family and the community. Advanced practice nurses (APNs) seek to improve the circumstances that contribute to poor population health by working with community members to modify or change their behaviors that may contribute to poor health outcomes. This type of collaboration has the potential to make or facilitate changes that improve health and reduce morbidity and mortality.

The APN should approach communities with an open mind and a focus on a comprehensive community health assessment (CHA) (see Chapter 9). A CHA helps the APN to gain an understanding of the community, its residents, their diversity, their goals, and aspirations for healthier lives, and the barriers to achieving these goals. People want a better life. They want to be healthier and they want to live longer, happier, and more productive lives. The challenge lies in changing the behaviors and attitudes of individuals and communities. For many, change is uncomfortable or difficult but is a necessary process for communities that want to make improvements. But a process of change is unlikely to be smooth if community members do not buy into this change and are not willing to take a risk or make a sacrifice for the unknown.

LEWIN'S STAGES OF CHANGE

Lewin's Stages of Change provides a brief but profound approach to change at the aggregate or community level (Allender, Rector, & Warner, 2010). In the role of a change agent, the APN begins by destabilizing the group or community by asking questions to generate hope and visions of something different, something possibly better. Perhaps the group or community is already experiencing a desire for something different. Disequilibrium in the current moment underscores the relevance and potential of change and of moving out of the current comfort zone.

Unfreezing

The first stage of change, *unfreezing*, may arise from the community's own self-assessment or it may be activated by the APN through motivation, health education, advocacy, or other strategies (Allender et al., 2010; Kurt Lewin, 2011). An APN may initiate unfreezing during the course of usual practice. For example, as part of a primary care practice, an APN may find that many adult patients want to increase their physical activity, but the lack of designated walking or biking trails is a barrier. The APN initiates a conversation with the head of the local farmers' cooperative and with the director of the county's agricultural extension office. A community meeting is planned, with broad attendance by local residents and representatives of other community organizations. Many express interest in increased physical activity, but doubt their ability to make changes to their community that will make it more "walker friendly." This meeting is the first of many opportunities to present the problem to the community and address possible solutions, and begin to build a bridge of confidence between the community and the healthcare provider. Focus groups (see Chapter 9) can also further this goal and provide more individual attention to the barriers while proposing possible solutions to address those concerns.

Changing, Moving, or Transition

The second stage in Lewin's model reflects an understanding that change is not a timed event, but an ongoing process that can be facilitated by the actions of the APN. This stage is known variously as *changing, moving,* or *transition* (Allender et al., 2010; Kurt Lewin, 2011). Community members begin individually and as a group to transition to new attitudes and behaviors as they acquire new skills and perspectives.

The combination of destabilizing the present state and the challenge of questioning the status quo of behaviors and attitudes can make the second stage the most difficult. The support role of the APN is very important, as the nurse must accept the community's attempts at change against the risk of early failures. The APN cannot necessarily direct community change, as community residents benefit from developing their own new patterns of behavior as these emerge from who they are and their past experiences. The APN can motivate and guide community members and help them build upon their experiences to make the changes necessary for success. Using the earlier example, the APN should provide encouragement about the value of change (e.g., an improvement in residents' physical activity levels leads to improved health—less need for medications, etc.), implement strategies to reduce fears (e.g., educate residents about other successful programs), develop skills to unlock new behaviors (e.g., encourage residents to work together as a peer support), provide prompts underscoring the importance of change attempts (e.g., use simple outcome measures for residents [i.e., step counters] to track progress and set goals), and remind residents about the benefits of the community's goal (e.g., a healthier community is a more productive community) (Allender et al., 2010; Kurt Lewin, 2011). As a result of regular community meetings, the rural community raises funds and constructs new walking trails on public land. A picnic shelter is also built to provide families and groups a place to gather after walking.

Refreezing

The third stage of *refreezing* (or *freezing*) reflects the restabilization of the community that follows after making change. This stage can require a period of time, as the change or transition that community members experience can lead to a change in their relationships and in their daily lives as they internalize what is now different. The system adapts to the impact of the change, and the community integrates the change into a newly stable and re-balanced present state. For example, the walking trails that were once seen as improbable are now embraced and accepted by the community. The APN can provide the community with additional tools to stabilize the change and to reinforce and maintain new community behaviors. Family and neighborhood events are encouraged to try out the new walking trail and to use the new picnic area for a healthy meal. Periodic reminders to area residents about the walking trails are included in local print and visual media.

The success of the change process can lead to an enhanced partnership between the nurse and the community with the potential for further collaboration. Ideally, over time, the rural community will increase its physical activity and may seek additional consultation, for example, on how to select and prepare nutritional meals. Two-way communication can identify and address resistance or barriers to change. The APN needs to identify potential problems or doubts, and reinforce the benefits and values of the changed behaviors. The emergence of a new equilibrium signals a potential exit point for the APN's engagement with the community (Allender et al., 2010; Lewin, 2011).

COMMUNITY ENGAGEMENT

Engagement

APNs are more likely to succeed in addressing community concerns when communities are prepared to engage in the process of change. *Engagement* is different from wishing or acknowledging that "something" needs to change in order to improve. According to the CDC, community *engagement* is "the process of working collaboratively with and through groups of people affiliated by geographic proximity, special interest, or similar situations to address issues affecting the well-being of those people" (as cited in McCloskey, McDonald, Cook et. al., 2011, p. 7). Before beginning a community engagement effort, the APN must carefully consider the target community/population. What are the results of the CHA and what is known about the community? What has been the history of this community during and following previous change and engagement efforts? How are the community and its various groups likely to perceive the APN and what is the potential for a successful engagement of community members (CDC/ATSDR Committee, n.d.)? Is the community prepared to engage in change? What about the community's social or physical environment may facilitate or impede change? During this assessment and initial contact, the APN needs to recognize the core principle of community self-determination and the limits of professional action. It is critical that the APN clearly recognize the principle that "No external entity should assume it can bestow to a community the power to act in its own self-interest" (CDC/ATSDR Committee, n.d., Principle 4). Community members will find their own power when they seek it in themselves and take action for themselves, their families, and their community.

Entering the community is a second important and necessary step in assessing the potential for engagement. The APN needs to establish relationships and build trust through contacts with community leaders and community organizations. As mentioned in earlier chapters, the community leaders are not always the political leaders, but rather can include leaders in the church, schools, charitable foundations, or any member of the community who is trusted as a leader. The successful engagement with the community will depend upon developing these relationships. Each community is distinctively unique; engaging with a community will require acknowledgment and inclusion of the cultures and diversity of that community in all steps of the engagement. Only by taking these steps can the APN fully identify and mobilize community assets and resources and lay the groundwork for building long-term change in the community. With that said, healthcare professionals must recognize the limits of professional control and the need and/ or cost of making a long-term commitment with the community and its residents (CDC/ATSDR Committee, n.d.) (Table 10.1).

TABLE 10.1   Principles of Community Engagement

Before starting a community engagement effort:

- Be clear about the purposes or goals of the engagement effort, and the populations and/ or communities you want to engage.
- Become knowledgeable about the community in terms of its economic conditions, political structures, norms and values, demographic trends, history, and experience with engagement efforts. Learn about the community's perceptions of those initiating the engagement activities.

For engagement to occur, it is necessary to:

- Go into the community, establish relationships, build trust, work with the formal and informal leadership, and seek commitment from community organizations and leaders to create processes for mobilizing the community.

(continued)

- Remember and accept that community self-determination is the responsibility and right of all people who comprise a community. No external entity should assume it can bestow to a community the power to act in its own self-interest.

For engagement to succeed:

- Partnering with the community is necessary to create change and improve health.
- All aspects of community engagement must recognize and respect community diversity. Awareness of the various cultures of a community and other factors of diversity must be paramount in designing and implementing community engagement approaches.
- Community engagement can only be sustained by identifying and mobilizing community assets and by developing capacities and resources for community health decisions and action.
- An engaging organization or individual change agent must be prepared to release control of actions or interventions to the community and be flexible enough to meet the changing needs of the community.
- Community collaboration requires long-term commitment by the engaging organization and its partners.

Note: From CDC/ATSDR Committee on Community Engagement. National Institutes of Health (2011). *Principles of community engagement: Applying principles to the community engagement process.* Retrieved from www.cdc.gov/phppo/pce/part3.htm

Gaining the Trust of the Community

When working with a community, population, or aggregate, the APN must include strategies to initiate, develop, and sustain trust between the APN and community leaders, community members, and stakeholders. Trust requires mutual intention and is characterized by reciprocity (Lynn-McHale & Deatrick, 2000). As a key element in social interaction, trust facilitates communication and mutual understanding. Trust is a basis for change, a constant connection that provides support when the change process destabilizes a known situation in favor of an unknown outcome. A focus on developing trust begins with the initial contact with community members (Macali, Galanowsky, Wagner, & Truglio-Londrigan, 2011). The resulting nurse-community relationship is a critical prerequisite to population intervention. Through a trusting relationship, the community member gains the security of the APN's stable presence as a prerequisite to risking the unknown.

Four categories of trust have been described: calculative, competence, relational, and integrated. In *calculative trust*, potential members of the community initiative estimate the balance of benefits and costs to be derived from a potential collaboration as well as each members' assets and linkages. *Competence trust* hinges on whether group members are capable of doing what they commit to do; this type of trust also underlies the development of mutual respect among the participants. *Relational trust* reflects the personal relationships that quickly arise among members of any group. Members may express the value of mutual exchanges and develop a sense of commitment to mutual goals. Taken together, these three categories of trust constitute *integrated trust*, the foundation of an ongoing partnership (Logan, Davis, & Parker, 2010).

Initiating trust is an essential first step in building a bond between the nurse and the community. The nurse's *presence* in the community is qualitative evidence of the intent to develop a professional relationship with the community and its members. The community's willingness to view this presence positively will hinge on the APN's clear communication of his or her role with the community. The APN should seek to frame his or her presence within the broader outlines of the consensus needs or goals of the community, to the extent that these are known.

Based on knowledge obtained from a CHA, the APN should interact appropriately with community members, for example, in relation to personal demeanor, communication patterns, cultural sensitivity, expressions of interest, and communication of knowledge about the community. Being "liked" by community members can be indefinable in its intent or as a goal, but either way it is nearly essential in practice. Acceptability by the community will lead to acceptance by its members, as the APN should always review and consider what the community needs or wants first. The nurse's expressions of interest in the community and its members are concrete indications of commitment and, to a certain extent, obligate the APN to the community and to assisting with the community members' priorities. If there is a specified time frame or funding for the program, the APN needs to share this limitation with the community and provide the community with the tools to sustain or build the program on their own.

Processes of Developing and Sustaining Trust

The process of developing trust between the APN and the community and its members will likely emerge from early collaborative efforts. In most cases, selecting small, achievable goals that can be met swiftly is recommended. The success of visible outcomes enhances the nurse's credibility and increases the community's willingness and openness to trust. Increasing the breadth and depth of community participation with these goals will also increase the proportion of community members who have had contact with the APN and will be an advantage as the nurse-community collaboration continues. It is likely that the community will embark on testing or probing the nurse's knowledge, behavior, and character for the sake of better understanding and will withhold open trust until the community's needs begin to be met. As the nature of the nurse-community relationship is constructed and evolves during this period of role negotiation, the APN must maintain commitment to the initial shared goals, demonstrate professional openness to engagement with the community, and continue visible and concrete participation in the community. As APNs share a community presence with the public health nurse, it is relevant to consider that "The less experience people have with trusting relationships and the less sense of personal power and control they have, the more time public health nurses must spend developing trust and strength" (Zerwekh, 1993, p. 1676).

Sustaining the community's trust is built on a record of commitment and ongoing interaction with the community and its members. The nurse's continuing presence within the community establishes a sort of continuity that is reinforced by reliable actions. Decisions by APNs that become predictable to the community build the community's independence in self-management. When community members can predict "what the nurse would do," they are well on their way to independent decision making for their health. As community members gain independence, the importance of the APN's leadership becomes less necessary. With increased community competence, the APN may face new challenges in sustaining the community's trust, and the APN's role as a leader will change. As a community gains self-efficacy and confidence in self-determination and in their individual perspectives, conflicts become more likely. Mutual participation in thoughtful resolution is essential. Sustaining the community's continued trust will depend upon the APN's personal and professional skills to modify relationships with the community and its members, and willingness to accept a new role as defined by a strengthened community.

Building Partnerships

If trust is an essential prerequisite for change, then partnerships are the essential underpinning for negotiating, planning, and implementing change. The long-lasting relationships that characterize some partnerships build on existing strengths even as new capacities are forged and developed. Themes of engagement, autonomy, and self-determination have shaped contemporary ideas of partnership since the mid-20th century. The Alma-Ata Declaration (1978) proposed a social model of health that underscored the need for "citizen's greater self-reliance and decisional control over their own health" (p. 152), and alerted national health systems to more formally involve citizens in healthcare decisions (Gallant, Beaulieu, & Carnevale, 2002). This is even more salient when addressing 21st century healthcare demands that require individual and community initiative to address and improve health promotion and disease prevention (Courtney, Ballard, Fauver, Gariota, & Holland, 1996).

Agency-Academic Partnerships

One long-standing approach to partnership is the bridging of health agencies and academic institutions through joint ventures. The University Public Health Nursing District (in Cleveland, Ohio, 1917–1962) linked local schools of nursing with an independent nursing agency that provided clinic services, public health services, and nurse home visiting (Farnham, 1964). Nursing students were assigned to the district for their public health nursing experiences. Assignments for diploma school students tended more to observation during a brief few weeks, compared to collegiate nursing students who became fully engaged over a semester in the breadth of public health nursing work. The key structural element was the public health nursing staff of the district who served as clinical educators for students, and direct care providers at other times.

More recently, the nursing center model has advanced a similar strategy. The Clemson University College of Nursing Center, for example, is a partner with the Pickens County Health Department (South Carolina) to place nursing faculty and students at a community-based center. Maternal-child services, acute and chronic disease screening, and home health services are some of the activities that have been provided to community members through this partnership. The exceptional benefits of this model have extended and diversified existing health services in the community (Barger & Crumpton, 1991).

As effective and contributory as these programs are, the agency-academic partnership model of collaboration between a health agency or primary care practice with a school of nursing will have a limited impact when community residents and the wider service-resource network remain uninvolved, and when services are delivered outside a collaborative planning process that includes community participants at the table from the beginning. Agency-academic partnership programs focus on delivering services and improving health, but do not address the critical underlying barriers to improving health. Changes in the community—both change that benefits community members and change that transforms the community's health—will only occur with the participation of community representatives, both community members and community leaders. One promising approach for successful academic-community partnerships uses the community-oriented primary care model to address the structural inequalities underpinning these challenges by placing a community-based organization in the central coordinating role for the partnership (Cherry & Shefner, 2004).

This discussion of agency-academic partnerships highlights the contrast between the APN as advocate or as catalyst when engaging with a community for health changes. In both the advocate and catalyst roles, the APN respects the community and its self-determination as a basis for developing strategies to assist or complement the community's efforts for health. The *advocate* understands "the world view, life circumstances, and priorities of those requesting or receiving care and exploring the possible options with them in light of their preferences" (Walker, 2011, p. 75). While recognizing the community partner's individuality and self-determination, the nurse advocate takes action on behalf of a community to alert or make change in policy, economic, or social systems affecting the community (Walker, 2011). This approach is closest to the APN role in the agency-academic partnership. In contrast, the APN as *catalyst* understands the community as containing "all the necessary qualities and resources for change" and focuses the APN role to provide "the spark that will initiate change, as desired by the community and on its terms" (Walker, 2011, p. 75). The catalyst role provides the framework for APN practice in sustainable partnerships and coalitions.

Sustainable Partnerships

Developing long-term relationships between the APN and community representatives and organizations is a necessary component for preparing communities for long-term change. Sustainable partnerships are characterized by a relationship process through which the nurse and partners "work and interact together" (Gallant et al., 2002, p. 153). Power is shared in a "power-with" approach "emphasizing the positive force created between partners and how this force sustains and propels a relationship forward" (p. 154). Win-win negotiation models are recommended in the clinical nursing context (Roberts & Krouse, 1990), and have value in the APN's collaborations with community leaders and members. Not only are all parties' views heard and valued, but also the power to make decisions is shared, leading to "a sense of responsibility and power" (Roberts & Krouse, 1990, p. 33). This is particularly important when establishing a context for the emergence of an empowered community.

Sustainable partnerships are supported by public participation that enhances decision making by reflecting the interests and concerns of partnership members, and by highlighting the underlying values guiding partnership operation. The community that is affected by a decision should be able to participate in influencing the decision, and should be included in a way that enables their full participation. Potential participants should be encouraged to use outreach strategies. Decisions are likely to be more sustainable when the needs, concerns, and interests of all parties are communicated. Communication strategies themselves should be open and negotiated to accommodate representative styles and approaches. Finally, feedback must be provided to all participants and the public about how the decision was made and the role of their input in making the decision (International Association for Public Participation, 2007; Rippke, Briske, Keller, & Strohschein, 2001).

Partnerships can only be characterized as such when certain conditions exist: Each partner must be recognized as having his or her own power and legitimacy, own purpose and goals, and own connection to that locale or community. At the same time, the work of the partnership itself must be or become more than any one partner's own goals. This is reflected in clear partnership objectives and mutual expectations. Regular patterns of feedback from and among all parties should be planned and shared. And finally, "all partners strive for and nurture the human qualities of open-mindedness, patience, respect, and sensitivity to the experiences of persons" representing every portion of the partnership (Labonte, 1997, p. 101).

Working With Community Leaders and Members: Building Coalitions

A coalition-building strategy can establish the groundwork and/or initiate intra-community relationships that contribute to an effective, sustained effort to identify and respond to community challenges and needs. Coalition building "promotes and develops alliances among organizations or constituencies for a common purpose. It builds linkages, solves problems, and/or enhances local leadership to address health concerns" (Keller, Strohschein, & Briske, 2008, p. 204). Coalitions bridge sectors, organizations, and constituencies to provide a benefit to the wider community. Coalitions provide a new means to listen to the community as they open new communication pathways. Coalitions "can be helpful in maximizing the influence of individuals and organizations, exploiting new resources, and reducing duplication of effort" (Butterfoss, Goodman, & Wandersman, 1993).

Coalitions are used widely in community interventions due to their flexibility and their "democratic appeal" (Parker et al., 1999, p. 182). For example, Healthy People coalitions at the county or city level study their community and develop several health promotion or disease prevention objectives. As these coalitions include health and social service professionals, business people, and religious and social organizations, they contain the expertise and connections that have an impact on a community's health. Coalitions are useful for many reasons. First, involving a broad range of community groups provides a diverse basis to address local problems and change community expectations. Second, health professionals believe that coalitions develop the capacity of local organizations; skills gained in one effort lead to organizational abilities that will later be applied to solve other problems. Third, coalitions can improve service coordination among community agencies resulting in reduced duplication and more effective use of resources (Parker et al., 1999). For example, when organizations exchange information as part of the coalition's work, organizational leaders may identify overlapping programs. The cost of duplicate efforts can then be reduced through cooperation across the agencies or consolidation at one host agency. Coalitions can also provide a springboard for community empowerment, "an enabling process through which individuals and communities take control of their lives and their environment" (Rippke et al., 2001, p. 212).

The APN should consider the use of a coalition as it can bring diverse resources together and assist in the community's recognition and response to health concerns. Even though coalitions have many important characteristics, the APN should consider whether devoting existing resources (such as time, energy, and commitment) to coalition building will lead to the best outcome. The decision also depends upon the availability and willingness of the right members for the coalition. Candidate members for the coalition should represent an organization or constituency, and they should have access to the members and resources of the groups they represent. Coalitions can include 12 to 18 members, but smaller groups are able to address more specialized interests, or more easily gain sufficient trust to permit mutual collaboration (Rippke et al., 2001). Many coalitions may need to add additional members as the coalition's focus broadens. Based on the coalition's program, additional groups may need to be added and additional resources may need to be requested from new partners. For example, a coalition meeting to address head injuries among children might refine its focus to promote safety helmet usage in activities such as bicycling and skate-boarding. This coalition might add the expertise of emergency department representatives and the resources of local store owners who sell bicycles or safety helmets.

The intent of a coalition is to assemble around a common interest in which each coalition member has a stake in the outcomes. As in any organization, coalitions require both structure and resources to achieve goals. As coalitions incorporate representatives of diverse organizations who hold diverse perspectives, it is important to facilitate good interpersonal dynamics and to develop reliable group processes for decision making (Rippke et al., 2001). A community coalition should be able to work together on a broad vision of what needs to be accomplished. A mission statement can be useful in providing formal guidance to the coalition effort, especially when a variety or range of perspectives exist among members. When developed collaboratively, this "common vision" can assist with formalization of the next steps (Wald, 2011).

The Process of Establishing Community Priorities

Most community leaders and members can easily identify a wide range of concerns or issues that reflect their wants or needs to improve their community's health. In strained economic times, such lists are likely to become even longer. During prioritization the available data and community information are reviewed by the coalition and community members to decide what to address and where resources should be targeted (Issel, 2004). The process of setting priorities includes selecting the most important concerns for attention by the coalition. Making this selection can be difficult or frustrating, because in many cases there are multiple problems that need to be addressed in the community. Some community leaders and members will approach this by advocating for the critical priorities affecting the community, while other coalition members will advocate their own personal priorities. Identifying a consensus priority will facilitate the coalition's purpose of finding a common vision or goal.

When considering what actions should receive high-priority attention, how can *wants* and *needs* be differentiated? *Needs* reflect an objective assessment or conform to a set of expected requirements, compared to *wants* that may be personal wishes or aspirations that fail to rise to the level of necessity. But it may be that the dividing line between wants and needs has more to do with *who* sorts wants from needs, rather than *how* the sorting is done. Wishes and needs for the same target community may differ based on the perspective of the viewer: Insiders and outsiders to the community may propose quite different lists. Rather than asking how to separate needs and wants, the better question may be: Should needs and wants be separated? Perhaps it is more constructive to view both as important and critical to address. For example, a group of health professionals concluded that the priority intervention for a neighborhood in a small, rural community in North Carolina should be to reduce infant mortality, based on significant epidemiological evidence. However, when neighborhood residents heard about the professionals' proposal, they insisted that their priority was a safe playground for their children—and it was built. This should not be considered a failure but rather a success. Although, one priority solution was sought another priority was identified and addressed leading to a positive outcome for the community.

The practice of priority setting is not purely quantitative; the highest ranking items do not have to be selected over lower ranked items. The process of decision making is interactive, perhaps even political. For example, the APN may believe that funding and personnel resources should be directed toward the most common diseases in a community. But what if the most frequent disease in a community is sinusitis? Should sinusitis receive attention above all other chronic diseases? Perhaps severity of illness should be an additional criterion. How should duration of illness be factored in? What about considering the possibility of recovery or rehabilitation as a criterion? And what about the actual cost of illness care? Perhaps immunizations are cost effective because they prevent morbidity and mortality at a very low cost. Through questions such as these and related community and partnership discussion, priority-setting discussions reveal much about the values and beliefs of the community and the coalition members.

Ordinarily, several priorities are selected by a coalition. Several of the selected priorities may require different resources and some priorities may separately seek external grant funding. Priority setting can be helpful in suggesting which items should be addressed first, and which should be discarded from the list due to lack of coalition interest or lack of confidence that the problem is solvable given existing resources (Blum, 1981). On the other hand, the availability of external resources or funding may justify selecting a priority, as it is most likely to be viable. In practice, the availability of funding often guides program decisions (Timmreck, 1995).

If a coalition priority requires financial support that is not immediately available, the coalition could make a decision: (1) to wait for a specified period of time until a funding source is willing to provide financial support; (2) to raise local funding specifically to support the coalition priority; or (3) to down-size the magnitude of the coalition's planned program by implementing a small pilot program or by initially implementing only a portion of the program. For example, a community seeks to address the low immunizations rates among pre-school children. The coalition's priority is to ensure adequate immunizations for all pre-school children in their community, but no funding is available for their larger goal. Because the coalition has some resources, they decide to develop a pilot program that focuses on improving influenza immunization for preschoolers. The coalition can begin their program immediately, which reinforces the success of the coalition's common goals and actions. The coalition will also gain a lot of information, as well as group, organizing, and technical skills through implementing the pilot program. Additionally, information on cost savings and health benefit should be obtained to further justify continuing and/or expanding the program. In some cases, coalitions can work with insurance providers to fund programs such as these to prevent or reduce costs incurred with emergency and hospital admissions. This skill acquisition, as well as the pilot program experiences and outcomes, will provide a strong foundation and justification when applying to fund a broader program to improve childhood immunizations rates.

Priority-Setting Approaches

The process of setting priorities is best conducted through a combination of qualitative and quantitative methods. Statistics about the frequency, duration, severity, disability, and mortality of certain health problems tell one story. Social understandings of health concerns and qualitative estimations of these health problems tell a different story. Priority setting allows for open discussion about perceptions, judgments, and understandings that can be the most valuable part of conducting a priority setting session. When the coalition discusses the community and its priorities, this furthers the coalition's work.

Criteria that are used to rate priorities can vary. A coalition's discussion is best served if it first decides which criteria are important to the group, and, second, applies these criteria to rank the community's issues and concerns. Coalition members will learn much about each others' preferences from both the first and second parts of the discussion, and subsequent decision making will be enhanced. Community members' viewpoints should also be incorporated; community forums or focus groups can be an effective means for involving community members. Those unable to attend a forum because of family obligations, work-shift timing, or disability can be contacted directly and their perspectives and opinions can still be included as input. For example, Dallas County, Texas, initiatives directed by Parkland Hospital's Community-Oriented Primary Care program employed a community prioritization approach that focused on "(1) leadership forums and (2) community advisory boards associated with each health center" (Pickens, Bombulian, Anderson, Ross, & Phillips, 2002, p. 1729).

Priority Chart

Several priority-setting approaches use a combination of quantitative and qualitative methods to provide comparative rankings that can highlight community concerns and issues that should receive attention. Tarimo (1991) includes a *Priority Chart* that incorporates several variables in a brief format suitable for discussion by nonprofessionals. Small groups are formed to evaluate the health problems (preferably no more than seven) or risk factors of concern in a population. The problems or factors are then listed and should relate to a single target population. Ranking is simplified when the list includes either health problems (heart disease, asthma, arthritis, adolescent pregnancy, etc.) or risk factors (tobacco use, high-fat diets, sedentary lifestyles, poor access to birth control methods, etc.). Small group members discuss and rank each health problem or risk factor using the following variables: frequency in the population, mortality in years of potential life lost, morbidity in years of reduced health, costs of solutions, and effectiveness of solutions (Tarimo, 1991, pp. 20–21). The priorities selected by the small groups are reported back to the larger group, tallied, and discussed. This approach can be powerful and instructive in the priority-setting process.

Problem Priority Criteria

Schuster and Goeppinger (2003) propose a more complex, mathematical system that shares some of Tarimo's *Priority Chart* assumptions. Their *Problem Priority Criteria* include the following: "(1) community awareness of the problem,

(2) community motivation to resolve or better manage the problem, (3) nurse's ability to influence problem solution, (4) availability of expertise to solve the problem, (5) severity of the outcomes if the problems are unresolved, and (6) speed with which the problem can be solved" (p. 362). Each criterion is independently rated on a 1 (low) to 10 (high) scale based on two questions: (1) How important is the criterion to problem solution? and (2) Does the partnership have the ability to resolve the problem? (pp. 362–363). In addition, a rationale for rating each parameter is documented. The two resulting numeric ratings (for problem importance and for ability to resolve) are multiplied to yield a problem ranking number (variable from 0 to 600). These steps are repeated for each separate problem that the group seeks to address (Shuster & Goeppinger, 2004). The community problems are then ranked from highest to lowest score. As this system requires detailed knowledge about each separate problem, it works best if those involved are highly familiar with the issues or concerns being prioritized, such as coalition leaders.

A "Skilled Planner" Approach

For setting priorities, Green and Kreuter (2005) recommend a series of key questions for use by "skilled planners" in "a process that balances the perceptions of stakeholder (sic) with objectively constructed descriptions of prevailing health problems and how these are distributed in the target population" (p. 99). Green and Kreuter's key questions reflect many of the themes of the two previous priority approaches, including comparison of relative mortality, morbidity, costs, and ease of solution. For example, one key question asks: "Which problems are most amendable to intervention?" (p. 99). Added themes included a concern for higher risk subpopulations (such as children, mothers, or ethnic minorities), and the disproportionate burden of the problem on the focus community compared to other communities. For example, a key question here is: "Which problem is not being addressed by other organizations in the community?" (Green & Kreuter, 2005, p. 99). This approach works well when professionals (the "skilled planners") conduct prioritization comparisons. Although this approach is less helpful in the APN's work with community coalitions, the "key questions" have the potential to add to or help guide discussions or reflections by coalition members or community residents.

The Hanlon Method and PEARL

The *Hanlon Method*, also referred to as the *Basic Priority Rating System* (Pickett & Hanlon, 1990, pp. 226–228; School of Public Health, 2004), is structured "to allow decision makers to identify explicit factors to be considered in setting priorities, to organize the factors into groups that are weighted relative to each other, and to allow the factors to be modified as needed and scored individually" (School of Public Health, 2004, p. 1). Three main components are independently rated on a scale for each candidate priority: (1) size of the problem, (2) seriousness of the problem, and (3) estimated effectiveness of the solution. The numeric results for each of the three variables are placed into an equation, and the results multiplied by the PEARL factor score to obtain the comparative rating (School of Public Health, 2004).

The *PEARL factors* are interpreted as strongly influencing whether or not a particular goal can be addressed in a specific community, even though the factors are not directly related to the health problem. *Propriety* (P) asks whether a proposed problem or program is consistent with the overall mission of the sponsoring organization. *Economic feasibility* (E) balances the costs of intervening or not intervening, including the economic outcomes of not intervening. *Acceptability* (A) addresses whether the community or program recipients will accept any intervention to address the goal. *Resources* (R) are assessed to determine if sufficient resources are available to address this goal? And last, *Legality* (L) poses the question of whether current laws will permit addressing this goal (School of Public Health, 2004).

The PEARL factors are scored individually as "possible" or "not possible" (i.e., each is rated as "one" or "zero"); given the mathematical formula, if even one of these qualifying factors is rated as "not possible" (i.e., as zero), then the Basic Priority Rating is zero, which indicates that the particular candidate priority should not be considered. At this point, a planning coalition may decide that their first step is to conduct community interventions that modify the PEARL factor rated as "not possible." For example, if an intervention is currently not acceptable to the population, steps might be taken to educate the population of the potential benefits of the intervention. If population opinion shifts and becomes more accepting of the intervention, it could be reconsidered and implemented (School of Public Health, 2004). Incorporating the PEARL factors into priority setting itself provides a stronger and more complex perspective, as part of the process is deciding which goal or program to select. The PEARL factors may also be an appropriate additional analysis in combination with any priority-setting approach, especially as it addresses the intervention component of a proposed need or program.

Selecting Goals to Address Prioritized Issues and Concerns

As a result of the priority-setting process, the community coalition identifies a ranked group of issues and concerns. The next question is: Should the coalition focus on a single goal or on multiple goals? Single goals do have an appeal of simplicity and require fewer resources. When a coalition focuses on multiple linked goals, it has more of an impact on the underlying causes of the problem, and more opportunity to draw community members into understanding these linkages. In the earlier example of creating walking trails, the combination of increasing physical activity and improving healthy food choices both address achieving an appropriate weight to prevent chronic disease. By linking these two health disease prevention behaviors through the walking trails intervention, it underscores the need for community members to combine several related actions to reduce their risks for poor health outcomes.

In fact, most community health issues and concerns are complex, multifaceted, and challenging to address. Based on the ecological model, multilevel planning models underscore the numerous sources of health problems. The *Multilevel Approach to Community Health* (MATCH) suggests that health problems will only be resolved when they are addressed simultaneously at the individual/family, organization, community, and government level, and this allows for a more effective modification of policy, practice, and behavior. Although this approach requires a potentially vast skill set, it can offer more efficient use of resources at a faster speed (Simons-Morton, Greene, & Gottlieb, 1995; Simons-Morton, Simons-Morton, Parcel, & Bunker, 1988). For example, it is not sufficient for the APN to convince a patient and his family that his sodium intake should be reduced. A broader approach should be taken to address the barriers in the community that make it difficult for an individual to make long-term changes. As in this case, the best patient teaching cannot easily overcome the barriers if local food stores carry only high-sodium food choices. The APN could participate in a community coalition to advocate for local food stores to stock healthier, low-sodium foods. County or state policy changes could persuade food stores that stocking low-sodium foods is to their advantage if, for example, they received a tax credit for the amount of healthier foods they carried and sold. Multilevel approaches provide more effective and sustainable changes, as these modify the underlying causes of current health problems and address the issues at a community and policy level.

The *Transtheoretical Model and Stages of Change* suggests that in any given population, individuals are at different points or stages in considering or implementing personal change (Prochaska, Redding, & Evers, 2008). Patients prescribed a lower-sodium diet will undergo a personal change process in deciding and acting on reducing dietary sodium. When a community coalition plans to modify personal health choices among community members, it will design interventions that simultaneously target residents at each of the stages of change. The intervention design will also support individuals and families in moving stepwise through the stages of change and in assisting backsliders to recommit to engaging in change.

In the *Diffusion of Innovations* model, the members of a population adopt new behaviors, new technologies, and so on, at predictable but very different rates and for very different reasons (Oldenburg & Glanz, 2008). In this case, to reach all members of the community, the coalition should target strategies at early, middle, and late points in the campaign to reduce dietary sodium. Those who are early adopters of the innovation respond to different approaches than those who are late adopters, and specific targeted approaches are employed based on their ability to change and stage of change.

Both the Stages of Change and the Diffusion of Innovations theories underscore the effectiveness of using multiple methods in modifying health-promoting behaviors among diverse community members. As a means to understand these complex relationships and to identify possible interventions, *The Guide to Community Preventive Services* provides intensive, highly developed recommendations for community-targeted health promotion and disease prevention programs (The Community Guide Branch, 2011). Given the complex nature of contemporary health promotion and disease prevention problems, theoretical and evidence-based approaches are critical in properly framing issues and concerns so that they can be addressed. For example, if an APN is planning a program to reduce dietary sodium, the *Nutrition Guidelines for Americans, 2010* (Center for Nutrition Policy, 2010) is an important resource to assist in this process.

Sustaining New Programs: Identifying Barriers in the Program Planning and Implementation Process

One challenge to sustaining new programs arises from existing problems or potential problems at the time the goal or program was selected as a focus by the coalition. Thorough, objective assessment of proposed community goals/programs will often yield doubts about implementation of a program or whether the implementation effort risks serious obstacles. The APN and the coalition's intervention team must both be carefully analytic and thoroughly honest. When potential problems are revealed, they must be acknowledged and addressed, as a "wait-and-see" approach is not effective. Barriers to program success can also emerge during implementation. Symptoms of potential problems include the following: delays in the implementation timeline, waning resources, disaffected partnerships, or recurring communication difficulties during coalition meetings. These challenges can be detected early by conducting an ongoing program review or formative evaluation. Both symptoms of problems and problems detected during program evaluation require the community intervention team to be honest about the presence of and need to address the barriers, and the importance of taking prompt action to address threats to the coalition's work. The APN brings problem-solving experience to these situations and should remind the coalition of the normative nature of the challenges to implementing a health promotion/disease prevention program.

Regardless of when in the process a barrier is identified, the characteristics of barriers can be grouped into: (1) characteristics of the goal/program; (2) characteristics of needed resources; (3) characteristics of community members, coalition members, and coalition leadership; (4) characteristics of the APN; or (5) a mismatch between community or coalition partners and the APN.

Barriers Due to Program Characteristics

Certain types of programs or goals may not be feasible to study in certain communities. Some goals may receive community support and have the weight of evidence behind their use, but are a violation of law (or illegal). For example, needle-exchange programs are effective in preventing the spread of blood-borne pathogens, but are illegal in some areas (Benjamin, O'Brien, & Trotter, 2002). In another case, the timeline necessary to achieve the stated program or goal may not match community expectations. For example, would the community's support wane before program goals are achieved? Will the community demand program outcomes immediately, but lack the means or resources to quickly achieve the goals? Air quality is an important quality of life issue, as well as being a short- and long-term health problem, yet modifying the sources of air pollution are time consuming and challenging (Yip, Pearcy, Garbe, & Truman, 2011). The community might not have patience to wait for change during successive law suits and environmental policy interventions over a prolonged period of time. For example, the challenges of sustaining a community coalition to address environmental health problems are illustrated in a case involving the pollution of the Love Canal neighborhood in Niagara Falls, New York (Blum, 2008).

Barriers Due to Unavailable Resources

Another barrier that is commonly encountered occurs when goals/programs may lack sufficient resources to succeed, perhaps because of inadequate financing, or because of insufficient, inadequate, or poorly trained leadership. Some groups may proceed to develop programs or goals even after the lack of resources has been recognized in the hope that sufficient personnel or financial resources will be secured. Not only are such programs initiated on unstable foundations, but existing resources that could be dedicated to program development are instead lost to failed attempts to explore and acquire needed resources.

Barriers Due to Human Factors

The leadership involved in the coalition can often be a barrier to their own success. Community or coalition partners, who participate in the development of community goals, may be unenthusiastic or disaffected in relation to the focus that was actually selected for implementation. Community partners may simply lack interest in the current priority and may wish to terminate their involvement in the coalition. Partners can also become disengaged or separated from coalition communications; they may disengage in working meetings or miss meetings all together. Given the contrasting possibilities, the APN and other coalition members need to assess the reasons these coalition members appear to be disaffected.

Partners can also become distracted by what is to them a more salient goal or concern, leaving little time and attention for coalition priorities. Reassessment of the goal or program should be carried out if it is deemed unlikely that these partners will change their minds. If they do change their minds, then one of the coalition's interventions should address recruitment and community awareness about program/goal benefits.

Apparent disinterest in coalition activities may also quietly signal that two or more subgroups in the coalition are unable to collaborate, even though both are necessary to the project's success. The APN and other coalition leadership should reach out to these subgroups to have a fuller picture of the difficulties and to support and counsel reinclusion of the subgroups. In this serious situation, negotiation between the conflicted subgroups may be possible, but the APN must be extremely diplomatic to avoid the appearance of siding with one group and further damaging the potential for collaboration.

The APN can also experience a lack of sustained interest in the program focus, perhaps because the selected program is only indirectly related to health concerns. Similar to community members or other coalition partners, the APN may find another goal more salient. It is difficult to consider, but important to acknowledge, if the nurse has become disengaged from the community and the coalition, whether because of circumstances in the nurse's personal life or because working with the community and/or the coalition has become difficult. The APN may find herself/himself overwhelmed with responsibilities that compete with other obligations. It can become difficult for the nurse to agree to a realistic timeline for goal or program implementation if it appears that there may be a prolonged timeline or the potential for a significant time commitment. The APN should acknowledge these personal challenges and seek support from within the coalition, or from elsewhere, to identify the barriers to participation and make a plan to reconstruct linkages with the coalition, or to make a decision to acknowledge the barriers and formally withdraw.

Barriers Due to the Nurse-Coalition Interface

Lastly, it may emerge that the community/coalition lacks the skills to partner with the APN. One appropriate step is to delay immediate programmatic work and focus efforts on skill building. This challenge is more likely to be revealed and addressed early if program implementation begins in an incremental way that permits skill and confidence building. In fact, incorporating these necessary elements as a first, planned stage of a larger program implementation is advantageous.

Preventing Problems in Collaborative Efforts

In the midst of hard work and complex organizing, some would suggest that some of these barriers could *not* have been anticipated or prevented. But on the whole, these problems should be foreseen by the coalition leadership and actions taken to prevent a negative impact on developing collaborative efforts. Three steps must be included in any initiative: First, during the planning stage, a coalition should dedicate time to honest reflection, anticipation, and identification of potential problems and barriers to any identified goals. Are coalition members genuinely "buying into" group plans? Is the coalition's roadmap realistic in its timeline and requirements for community participation? Second, every coalition should periodically reassess its goals and plans. Depending upon the nature and composition of the coalition, this reassessment can be conducted by the leadership (in its broadest, most representative, and diverse sense). In addition, a community meeting will generate an even better understanding of the current status of the coalition's efforts. The community meeting provides a forum for recognizing and acknowledging success to date, celebrating the success, and focusing/refocusing on next steps. Honest reflection on symptoms and suggestions of problems with goals should lead to specific strategies to further understand and address the issues and concerns to minimize negative consequences on the larger coalition and the initiative itself. Third, if issues and concerns are revealed, the coalition leadership should make a judgment about the nature and process of the initiative. Should the initiative continue as currently planned, or should changes be made? Would it be better to modify or eliminate a goal, or would this lead to a coalition member dropping out? Coalition leaders might decide to face a conflict and openly discuss the challenge and its many facets, and by identifying a solution, strengthen the overall initiative and the coalition itself.

In sum, "side-stepping" the problems means that the APN and the coalition can and should be alert to potential challenges. Regular reassessment of the program and early awareness of potential problems are essential for success as is finding a prompt solution. Early success in any effort builds the collaborative and spurs efforts forward. Conflicts and confusion that drain energy from the coalition partners should be prevented if possible or at least minimized. Facing confusion and/ or conflicts can strengthen collaborative work and model problem-solving strategies that can result in increasing community capacity to address future challenges.

Developing Outcomes for Coalition Work

The priority-setting discussions should identify at least one, but likely several issues or concerns for the APN and the coalition's project. The next step is to develop outcomes and related means to achieve these outcomes, based on the selected priorities. Identifying outcomes is essential to later work including program evaluation.

The process of defining outcomes or even revising outcomes can be daunting. This process can be a critical step in program development that lays the groundwork for successful and sustainable programs. Even when all of the constituencies in the coalition have previously agreed on the priorities for the community's health, establishing outcomes for these priorities can lead to unforeseen barriers. First, traditional academic/professional configuration of outcomes may be unfamiliar to community members within the partnership; consideration of alternative means to present these ideas, steps to achievement, and a related timeline can facilitate the process. Outcomes should remain in a contextual format that is appropriate for the target community for the duration of the project. Second, well-defined outcomes that are clearly stated may be the first indication to coalition partners of the extensive work ahead. Presenting the outcomes with a clear timeline and delineation of the steps needed to achieve these goals is a way to demonstrate a well thought out plan that addresses the process that is necessary to achieve these outcomes. It also can facilitate a sense of community efficacy, as it sets up the framework to show these goals are achievable. Generating these steps is an appropriate focus for the coalition at the time the outcome statements are presented to the group.

When the APN and coalition members have agreed on the stated outcomes, the next step is to commit to work toward their resolution. As coalition members represent their constituencies, these members should take responsibility for communicating with their organizations or neighborhoods about the coalition's plans. The APN can assist coalition members to design campaigns to involve their constituencies. These campaigns can assist coalition members to facilitate adoption of both the outcomes and the steps to achieve the outcomes among their constituents. Focused organizational or neighborhood meetings/gatherings are useful in accomplishing this. The overall goal is to achieve a "buy-in" and commitment to work on the goals among the constituents and the coalition partners.

To support the coalition members, the APN and the coalition as a whole should set a "launch date" for the planned program and have a celebration to develop energy and reflect the commitment of the wide variety of coalition partners. Coalition efforts to recruit and retain the dedication and interest of constituency members will also validate the leadership role of each constituency's representative within the coalition. This results in strengthening the leader roles of coalition representatives in their community. APN activities in coalitions can often include leadership development of the coalition members.

Continued work toward achieving the planned outcomes will likely have both periods of accomplishment and periods with minimal progress. The APN can remind the coalition of the previously identified interim markers of progress toward the selected coalition outcomes. Achievement of each significant step should be recognized and celebrated. A good example of marking progress is the pictures that are posted in fund-raising campaigns that show increases in donations using an oversized thermometer posted in a visible location. Visible indicators or a giant "check-list" can convey to community members the status and growing impact of the coalition's efforts. Small rewards or giveaways such as a celebratory balloon or a coalition-emblazoned key chain can also be used to signal progress toward outcomes.

The APN and the coalition members should plan periodic formative evaluations of the progress in attaining outcomes, as well as summative evaluations of those elements of the overall plan that have been completed. Marking success and progress is important for the coalition efforts as well, and offers possibilities for events that build the coalition team and the interpersonal relationships among coalition representatives. When the APN breaks down the program into do-able steps, the efficacy of community members and retention of coalition partners is enhanced.

Sustaining Programs and Initiatives

As programs and initiatives gain strength and the coalition sees their planning lead to better health outcomes in the community, the APN should consider ways to keep the work going and to establish it as a permanent element of that community. To do this, the APN and the coalition must take steps to institutionalize the initiative. These plans will ensure the continuity of the work and, with increased duration of the program, will increase the potential for achieving the identified outcomes. The APN will introduce and guide the coalition first through a careful strategic plan for institutionalization. This will focus the coalition on what is needed. In fact, consideration of sustaining or institutionalizing an initiative should begin when it is first conceptualized, or at least when clear outcomes have been identified and are beginning to be implemented (Community Toolbox, 2011a). The importance of the institutionalization plan underscores the APN's key role in guiding program development and in guiding the team to an understanding about what steps are necessary at which phase in the program planning and implementation.

Planning for Institutionalization

How should the APN guide the coalition in planning for institutionalization? A first step is to acknowledge that what it does is important and that the coalition's program is worth continuing. In that light, it will make sense to ensure that the program's mission, staffing, and resources are adequate. Given continued confidence in its planned outcomes, noting program accomplishments will provide the coalition with motivation to continue to build. Publicizing the coalition's successes will solidify both the coalition and its constituencies and, more importantly, can draw the public into the coalition's mission and work. Community members are key players in long-term sustainability and can assist in the institutionalization process. When programs involve more people, their staying power increases (Community Toolbox, 2011b). Perhaps a nearby community would like to develop a similar program? Perhaps outsiders would like to learn about how the program operates and how it achieves its goals? Enhancing the connections and respect for the program and spreading the coalition's programs to new neighborhoods improve how others see the program, and this translates into more support for the program.

Funding: A Major Barrier to Sustainability

The major barrier to sustainability and to institutionalization is adequate financing, which for many organizations is an ongoing challenge to accomplishing the planned outcomes. As with other factors that support sustainability planning for future financial security, it is best addressed from the start of program inception. A place to begin is to market the organization by letting others know what the coalition's program has accomplished. The APN and coalition members will build its image and community relations, develop members and friends, and actively deliver the coalition's message for health and personal/community change.

Existing financial resources may go further if staff positions are shared with another compatible organization. Or the coalition's program may become so successful that a larger organization would like to support it, or perhaps even assume responsibility for the coalition, its identified outcomes, and its programs in operation. Grants, fund-raising functions, third-party funding, public funding, a fee-schedule, and in-kind support may also assist with financing (Community Toolbox, 2011c). Community health programs can be particularly attractive to academic partners such as nursing, public health or medical schools and universities, which the APN can assist in recruiting or relationship building. Personnel resources may be available in the form of educational programs in nursing, medicine, social work, public health, and other professions.

Stabilization and Reassessment

The role of the APN with the coalition and the change process is very active, but this role draws to an end during the step in Lewin's Stages of Change known as refreezing. During this step, reassessment and stabilization are typical and expected, which focuses "the change agent's and actor's attention and energy on progress and continuity for the change" (Kettner, Dailey, & Nichols, 1985, p. 288). The APN may or may not continue with the community coalition. But even when the APN continues, the role of change agent is less necessary and begins to fade as the change is institutionalized or stabilized. But rather than immediately separating from a successful coalition program, the APN should emphasize the autonomous functioning and continued survival of the program (Kettner et al., 1985).

The APN should initiate a reassessment of the change process and the coalition's work. Input is sought from all participants about whether the impact of the coalition's changes is meeting their needs. Members of the community coalition itself give feedback, as do a sample of their constituents who are recruited to reflect on the practical consequences and the meaning of the change effort. To what extent has the change been accepted, approved, and adopted among coalition members, their constituents, stakeholders, and other community members? A careful review of whether the community coalition's goals were met should be included. Though perhaps challenging to anticipate, this step will be easier if early in the project the APN guides the community coalition to accompany their specification of outcomes with clear descriptors for outcome achievement.

The APN will also assist and explore with the community coalition appropriate means to share their experiences with a wider audience through oral presentations, visual and audio media publicity, and articles for publication in magazines, journals, community newspapers, and online postings. The APN and coalition members may offer assistance to other community groups who are in the early stages of planning similar efforts. Coalition members may take the strengths of this coalition experience, with their new skills and abilities, and apply what they have gained to other issues in support of their own communities.

SUMMARY

The APN's ability to employ the change process is an essential component of reaching beyond the clinical encounter to address the community context and conditions that lead to poor health in individuals and families. The community encounter engages the APN and community partners in an ongoing process of increased understanding and skill/ability development.

The APN who sets out to engage communities in change requires many skills. Foremost is the ability to strategically and successfully introduce the need for change to improve population health. At any one time, the APN may be called upon to moderate a focus group, diplomatically defuse a situation, collect data in order to identify targets for intervention and to measure change, and help in the identification and construction of achievable outcomes. Although the initial role of the APN is leader, he or she must also be prepared to step aside and allow members of the community to identify priorities for change. It is paramount that the APN understands that it is community members who make final decisions about health priorities. An important role of the APN is helping community members to acquire the necessary skills to make changes and to create a sustainable environment. It requires a true partnership between the APN and the community to create meaningful change and it is through helping communities to sustain those changes and become leaders themselves that those changes will become embedded in the community.

Extending APN practice into the community improves clinical outcomes directly because as community problems are identified and managed this complements the APN's efforts to reduce individual and family health problems. Sustaining the coalitions and programs that develop as a result of the APN's partnership with community members has the potential to achieve far reaching improvements in population health.

EXERCISES AND DISCUSSION QUESTIONS

Exercise 10.1   What ethical principles apply when working with communities? Conduct a personal skills inventory. Of the ethical principles that you have identified, which ones do you have sufficient skills in to be able to work effectively with a community coalition? Are there areas where you would like to develop stronger abilities? How would you go about developing the skills and knowledge to do so?

Exercise 10.2   Consider a community known to you. If you were working with a partnership group to set priorities for community collaboration, which priority-setting criteria would you recommend for use by your group?

Exercise 10.3   What factors would you consider before you made an implicit/explicit commitment to engage with a community or neighborhood to improve residents' health status? How would you specifically engage with the community to negotiate your role?

Exercise 10.4   Consider a community known to you. You wish to take initial steps to build a partnership with the community. What data and information will you have analyzed/considered before you contact community leaders/members/organizations? Which area leaders/members/organizations would you contact initially, to introduce the idea of a partnership?

Exercise 10.5   Obtain a copy of the Tarimo (1991) *Priority Chart* (see the reference list). With others, select six or seven community issues or concerns and rank these using the tool. What did your group agree about? Disagree about? In what ways would your group consider modifying the tool?

REFERENCES

Allender, J. A., Rector, C., & Warner, K. D. (2010). *Community health nursing: Promoting and protecting the public's health* (7th ed.). Philadelphia, PA: Wolters Kluwer/Lippincott Williams & Wilkins.

Barger, S. E., & Crumpton, R. B. (1991). Public health nursing partnership: Agencies and academe. *Nurse Educator, 16*(4), 16–19.

Benjamin, G., O'Brien, D. J., & Trotter, D. (2002). Do we need a new law or regulation? The public health decision process. *The Journal of Law, Medicine & Ethics, 30*(3), 45–47.

Blum, E. D. (2008). *Love Canal revisited: Race, class, and gender in environmental activism.* Lawrence, Kansas: University Press of Kansas.

Blum, H. L. (1981). *Planning for health: Generics for the eighties* (2nd ed.). New York, NY: Human Sciences Press.

Butterfoss, F. D., Goodman, R. M., & Wandersman, A. (1993). Community coalitions for prevention and health promotion. *Health Education Research, 8*(3), 315–330.

CDC/ATSDR Committee on Community Engagement. (n.d.). Principles of community engagement. Retrieved from http://www.cdc.gov/phppo/pce/

Center for Nutrition Policy and Promotion, United States Department of Agriculture. (2010). *Dietary guidelines for Americans, 2010.* Retrieved from www.cnpp.usda.gov/DGAs2010-PolicyDocument.htm

Cherry, D. J., & Shefner, J. (2004). Addressing barriers to university-community collaboration: Organizing by experts or organizing the experts? *Journal of Community Practice, 12*(3), 219–233. doi:10.1300/J125v12n03_13

Courtney, R., Ballard, E., Fauver, S., Gariota, M., & Holland, L. (1996). The partnership model: Working with individuals, families, and communities toward a new vision of health. *Public Health Nursing, 13*, 177–186.

Farnham, E. (1964). *Pioneering in public health nursing education: The history of the University Public Health Nursing District, 1917–1962.* Cleveland, OH: Press of Western Reserve University.

Gallant, M. H., Beaulieu, M. C., & Carnevale, F. A. (2002). Partnership: An analysis of the concept within the nurse-client relationship. *Journal of Advanced Nursing, 40*, 149–157.

Green, L. W., & Kreuter, M. W. (2005). *Health program planning: An educational and ecological approach* (4th ed.). Boston, MA: McGraw-Hill.

International Association for Public Participation. (2007). *IAP2 core values of public participation.* Retrieved from http://www.iap2.org/displaycommon.cfm?an=4

Issel, L. M. (2004). *Health program planning and evaluation: A practical systematic approach for community health.* Sudbury, MA: Jones and Bartlett Publishers.

Keller, L. O., Strohschein, S., & Briske, L. (2008). Population-based public health nursing practice: The intervention wheel. In M. Stanhope & J. Lancaster (Eds.), *Public health nursing: Population–centered health care in the community* (7th ed., pp. 187–214). St. Louis, MO: Mosby Elsevier.

Kettner, P. M., Daley, J. M., & Nichols, A. W. (1985). *Initiating change in organizations and communities: A macro practice model.* Monterey, CA: Brooks/Cole Publishing Company.

Kurt Lewin Change Management Model. (2011). Retrieved from http://www.change-management-coach.com/kurt_lewin.html

Labonte, R. (1997). Community, community development, and the forming of authentic partnerships: Some critical reflections. In M. Minkler (Ed.), *Community organizing and community building for health* (pp. 88–102). New Brunswick, NJ: Rutgers University Press.

Logan, B. N., Davis, L., & Parker, V. G. (2010). An interinstitutional academic collaborative partnership to end health disparities. *Health Education and Behavior, 37,* 580–592. doi:10.1177/1090198110363378

Lynn-McHale, D. J., & Deatrick, J. A. (2000). Trust between family and health care provider. *Journal of Family Nursing, 6,* 210–230.

Macali, M, Galanowsky, K., Wagner, M., & Truglio-Londrigan. (2011). Hitting the pavement: Intervention of case finding. In M. Truglio-Londrigan & S. B. Lewenson (Eds.), *Public health nursing: Practicing population-based care* (pp. 185–219). Sudbury, MA: Jones & Bartlett Publishers.

McCloskey, D.J., McDonald, M.A., Cook, J., Heurtin-Roberts, S. Updegrove, S., Sampson, D., Gutter, S. & Eder, M. (2011). *Community engagement: Definitions and Organizing Concepts from the Literature.* In National Institutes of Health. (NIH Publication No. 11-7782). Retrieved from http://www.atsdr.cdc.gov/communityengagement/pdf/PCE_Report_508_FINAL.pdf

National Institutes of Health. (2011). *Principles of Community Engagement* (2nd ed) (NIH Publication No. 11-7782). Retrieved from http://www.atsdr.cdc.gov/community engagement/pdf/PCE_Report_508_FINAL.pdf

Oldenburg, B., & Glanz, K. (2008). Diffusion of Innovations In K. Glanz, B. K. Rimer, & K. Viswanath (Eds.), *Health behavior and health education: Theory, research, and practice* (4th ed., pp. 313–333). San Francisco, CA: Jossey-Bass.

Parker, E. A., Eng, E., Laraia, B., Ammerman, A., Dodds, J., Margolis, L., & Cross, A. (1999). Coalition building for prevention, In R. C. Brownson, E.A. Baker, & L. F. Novick (Eds.), *Community-based prevention: Programs that work* (pp. 182–198). Gaithersburg, MD: Aspen Publishers.

Pickens, S., Boumbulian, P., Anderson, R. J., Ross, S., & Phillips, S. (2002). Community-oriented primary care in action: A Dallas story. *American Journal of Public Health, 92,* 1728–1732.

Pickett, G., & Hanlon, J. J. (1990). *Public health: Administration and practice* (9th ed.). St. Louis, MO: Times Mirror/Mosby College Publishing.

Prochaska, J. O., Redding, C. A., & Evers, K. E. (2008). The transtheoretical model and stages of change. In K. Glanz, B. K. Rimer, & K. Viswanath (Eds.), *Health behavior and health education: Theory, research, and practice* (4th ed., pp. 97–121). San Francisco, CA: Jossey-Bass.

Rippke, M., Briske, L., Keller, L. O., & Strohschein, S. (2001). *Public health interventions: Applications for public health nursing practice.* St. Paul, MN: Minnesota Department of Health.

Roberts, S. J., & Krouse, H. J. (1990). Negotiation as a strategy to empower self-care. *Holistic Nursing Practice, 4*(2), 30–36.

School of Public Health, University of Illinois at Chicago. (2004). *Guide for establishing public health priorities* (rev'ed). Retrieved from http://www.uic.edu/sph/prepare/courses/ph440/mods/bpr.htm

Schuster, G. F., & Goeppinger, J. (2004). Community as client: Assessment and analysis. In M. Stanhope & J. Lancaster (Eds.), *Community and public health nursing* (6th ed., pp. 342–373). St. Louis, MO: Mosby.

Simons-Morton, B. G., Greene, W. H., & Gottlieb, N. H. (1995). *An introduction to health education and health promotion* (2nd ed.). Prospect Heights, IL: Waveland Press.

Simons-Morton, D. G., Simons-Morton, B. G., Parcel, G. S., & Bunker, J. F. (1988). Influencing personal and environmental conditions for community health: A multilevel intervention model. *Family and Community Health, 11*(2), 25–35.

Tarimo, E. (1991). *Towards a healthy district.* Geneva, Switzerland: World Health Organization. Retrieved (in pdf) from http://www.eric.ed.gov/ERICWebPortal/contentdelivery/servlet/ERICServlet?accno=ED337548

Timmreck, T. C. (1995). *Planning, program development, and evaluation: A handbook for health promotion, aging and health services.* Boston, MA: Jones and Bartlett Publishers.

The Community Guide Branch, Centers for Disease Control and Prevention. (2011). *The guide to community prevention services.* Retrieved from www.thecommunityguide.org/index.html

The Community Toolbox. (2011a). *Our model of practice: Building capacity for community and system change.* Retrieved from http://ctb.ku.edu/en/tablecontents/sub_section_main_1002.aspx

The Community Toolbox. (2011b). *Strategies for the long-term institutionalization of an initiative: An overview.* Retrieved from http://ctb.ku.edu/en/tablecontents/sub_section_main_1329.aspx

The Community Toolbox. (2011c). *Strategies for sustaining the initiative.* Retrieved from http://ctb.ku.edu/en/tablecontents/sub_section_main_1330.aspx

Wald, A. (2011). Working together: Collaboration, coalition building, and community organizing. In M. Truglio-Londrigan & S. B. Lewenson (Eds.), *Public health nursing: Practicing population-based care* (pp. 267–283). Sudbury, MA: Jones & Bartlett Publishers.

Walker, S. S. (2011). Ethical quandaries in community health nursing. In E. T. Anderson & J. McFarlane (Eds.), *Community as partner: Theory and practice in nursing* (6th ed., pp. 73–85). Philadelphia, PA: Wolters Kluwer/Lippincott Williams & Wilkins.

Yip, F. Y., Pearcy, J. N., Garbe, P. L., & Truman, B. I. (2011). Unhealthy air quality—United States, 2006–2009. *Morbidity and Mortality Weekly Report, 60*(1). Retrieved from http://www.cdc.gov/mmwr/preview/mmwrhtml/su6001a5.htm?s_cid=su6001a5_w

Zerwekh, J. V. (1992). Commentary: Going to the people—Public health nursing today and tomorrow. *American Journal of Public Health, 83,* 1676–1678.

Index